Hemostasis and Thrombosis

Thomas G. DeLoughery

Editor

Hemostasis
and Thrombosis

Fourth Edition

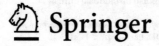

Editor
Thomas G. DeLoughery
Division of Hematology/Medical Oncology
Oregon Health & Sciences University
Portland, OR
USA

ISBN 978-3-030-19329-4   ISBN 978-3-030-19330-0   (eBook)
https://doi.org/10.1007/978-3-030-19330-0

This Springer imprint is published by the registered company Springer Nature Switzerland AG
The registered company address is: Gewerbestrasse 11, 6330 Cham, Switzerland

Contents

Contributors

Molly M. Daughety, MD Division of Hematology and Oncology, Duke University Medicine Center, Durham, NC, USA

Thomas G. DeLoughery, MD MACP FAWM Division of Hematology/Medical Oncology, Department of Medicine, Pathology, and Pediatrics, Oregon Health & Sciences University, Portland, OR, USA

Kristina Haley, DO Department of Pediatrics, Division of Pediatric Hematology/Oncology, Oregon Health & Sciences University, Portland, OR, USA

Bethany T. Samuelson Bannow, MD Division of Hematology and Oncology, Duke University Medicine Center, Durham, NC, USA

The Hemophilia Center, Oregon Health & Science University, Portland, OR, USA

Joseph Shatzel, MD Division of Hematology/Medical Oncology, Department of Medicine and Biomedical Engineering, Oregon Health & Sciences University, Portland, OR, USA

Basics of Coagulation

Thomas G. DeLoughery

The basic mechanics of hemostasis must be grasped in order to understand the disorders of hemostasis and the therapies designed to alter coagulation. Generally, coagulation is divided into fibrin formation, fibrinolysis, platelet function, and natural anticoagulants.

Formation of Fibrin

The coagulation cascade is a series of enzymatic steps designed to amplify the insult of initial trauma into the formation of a fibrin plug. Recent research has revealed how fibrin formation occurs in vivo rather than how it occurs in the test tube. The in vivo pathway for the purposes of this book is called the "new pathway" of coagulation. Unfortunately, the two most common laboratory tests for coagulation and many books are still based on the test tube models of coagulation. It is important to learn (a little bit) about the older models of coagulation to understand these two laboratory tests and much of the classic literature (Fig. 1.1).

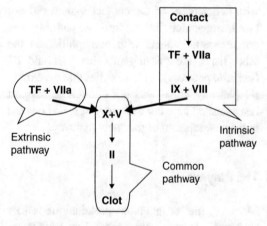

Fig. 1.1 Coagulation cascades

T. G. DeLoughery (✉)
Division of Hematology/Medical Oncology,
Department of Medicine, Pathology, and Pediatrics,
Oregon Health & Sciences University,
Portland, OR, USA
e-mail: delought@ohsu.edu

The Old Pathways

In the test tube, tissue factor (TF) +VIIa is much more effective in activating factor X than factor XI. This pathway is initiated by adding bits of tissue ("tissue thromboplastin," usually minced animals' brains) to plasma. The brain tissue was used in these studies because it is an excellent source of both phospholipids and tissue factor. Since an extrinsic initiator, brain, was added, this pathway is known as the *extrinsic pathway*. The second pathway is triggered when blood is exposed to glass. Since nothing is added (except the glass surface) this is called the *intrinsic pathway*. This pathway is dependent on a different set of enzymes that result in factor XII activating factor XI. Since both pathways are the same once Factor X is formed, the path from factor X to fibrin formation is known as the "common" pathway.

To recap:

Extrinsic pathway: **TF+VIIa**→Xa+V→IIa→clot
Intrinsic pathway: **Contact system→IXa+VIII** →Xa+V→IIa→clot
Common pathway: →**Xa+V→IIa→clot**

These pathways explained laboratory findings but did not match clinical observations. Patients with deficiencies of the contact system did not bleed, suggesting that the intrinsic pathway was not relevant. Patients with hemophilia, on the other hand, are missing proteins VIII and IX (intrinsic pathway), which implies that the extrinsic pathway alone was not enough to support hemostasis. These contradictory observations led to the development of the "new pathway."

The Players

Most of the coagulation proteins are either enzymes (serine proteases) or cofactors

(Table 1.1). A coagulation protein is a framework consisting of a serine protease with different protein domains added to it. The purpose of these domains is to add different capabilities to the clotting proteins.

Factors II, VII, IX, and X, protein C, protein S, and protein Z have vitamin K-dependent glutamic acid (GLA) domains on the amino terminus of the protein. These domains contain 9–11 glutamic acids modified to form gamma-carboxyglutamic acid (GLA) (Fig. 1.2). This modification allows calcium to bind to these proteins. The binding of calcium changes the conformation of the proteins and serves to bind them in turn to phospholipid surfaces. The hepatic GLA redox reaction is dependent on vitamin K ("*K*oagulation"). Without this vitamin, dysfunc-

Table 1.1 Coagulation proteins

Enzymes	Cofactors	Miscellaneous
Factor IIa	Tissue factor	Fibrinogen
Factor VIIa	Factor V	Factor XIII
Factor IXa	Factor VIII	Alpha$_2$-antiplasmin
Factor Xa	Protein S	PAI-1
Factor XIa		Antithrombin
Protein C		
tPA		
Plasmin		

Fig. 1.2 Function of GLA domains

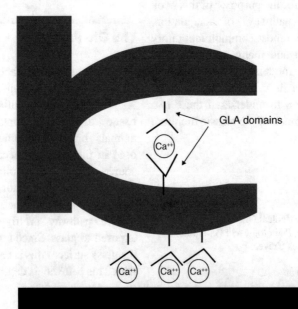

Fig. 1.3 Lysine residues and kringle domains

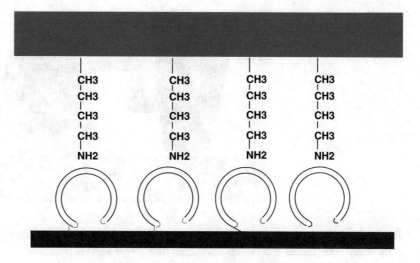

tional coagulation proteins are produced which function poorly in coagulation reactions. The drug warfarin blocks the recycling of vitamin K and leads to a reduction in functional coagulation factors.

Factor II, tissue plasminogen activator (tPA), and plasminogen contain "kringle" regions (named after a Danish pastry). The kringle domains help these proteins bind to fibrinogen (Fig. 1.3).

The cofactors V and VIII are very similar molecules and require activation by thrombin. The mechanism underlying their cofactor function is unknown. The presence of these two cofactors enhances the efficiency of the coagulation factors by at least 100,000-fold.

"Quaternary Complex"

Most coagulation reactions have four components, starting with the *enzyme* binding to a *cofactor* that is bonded by *calcium* to a *surface* (Table 1.2). This serves to make a little "coagulation factory" on the surface and improves the efficiency of the reaction by bringing the components together (Fig. 1.4).

- *Enzyme*: (VIIa, XIa, Xa, IIa, protein C)
- *Cofactor*: (V, VIII, tissue factor, protein S) — speeds up reactions by orders of magnitude
- *Calcium*: binds protein to surfaces

Table 1.2 Key coagulation reactions

Key reactions	
The new pathway	
TF+VIIa--->IXa+VIII-->Xa+V-->IIa-->Clot	
The old pathway	
Intrinsic pathway	**Contact system** →IXa+VIII→Xa+V→IIa→clot
Extrinsic pathway	**TF+VIIa**→Xa+V→IIa→clot
Common pathway	→**Xa+V**→**IIa**→**clot**
Fibrin formation	
Fibrinogen-(*thrombin*) →fibrin monomer→ fibrin polymer --(*factor XIII*) →fibrin clot	

- *Phospholipid surface*: Has a negative charge and speeds reactions by bring proteins closer to each other

Initiation of Coagulation

Overview: **TF+VII→IX+VIII→X+V→II**

The key step in the initiation of coagulation is exposure of tissue factor (TF). TF is a transmembrane surface molecule that is more or less on all cell surfaces except endothelial cells and circulating blood cells. Thus, flowing blood under normal conditions is never exposed to TF. With trauma, blood spills out of the vessel and contacts TF. This is what initiates the coagulation cascade.

TF binds factor VII. This reaction would stop immediately without active factor VII (VIIa) to cleave factor IX. However, a tiny bit (0.1%) of

Fig. 1.4 Role of cofactors

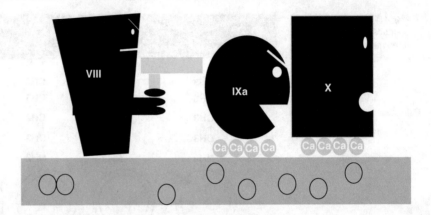

factor VII circulates in the active form. This bit of VIIa from the blood binds TF and then the TF-VIIa complex activates surrounding TF-VII complexes and these complexes start converting factor IX into IXa ("intrinicase") and X into Xa ("extrinsicase").

When factor IXa is formed, it, along with cofactor VIIIa, converts X into Xa. The presence of VIIIa is crucial for the function of the Xa complex. While VIIa activation of X is the initial step in coagulation, soon XIa generation becomes the predominant pathway for Xa generation. Of note, the underlying pathology of the two most common forms of hemophilia is the absence of the two proteins in this reaction (IX and VIII).

Factor Xa (generated by either VIIa or IXa) binds with cofactor Va to generate thrombin (IIa) from prothrombin (II). The production of thrombin is the final step in the initiation of coagulation and is the single most crucial step in hemostasis.

Thrombin

Thrombin is a multifunctional molecule. It functions to:

- Cleave *fibrinogen* into fibrin
- Activate *factors V and VIII*
- Activate *factor XIII*

- Activate *factor XI*
- Activate *platelets*
- Activate *thrombin activatable fibrinolysis inhibitor (TAFI)*
- Activate *fibrinolysis*
- Activate *protein C*

Thrombin is unique in several ways. It does not require a cofactor for enzymatic function. When it is activated, it separates from its GLA domain so it can float around to promote clotting. Thrombin also provides both *positive feedback* by activating factors V, VIII, XI, and XIII and TAFI and *negative feedback* by activating protein C and promoting fibrinolysis. Thrombin activation of factor XI provides a further positive feedback loop. Active factor XI activates IX, eventually leading to more thrombin generation.

Fibrin Formation

Fibrin is formed by turning soluble circulating fibrinogen into an insoluble fibrin thrombus (Fig. 1.5). This is done in two steps. In the first step, thrombin converts fibrinogen into fibrin monomers which spontaneously polymerize to form fibrin polymers. In the second step, factor XIII stabilizes the clot by forming amide bonds between different fibrin polymers:

Fibrinogen → fibrin monomer → fibrin polymer → fibrin clot

Fig. 1.5 Formation of fibrin from fibrinogen

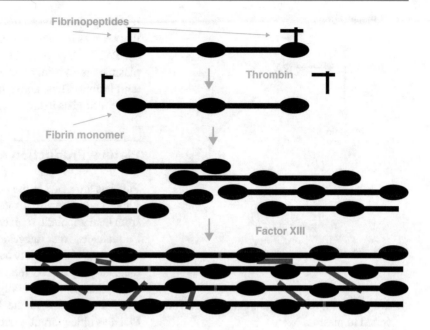

Thrombin acts on fibrinogen and clips off two peptides (fibrinopeptides A and B). This produces the *fibrin monomer*. The act of thrombin clipping off these peptides exposes polymerization sites that can bind to other fibrin monomers. The monomers polymerize together to form a loose clot. *Factor XIII* then solidifies the bond by forming glutamyl-lysine bridges between the side chains of the fibrin monomers. Note that factor XIII is the only coagulation enzyme that is *not* a serine protease.

In addition, thrombin promotes coagulation by activating thrombin activatable fibrinolysis inhibitor (TAFI). TAFI cleaves the lysine residues to which many fibrinolytic enzymes bind, rendering the clot less likely to be dissolved.

Propagation

Thrombin can activate factor XI which acts as positive feedback as factor XIa. This activated factor generates more IXa. This then leads to more thrombin generation. More thrombin formation leads to activation of TAFI. This theory is consistent with the finding that patients lacking factor XI often have bleeding in sites of fibrinolytic activity such as the mouth after oral surgery.

As discussed later in the chapter, tissue factor pathway inhibitor (TFPI) inhibits the TF-Xa pathway. This results in continuing thrombin generation that is dependent on thrombin activation of XI.

Fibrinolysis

The fibrinolytic system is responsible for breaking down blood clots once they have formed. Obviously, this is an important process to prevent thrombi from getting too large, to aid wound healing, and to prevent thrombosis in an undesirable place. Recent research has also implicated roles for proteins from the fibrinolytic system in diverse processes such as cancer metastasis and memory.

Fibrinolytic Proteins

The key proteins in the fibrinolytic system are (Fig. 1.6):

- *Plasmin*: This is a serine protease produced by the liver which cleaves bonds in fibrin and fibrinogen. Normally it circulates as an inac-

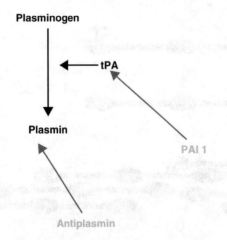

Fig. 1.6 Fibrinolysis

tive precursor *plasminogen, but* it can be converted to plasmin by:
- *Tissue plasminogen activator (tPA)*: This is produced by endothelial cells. tPA is the physiologic activator of plasminogen.
- *Urokinase (UK)*: This is secreted in the urine (hence its name) and in many other cells. It is also a potent activator of plasminogen.

Several inhibitors of fibrinolysis are present to keep the fibrinolytic system in balance:

- *Plasminogen activator inhibitor (PAI-1)*: PAI-1 is made by the liver and endothelial cells. It binds and inactivates tPA.
- *Alpha₂ antiplasmin*: This is made by the liver. It binds and inactivates plasmin.

Fibrinolysis: The Process

The effectiveness of tPA to cleave plasminogen to plasmin is far greater when plasminogen and tPA are *both bound* to the fibrin clot. Moreover, when plasmin is bound to fibrin, it is protected from the action of circulating alpha₂-antiplasmin.

A formed thrombus carries with it the seeds of its own destruction by incorporating plasminogen into the clot. tPA released from nearby endothelial cells percolates into the clot. The tPA binds to fibrin and then converts plasminogen to plasmin, which lyses the clot. Any excess tPA that escapes into the plasma is rapidly inactivated by PAI-1. Any plasmin that escapes into the plasma is rapidly inactivated by alpha₂-antiplasmin. Thus, active fibrinolysis is confined to the thrombus itself.

Platelet Production and Life Span

Platelets are made in the bone marrow (Fig. 1.7). Large cells known as megakaryocytes (derived from hematopoietic stem cells) are the precursors to platelets; one megakaryocyte can produce 2000 platelets. Platelets bud off the edges of the megakaryocytes and the megakaryocyte eventually perishes by literally "evaporating." The platelet circulates in the blood for 7–10 days. Platelets either circulate freely or are sequestered in the spleen. At any given time, one-third of the platelets are located in the spleen.

Thrombopoietin (TPO)

Discovered in 1994, TPO is the main growth and maturation factor for megakaryocytes. One-half of the TPO molecule is very similar to erythropoietin. TPO can make early precursor cells differentiate into megakaryocytes and can induce generation of platelets by megakaryocytes. TPO and molecules with TPO-like activity are currently used in therapy of immune thrombocytopenia and aplastic anemia as they are able to stimulate stem cells.

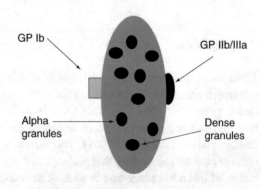

Fig. 1.7 Platelet structure

Fig. 1.8 Function of von Willebrand factor

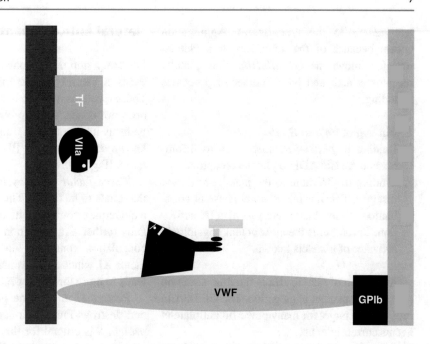

Functions of Platelets

Platelets do four things:

1. *Adhere* to damaged endothelium
2. *Store* ADP and proteins
3. *Aggregate* with other platelets
4. *Provide a surface* for coagulation reactions

Platelet Adhesion

Damage to a blood vessel exposes *collagen* that is wrapped around the vessel. The exposed collagen reacts with and binds a large multimeric protein known as *von Willebrand factor* (vWF). Once it is bound, von Willebrand factor changes in conformation at one end so that it now can bind to platelets. The von Willebrand factor attaches to the platelet receptor *Glycoprotein (Gp) Ib*. Platelet adhesion by von Willebrand factor creates a platelet monolayer over an injured surface. The binding of von Willebrand factor to Gp Ib leads to physiological changes called platelet activation.

About von Willebrand Factor

Von Willebrand Factor (vWF) is a huge molecule, up to 20 million daltons in molecular weight. It serves another role in hemostasis by carrying and protecting coagulation factor VIII. Patients who completely lack vWF also lack factor VIII, which results in a severe bleeding disorder (Fig. 1.8).

Summary of Platelet Adhesion
Platelet adhesion is initiated by exposed *collagen*, which leads to the binding of *von Willebrand factor* (the glue) to the platelet receptor *GP Ib*.

Platelet Storage

Platelets are filled with granules that store ADP and other proteins released when platelets are activated. *Alpha* granules store proteins, and *dense* granules store chemicals. Alpha granules contain proteins such as vWF and factor V. *Dense* granules contain chemicals such as serotonin and ADP which, after release, activate nearby platelets. Platelet activation also leads to production of thromboxane A_2, a key activator of platelets (recall that thromboxane A_2 synthesis is blocked by aspirin).

Platelet Aggregation

Platelet aggregation is the binding of platelets to *each other* (as opposed to adhesion where platelets *adhere* to the *vasculature*). Aggregation occurs because of the activation of a platelet receptor known as *GP IIb/IIIa*. This platelet receptor is activated by a number of processes including:

1. Binding of *vWF* to *Gp Ib*.
2. Binding of *platelet agonists* such as thromboxane A2 and ADP to platelet receptors.
3. Binding of thrombin to the platelet *thrombin* receptor. This ties the humoral phase of coagulation (tissue factor, etc.) to platelet activation. Thrombin is the *most* potent physiologic activator of platelets known.

Activation of GP IIb/IIIa is the final common pathway for platelet aggregation. The GP IIb/IIIa receptor is a target for many powerful antiplatelet agents currently in use.

After the platelets have formed a monolayer on an injured surface, they release platelet agonists such as ADP. This activates nearby platelets, causing them to activate their own GP IIb/IIIa. Fibrinogen (abundant in the plasma) then binds to all the active Gp IIb/IIIa exposed on the platelet surface. The glue for platelet aggregation is *fibrinogen*. This acts to clump platelets together into a large mass, forming a platelet plug that stops the bleeding.

Platelet Surface

Coagulation reactions take place on *surfaces*. This allows all the coagulation factors to be close to one another and increases the efficiency of the reactions. When platelets are activated, they expose a negatively charged phospholipid— *phosphatidylserine*. Phosphatidylserine augments the binding of coagulation factors to injured surfaces. Since platelets are found at the site of injury, their surfaces provide a platform for coagulation. When platelets are activated, little blebs (called platelet *microparticles*) bubble off the surface. These microparticles increase the surface area available for coagulation reactions many times over.

Natural Anticoagulants

For every step of the coagulation cascade, there exists a natural protein inhibitor of that step. These proteins ensure that excess thrombosis does not occur. These proteins are tissue factor pathway inhibitor (TFPI), antithrombin (formally known as antithrombin III), protein C, and protein S (Fig. 1.9).

Tissue factor pathway inhibitor is a protein that binds to factor Xa. This complex then forms a quaternary complex with tissue factor-VIIa and halts further IXa formation. It is speculated that coagulation continues via thrombin activating factor XI which in turns activates factor IX and leads to more thrombin generation.

Protein C is a serine protease that cleaves and destroys factors Va and VIIIa. Its cofactor *protein S* is crucial for this function. Both proteins C and S are vitamin K dependent. Protein S has two unusual features. First, it is not a serine protease. Second, it circulates in two forms in the plasma, a free form and a form bound to C4B-binding protein. Only the free form can serve as a cofactor to protein C. Normally about 40% of protein S exists in the free form. Alterations in this ratio, either acquired or genetic, are responsible for many of the hypercoagulable states.

Antithrombin is a serine protease inhibitor that binds and inactivates all the serine proteases of the coagulation cascade. Its function is greatly

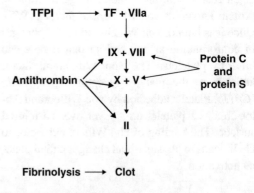

Fig. 1.9 Natural anticoagulants

augmented by either natural heparan or exogenous heparin. The addition of these complex polysaccharides leads to a dramatic increase in antithrombin's ability to bind and neutralize serine proteases.

Suggested Reading

Chapin JC, Hajjar KA. Fibrinolysis and the control of blood coagulation. Blood Rev. 2015;29(1):17–24. https://doi.org/10.1016/j.blre.2014.09.003.

Estevez B, Du X. New concepts and mechanisms of platelet activation signaling. Physiology (Bethesda). 2017;32(2):162–77.

Long AT, Kenne E, Jung R, Fuchs TA, Renné T. Contact system revisited: an interface between inflammation, coagulation, and innate immunity. J Thromb Haemost. 2016;14(3):427–37.

O'Donnell JS, O'Sullivan JM, Preston RJS. Advances in understanding the molecular mechanisms that maintain normal haemostasis. Br J Haematol. 2019.

Smith SA, Travers RJ, Morrissey JH. How it all starts: initiation of the clotting cascade. Crit Rev Biochem Mol Biol. 2015;50(4):326–36.

Ten Cate H, Hackeng TM, García de Frutos P. Coagulation factor and protease pathways in thrombosis and cardiovascular disease. Thromb Haemost. 2017;117(7):1265–71.

Vojacek JF. Should we replace the terms intrinsic and extrinsic coagulation pathways with tissue factor pathway? Clin Appl Thromb Hemost. 2017;23(8):922–7.

Witkowski M, Landmesser U, Rauch U. Tissue factor as a link between inflammation and coagulation. Trends Cardiovasc Med. 2016;26(4):297–303.

Tests of Hemostasis and Thrombosis

Thomas G. DeLoughery

A routine laboratory test once well-established is often slavishly adhered to, with little further thought about how it originated, why it is done or what it means. To justify it, the phrases 'for the record' and 'for protection' are often heard. Tests done only for these reasons not only are generally a waste of time and money but can also be quite misleading, and may give to the physician a false sense of security, or produce worry and concern over a potentially serious disorder when no disease actually exits.

–Diamond and Porter, *NEJM* 1958.

Testing of hemostasis is done for three reasons: to screen for coagulation disorders, to diagnose these disorders, and to monitor therapy. Tests of hemostasis and thrombosis are performed on nearly every patient in the hospital.

Bleeding Disorders

Bleeding History

The bleeding history is the strongest predictor of bleeding risk with any procedure. It is essential that the history includes more questions than just

T. G. DeLoughery (✉)
Division of Hematology/Medical Oncology,
Department of Medicine, Pathology, and Pediatrics,
Oregon Health & Sciences University,
Portland, OR, USA
e-mail: delought@ohsu.edu

"are you a bleeder?" A good history for bleeding can be obtained in minutes by asking a few specific questions as outlined in Chap. 3. Bleeding due to coagulation defects is unusual, recurrent, and excessive, but rarely spectacular.

The use of "bleeding assessment tools" to provide more quantitative assessment of bleeding is increasingly common. An example that is frequently used is the ISTH-SSC form (https://bleedingscore.certe.nl/). These tools are particularly useful in clinical studies of bleeding disorders.

Specific Assays for Bleeding Disorders (Tables 2.1, 2.2, and 2.3)

Prothrombin Time (PT)

The PT measures the amount of time it takes the VIIa to form a complex with tissue factor and proceeds to clot formation. The test is performed by adding tissue thromboplastin (tissue factor) to plasma. Prolongation of only the PT most often indicates isolated factor VII deficiency. Combined prolongation of PT and activated partial thromboplastin time (aPTT) indicates either factor X, II, or V deficiency or multiple defects. However, depending on the reagent, occasionally mild (~50% of normal) deficiency in factors V or X can present with only modest elevation of the PT. The major clinical use of PT is to monitor

© Springer Nature Switzerland AG 2019
T. G. DeLoughery (ed.), *Hemostasis and Thrombosis*,
https://doi.org/10.1007/978-3-030-19330-0_2

Table 2.1 Prothrombin time/INR

Plasma + calcium + tissue thromboplastin
TF+VIIa→Xa+V→IIa→clot

Table 2.2 Activated partial thromboplastin time

Plasma + calcium + kaolin + phospholipids
Contact →XIa→IXa+VIII→Xa+Va→IIa→clot

Table 2.3 Interpretations of elevated PT and/or aPTT

PT only:
Factor VII deficiency
Congenital
Acquired
Vitamin K deficiency
Liver disease
Factor VII inhibitor
Rarely in patients with modest decreases of factor V or X
PTT only
Contact factor XI, IX, VIII deficiency
Contact factor XI, IX, VIII specific factor inhibitor
Heparin contamination
Antiphospholipid antibodies
Both
Factor X, V, or II deficiency
Factor X, V, or II inhibitor
Improper anticoagulant ratio (hematocrits >60 or < 15)
High doses of heparin (elevation of aPTT greater relative to PT)
Large warfarin effect (elevation of PT greater relative to APTT)
Low fibrinogen (<80 mg/dl)

warfarin therapy. Since different laboratories use different reagents, the consistent way to monitor warfarin therapy is to use the international normalized ratio (INR).

The INR is a method of standardizing prothrombin times obtained from different laboratories. The INR is derived by dividing the patient's prothrombin time by the laboratory control and raising this to the international sensitivity index (ISI). The ISI is known for each prothrombin time laboratory reagent, and it adjusts the prothrombin time for the differing sensitivities of reagents. Using the INR instead of the prothrombin time has resulted in more accurate monitoring of warfarin dosage. Many laboratories now only report the INR and not the prothrombin time.

It is important to remember the INR is only standardized for patients on chronic warfarin therapy. Frequently patients – especially those who are critically ill – will have minor elevations of the INR (1.2–1.6 range) which is of no clinical significance. In patients with liver disease, the INR is not consistent between different laboratories; this may lead to variation in scoring of the liver disease severity.

Evaluation of an elevated PT (INR) If an elevated PT is the only laboratory abnormality, this indicates a factor VII deficiency and usually confers no additional risk of bleeding since one needs only 5–10% of normal factor VII levels to support hemostasis. Congenital factor VII deficiency is very rare and presents with childhood bleeding. Heterozygotes for factor VII deficiency present with no bleeding but an elevated prothrombin time (INR 1.5–2.0).

The most common acquired etiology of an elevated PT is vitamin K deficiency due to warfarin use or inadequate vitamin K intake. Liver disease is the next most common acquired cause. Since factor VII has the shortest half-life, its synthesis (and level) will drop first with liver disease. In combined elevations of the PT and aPTT, the differential is either the rare factor V, X, or II deficiency or multiple acquired defects such as those occurring with disseminated intravascular coagulation (DIC). In very sick patients, levels of factor VII often fall, causing a modest prolongation of the PT (INR up to 3.0). Some direct oral anticoagulants such as rivaroxaban can result in INR elevations.

Activated Partial Thromboplastin Time (aPTT)

The aPTT is performed by adding an activator such as clay to plasma. The aPTT measures the speed of the contact pathway (XII, kallikrein, XI)→IXa+VIIIa→Xa+Va→IIa→clot.

In patients with elevated levels of factor VIII, the aPTT can be shortened due to increased efficiency of the coagulation reactions. This is seen in inflammatory states, uremia, in patients on cyclosporine, and in pregnancy.

There are four etiologies to consider when the aPTT is elevated:

1. *Factor deficiency*. The aPTT does not rise until the plasma level of a single coagulation factor is below 30–40%. However, only mild decrements (60–70% range) in multiple factors will prolong the aPTT.
2. *Lupus inhibitors (antiphospholipid antibodies [APLA])*. Antiphospholipid antibodies (APLA) are antibodies that react with certain phospholipids in the body. They will also react with the phospholipid in the test reagent for the aPTT. Thus, they will artifactually prolong the aPTT. The presence of these antibodies may indicate, paradoxically, a higher risk of thrombosis and not bleeding. They may be found as part of an autoimmune disease, as a sequela after infections, with intake of certain medicines, and they can occur in low titers in up to 30% of the population.
3. *Factor inhibitors*. These are antibodies to specific coagulation factors such as factor VIII. These inhibitors are usually found in hemophiliacs, or they may be acquired in the elderly, or after pregnancy. Presence of these inhibitors is usually associated with severe bleeding, often with large ecchymoses.
4. *Heparin or other anticoagulants*. Heparin, even minute amounts, can prolong the aPTT. This most often occurs when blood for the aPTT is drawn from catheter lines. The use of direct oral anticoagulants can also lead to PTT elevations.

How to tell 1–4 apart   The simplest way to avoid heparin contamination is always to draw blood from peripheral sites. In addition, the thrombin time (see below) will always be prolonged with heparin and direct thrombin inhibitors. Many labs are also performing anti-Xa levels to rule out heparin or factor Xa inhibitors. The 50:50 mix will differentiate the rest (Tables 2.4 and 2.5). The 50:50 mix is performed by making a mixture of the patient's plasma and normal pool plasma and performing aPTT on the mix. The mixture is incubated for a period of time (usually 60 or 120 minutes) and the aPTT's are performed at those times. Each of the three major differential

Table 2.4   Four causes of elevated APTT and response to 50:50 mix

1. Factor deficiency – corrects
2. Antiphospholipid antibodies – does not fully correct
3. Factor inhibitors – corrects at time 0 but then prolongs
4. Heparin, direct anticoagulants – does not correct (usually obvious from history)

Table 2.5   Examples of 50:50 mixes

1. Factor VIII deficiency
2. Antiphospholipid antibodies
3. Factor VIII inhibitor

Time	0	30	60	120
Normal	30	32	33	34
Patient's	50	52	55	53
50:50-def (1)	30	32	33	34
50:50-apla (2)	40	38	42	39
50:50-inhib (3)	30	40	45	65

etiologies of an elevated aPTT (ideally) will provide different results in the 50:50 mix:

1. *Factor deficiency*. An initially elevated aPTT will correct to normal at time 0 and stays in the normal range on each of the time points. Since it takes only 30–40% of normal coagulation factors to normalize the aPTT, even with a complete lack of a factor, the mixing in of the normal pool will raise this level to 50% and normalize the aPTT.
2. *APLA*. The aPTT does not correct to normal at time 0 or any time point. The aPTT may actually prolong further with addition of patient's plasma (lupus cofactor effect). The crucial point is that the aPTT will not *fully* correct with the 50:50 mix.
3. *Factor inhibitors*. The aPTT may correct to normal at time 0 but then prolongs with further incubation. This demonstrates the importance of the incubation step in performing the 50:50 mixing test. Strong inhibitors may prolong the 50:50 mix aPTT even at time 0, but the aPTT will be more prolonged with longer incubation.

Specific Factor Assays

The standard method for measuring coagulation factors is by assaying their activity level. Many bleeding defects are due to abnormal factors and not absent ones. Furthermore, measuring activity levels is easier than directly measuring levels.

The assays are performed by mixing the patient's plasma with sample plasma that is missing a specific coagulation factor. For example, if someone is factor VIII deficient and their plasma is mixed with a factor IX deficient plasma, the clotting time will correct. If, however, the patient's plasma is mixed with a factor VIII deficient plasma, the clotting time will remain prolonged. To measure the exact level of factor deficiency, the clotting time with the deficient plasma is compared with a series of clotting times done with known factor levels. For example, if the plasma has a clotting time of 45 seconds, look on a standard curve and note the clotting time for 10% factor VIII is 42 seconds and the time for 5% factor VIII is 47 seconds. By extrapolation the patient has only 7% factor VIII.

Platelet Function

Bleeding Time

Once a standard screening test, the bleeding time is now rarely performed. It is best viewed as sensitive but not specific. If a patient has a normal bleeding time, then their risk of bleeding with a procedure is low. Unfortunately, a prolonged bleeding time does not reliably predict bleeding with a procedure. Measuring the bleeding time before procedures is not useful in otherwise asymptomatic patients who do not have a bleeding history. Prolongation of bleeding time can occur with platelet disorders, with von Willebrand disease, and with connective tissue defects. The bleeding time lacks diagnostic specificity as a screening test. It is best used in the evaluation of patients with a history suggestive of a bleeding disorder.

Platelet Function Analysis

Recently, a number of laboratory platelet tests have been developed to improve on the bleeding time. The most popular of these tests is the PFA-100. Whole blood is used for this assay and is exposed to either collagen/ADP or collagen/epinephrine surrounding a small hole. The endpoint of the test is closure of this hole due to platelet aggregation. The test appears to be more sensitive than the bleeding time for congenital bleeding disorders, but like the bleeding time, it is not useful for mass screening of patients. The major advantages of the PFA-100 are that it is not as dependent on technical factors and is reproducible.

The VerifyNow assay is designed to assess level of platelet inhibition by antiplatelet agents. There are specific assays for aspirin and for ADP receptor inhibitors such as clopidogrel. Although this assay can find evidence of aspirin or clopidogrel resistance in many patients, it is still controversial as to whether these findings will change clinical outcomes.

Flow Cytometry

Increasingly, the use of flow cytometry has become important in hemostasis diagnostics. Flow cytometry can be used to assess for platelet dense granules and for the presence of platelet glycoproteins such as Gp IIb/IIIa in order to specifically diagnose disease such as Glanzmann thrombasthenia.

Specific Platelet Studies

The platelet aggregation assay is performed by mixing platelets with specific agonists such as ADP or thrombin. Light is shone through the test tube containing the platelets, and if they aggregate, more light is transmitted allowing measurement of platelet aggregation. Advantages of platelet aggregation assays are that specific defects can be identified such as Bernard-Soulier disease. However, the downsides are lack of standardization and limited availability since freshly drawn platelets have to be used for the assay.

Electron microscopy of the platelet can reveal such defects as dense granulate deficiency, but it is not widely available and interpretation is not standardized.

There is a growing use of specific molecular panels (next-generation sequencing) to diagnose platelet disorders. In some studies, up to 50% of patients with a history or testing suggestive of a platelet disorder will have abnormal findings on this assay. Currently, lack of standardization, the finding of genetic variation of uncertain significance, and cost hinder more widespread use.

Test for DIC

Simply put, DIC is inappropriate activation of thrombin (IIa). As discussed in Chap. 8, this leads to the following: (1) conversion of fibrinogen to fibrin, (2) activation of platelets (and their consumption), (3) activation of factors V and VIII, (4) activation of protein C (and degradation of factors Va and VIIIa), (5) activation of endothelial cells, and (6) activation of fibrinolysis.

There is no one test that will diagnosis DIC; one must match the testing to the clinical situation.

Screening tests The PT and aPTT are usually elevated in acute DIC with severe depletion of coagulation factors, but these tests may be normal or even shortened in chronic forms where increased coagulation factor synthesis can compensate for factor depletion. One can see a shortened aPTT in DIC for two reasons: in patients with severe DIC, a large amount of activated II and factor X is "bypassing" the contact pathway, and aPTTs as short as 10 seconds have been seen in acute DIC. In chronic DIC, the high levels of factor VIII lead to a shortened aPTT. The platelet count usually falls but may be normal in chronic DIC. Serum fibrinogen is low in DIC but again may be in the "normal" range in chronic DIC.

Specific tests for DIC These are a group of tests which allow one to deduce that abnormally high concentrations of IIa are present (Table 2.6).

Ethanol gel and protamine tests Both of these older tests detect circulating fibrin monomers.

Table 2.6 Specific tests for DIC

D-dimers: fibrin degradation products
FDP: Fibrin *and* fibrinogen degradation products
Protamine sulfate/ethanol gel: detects circulating fibrin monomers (DIC)

Circulating fibrin monomers are present when IIa acts on fibrinogen. Usually the monomers polymerize with the fibrin clot but when there is too much IIa, these monomers can circulate. Detection of circulating fibrin monomers means there is too much IIa and therefore DIC.

Fibrin degradation products (FDP) When plasmin acts on the fibrin/fibrinogen molecule, it cleaves the molecule in specific places. Thus, FDP levels will be elevated in situations of increased fibrin/fibrinogen destruction (DIC, fibrinolysis). Fibrinogen degradation products result from destruction of circulating fibrinogen and fibrin breakdown products from a fibrin clot. High levels of FDP are also seen in dysfibrinogenemias. This is because the first step of the test causes all the fibrinogen to clot and then reagents are used to detect any leftover fragments. Since abnormal fibrinogen cannot clot, it will also be detected. This is one reason that elevated "FDPs" are often seen in liver disease and dysfibrinogenemias.

D-dimers When fibrin monomers bond to form a thrombus, factor XIII acts to bind their "D" domains together. The resulting bond is resistant to plasmin; the degradation fragment is called the "*D-dimer.*" Elevated levels of D-dimer indicate that (1) thrombin has acted on fibrinogen to form a fibrin monomer that bonded to another fibrin monomer by factor XIII, and (2) this clot was lysed by plasmin.

To summarize, since high levels of plasmin can destroy both fibrinogen and fibrin, clinicians need to distinguish between *fibrin* and *fibrinogen* degradation products. The difference between these two is that when a clot is formed, factor XIII stabilizes the clot by forming peptide bonds between the fibrin monomers. The distal end of the fibrinogen molecule is called the "D-domain." Plasmin cannot break the bond linking the adjacent two D-domains, which can then be detected

Table 2.7 The thrombin time

Add thrombin to plasma→clot
Elevated in:
1. Direct thrombin inhibitors (dabigatran, etc.)
2. DIC
3. Dysfibrinogenemia
4. Heparin use
5. Low fibrinogen levels
6. High fibrinogen levels
7. Uremia

Table 2.8 Thromboelastography

TEG parameter	Interpretation	Direction – products
R time	Reaction time – time to fibrin formation	Increased – FFP
K time	Kinetics – time 2–20 mm of amplitude	Increased – cryoprecipitate
Alpha angle	r/k slope of tracing–increase in thrombus strength, fibrinogen concentration	Decreased – cryoprecipitate
Maximal amplitude	Strength and stability of the thrombus	Decreased – platelets
Whole blood lysis index	Fibrinolysis	Increased – antifibrinolytic

by the fibrin degradation product test, i.e., the D-dimer assay.

Thrombin time (Table 2.7) This test is performed by adding thrombin to plasma. The added thrombin directly clots fibrinogen. The thrombin time is only affected by factors that interfere with thrombin or fibrinogen. The thrombin time is elevated in (1) DIC (FDP's interfere with polymerization), (2) low fibrinogen levels, (3) dysfibrinogenemia, and (4) the presence of heparin or direct thrombin inhibitors (very sensitive).

Reptilase time This is the same as thrombin time but is performed with a snake venom (*Bothrops atrox*) that cleaves fibrinogen and is insensitive to heparin. The reptilase time is elevated in the same conditions in which the thrombin time is elevated, but the reptilase time is not affected by heparin. Thrombin time and reptilase time are most useful in the evaluation of dysfibrinogenemia.

Ecarin Time The ecarin time is performed by using snake venom from *Echis carinatus* (saw-tooth viper). This venom directly activates prothrombin, leading to clot formation. It is inhibited by direct thrombin inhibitors and is useful for monitoring the antithrombin class of antithrombotic agents such as dabigatran and argatroban.

Fibrinogen Levels Fibrinogen activity levels are assayed by using a modified thrombin time. The causes of a low fibrinogen level are:

- Liver disease
- Disseminated intravascular coagulation
- Dilution (i.e., massive transfusions)
- Dysfibrinogenemia or afibrinogenemia

Thromboelastography (TEG) (Table 2.8)

TEG is a unique laboratory test that examines whole blood thrombus formation and lysis. TEG is performed by placing a 0.35 ml of whole blood into an oscillating container with a pin that measures the force of thrombus formation. TEG measures five parameters (Table 2.8):

- R time: time from starting TEG until clot formation
- K time: time between tracing going from 2 to 20 mm
- Alpha angle: slope of tracing between r and K time
- MA: greatest amplitude of TEG tracing
- Blood lysis: amplitude of tracing 30–60 minutes after MA

Most modern TEG machines automatically calculate these parameters. In addition, some TEG has a heparinase container for use in patients on heparin. Currently, the main use of TEG is with liver transplantation, cardiac surgery, and trauma patients. TEG allows rapid point-of-care testing of coagulation and is particularly useful in assessing fibrinolysis and hemostasis in patients with liver disease

Thrombotic Disorder

As with bleeding disorders, the history is important for evaluation of thrombotic disorders. Patients need to be quizzed not only about obvious thrombosis but also about episodes of leg swelling, shortness of breath, and diagnoses of "walking pneumonia." The family history is also crucial. Like bleeding disorders, hypercoagulable states are often heritable but with incomplete penetrance so one needs to be persistent in questioning.

Tests for APLA

APLAs are important to detect because in certain patients they are associated with a syndrome that may include a hypercoagulable state, thrombocytopenia, fetal loss, dementia, strokes, Addison's disease, and skin rashes. There are two main tests for APLAs: testing for presence of antibodies to cardiolipin and the coagulation-based tests for APLA.

Coagulation-based tests   As noted above, APLA reacts with phospholipid. The phospholipids provide a surface where the coagulation reactions take place. The basis for all the coagulation-based tests is that antibodies on the phospholipid will prolong the coagulation reactions and thus the test time. Once an elevated aPTT is found, one must verify it by showing it does not fully correct with a 50:50 mix. To prove the inhibitor is dependent on phospholipids, one then adds phospholipid derived from platelets or hexagonal phase phospholipids. APLA reacts strongly with these phospholipids, and addition of these will correct the coagulation tests by absorbing out the APLA.

To summarize, one screens for APLA with coagulation-based tests to see if any clotting times are prolonged. If a test result is elevated, then a 50:50 mix is done to ensure the elevation is not due to a specific factor deficiency. If no factor deficiency, then one uses a phospholipid source to correct the clotting time and verify the presence of APLA.

Specific Assays

aPTT   The routine aPTT only detects 30% of patients with APLA and is inadequate as a single test for APLA screening. One can increase sensitivity by using different aPTT reagents.

Kaolin clotting time   This test uses no added phospholipid and is a sensitive test to detect APLA. However, it is technically demanding to do properly.

Platelet neutralization test   This test takes a coagulation reaction that is prolonged by plasma and does not correct with a 50:50 mix. Extracts of platelet phospholipids are added to the plasma and an aPTT is performed. The platelet phospholipid is very avid for APLA, "soaks up" the antiphospholipid antibody, and corrects the aPTT. If the aPTT corrects with addition of platelets, this is diagnostic for APLA.

Hexagonal phospholipid neutralization   This test is based on the same principle as the platelet neutralization test, but it uses t hexagonal phospholipid which is more specific for antiphospholipid antibodies. Current test kits that use hexagonal phospholipids also have added plasma and inhibitors of heparin. The additional reagents allow this assay for lupus inhibitors to be performed on anticoagulated patients. The test is reported as the time in seconds between the PTT with and without added phospholipids.

Silica clotting time   This test uses silica to activate coagulation and a reagent with very low levels of phospholipids. If the test is prolonged, then it's repeated with a high phospholipid reagent. If the PTT prolongation was due to antiphospholipid then the addition of high phospholipid reactant will correct the prolongation. This test is reported as a ratio between the PTT with and without added phospholipids.

Dilute Russell viper venom time (dRVVT)   This test is very sensitive to any interference with phospholipids and is very sensitive to APLA. It is performed by initiating the coagulation cascade with Russell Viper venom which directly activates factor X and is very sensitive to phospholipids. dRVVT will also be increased in warfarin patients and with deficiencies of X, V, or II. There is a phospholipid neutralization step used to derive a dRVVT ratio (without/with phospholipids) to find antiphospholipid antibodies.

The use of any direct oral anticoagulant can lead to false positive (and in some cases false negative) testing for lupus inhibitors. Patients taking these drugs should not have inhibitor testing performed, and as noted, many labs are now screening samples for these drugs before performing specialized coagulation testing.

Anticardiolipin antibodies (ACLA) This is an ELISA test for antibodies to cardiolipin. Therefore, it can be performed on plasma that has been anticoagulated. Test results are reported in arbitrary units. Tests are also reported as specific isotypes (IgG, IgA, IgM). It is still debated whether specific isotypes indicate specific diseases, but most "secondary" (i.e., associated with infection) ACLA tend to be IgM subtypes. Only high titers (>40 units) are associated with APLA.

Anti-beta2 glycoprotein antibodies Although "APLA" are named for antibodies to phospholipids, the real targets are phospholipid-protein combinations. For anticardiolipin antibodies the protein target is beta$_2$-glycoprotein (B$_2$GP). It appears that anti-B$_2$GP antibodies may be more specific for pathogenic APLA, as they are usually negative in infection-associated APLA and other APLAs not associated with thrombosis. Currently, anti-B$_2$GP testing is most useful in evaluation of the low-titer ACLA.

Approach to the patient suspected of having APLA Unfortunately, no single test can screen a patient for APLA. One must perform the *entire* panel on patients suspected of having APLA. The panel would include:

- Anticardiolipin antibodies
- Anti-beta2 glycoprotein antibodies
- Lupus inhibitor screen (with at least two different testing methods such as dRVVT and hexagonal phospholipid)

Hypercoagulable States

There are several tests to detect inherited or acquired hypercoagulable states as outlined in Chaps. 17 and 18. The best method is, again, to perform activity assays. Activity assays can be performed for the major inherited disorders including protein C, protein S, antithrombin III deficiencies, and hereditary resistance to activated protein C. Since proteins C and S are vitamin K-dependent proteins, their levels will be falsely low in patients taking the vitamin K-blocking blood-thinner warfarin. Any of the coagulation-based thrombophilia tests also have the potential to be interfered with by the direct oral anticoagulants, and patients should not be on these agents if this testing is to be performed.

Suggested Reading

Hayward CPM. How i investigate for bleeding disorders. Int J Lab Hematol. 2018;40(Suppl 1):6–14.

Khair K, Liesner R. Bruising and bleeding in infants and children--a practical approach. Br J Haematol. 2006;133(3):221–31.

Lassila R. Platelet function tests in bleeding disorders. Semin Thromb Hemost. 2016;42(3):185–90.

Levi M, Meijers JC. DIC: which laboratory tests are most useful. Blood Rev. 2011;25(1):33–7.

Loizou E, Mayhew DJ, Martlew V, Murthy BVS. Implications of deranged activated partial thromboplastin time for anaesthesia and surgery. Anaesthesia. 2018;73(12):1557–63.

Mezzano D, Quiroga T. Diagnostic challenges of inherited mild bleeding disorders: a bait for poorly explored clinical and basic research. J Thromb Haemost. 2019;17(2):257–70.

Pengo V, Tripodi A, Reber G, Rand JH, Ortel TL, Galli M, De Groot PG, Subcommittee on Lupus Anticoagulant/Antiphospholipid Antibody of the Scientific and Standardisation Committee of the International Society on Thrombosis and Haemostasis. Update of the guidelines for lupus anticoagulant detection. Subcommittee on Lupus Anticoagulant/Antiphospholipid Antibody of the Scientific and Standardisation Committee of the International Society on Thrombosis and Haemostasis. J Thromb Haemost. 2009;7(10):1737–40.

Rimmer EK, Houston DS. Bleeding by the numbers: the utility and the limitations of bleeding scores, bleeding prediction tools, and bleeding case definitions. Transfus Apher Sci. 2018;57(4):458–62. https://doi.org/10.1016/j.transci.2018.07.004. Epub 2018 Jul 21.

Bleeding Disorders: A General Approach

3

Thomas G. DeLoughery

Patients with bleeding disorders may present in a variety of ways. Using the history and basic screening tests, one can narrow the differential considerably. Key questions to ask are (Table 3.1):

1. *Is the bleeding real?* Patient perception of bleeding is not always useful in diagnosing a bleeding disorder. One should specify in detail the history of bleeding. The following questions are helpful in obtaining a bleeding history:
   1. Have you ever had a nosebleed? How frequently do these occur? Has any required a trip to the hospital?
   2. Have you ever had bleeding with dental work? Did it require stitching or packing due to the bleeding? Did it bleed the next day?
   3. What surgeries have you undergone? Did any of them require transfusions? Did your surgeon comment on excessive bleeding?
   4. What is the biggest bruise you ever had? How did it happen?
   5. How long are your menstrual periods? Have you ever been so anemic you needed

Table 3.1 The key questions

1. Is the bleeding real?
2. Is it platelet type bleeding or coagulation defect bleeding?
3. Is it acquired or congenital?
4. What tests do I perform and how do I interpret them?

   to be on iron replacement? Did you have excessive bleeding after childbirth or require a transfusion then?
   6. Have you ever had bleeding when you urinated, have you ever vomited blood, or have you seen blood in the toilet from your bowels?
   7. Do your gums bleed when you brush or floss your teeth?

Bleeding with coagulation disorders is excessive for the situation, prolonged, and recurrent. For example, a patient with hemophilia will bleed for several hours from a minor wound before a clot forms and then the bleeding may recur for days. Patients with mild bleeding disorders will manifest bleeding with dental extractions and surgeries. However, some patients with von Willebrand disease (due to the variability of the disease) may have had previous hemostatic challenges and not suffered significant bleeding.

As noted in Chap. 2, "Bleeding Assessment Tools" are now available and may be used to provide a more quantitative assessment of bleeding. An example that is frequently used is the ISTH-SSC

T. G. DeLoughery (✉)
Division of Hematology/Medical Oncology,
Department of Medicine, Pathology, and Pediatrics,
Oregon Health & Sciences University,
Portland, OR, USA
e-mail: delought@ohsu.edu

© Springer Nature Switzerland AG 2019
T. G. DeLoughery (ed.), *Hemostasis and Thrombosis*,
https://doi.org/10.1007/978-3-030-19330-0_3

form (https://bleedingscore.certe.nl/). These tools are particularly useful in clinical studies of bleeding disorders. For better quantitation of menstrual bleeding, the Philipp score is helpful: https://www.cdc.gov/ncbddd/blooddisorders/women/documents/menorrhagiafortesting.pdf

2. *Is the bleeding due to factor deficiencies or platelet defects?*

Patients with bleeding due to platelet defects (and von Willebrand disease) will manifest mainly mucocutaneous bleeding. They will have excessive bruising, gingival bleeding, and frequent nose bleeds. Patients with coagulation factor deficiencies will tend to have muscle and joint bleeds. Both groups of patients will bleed excessively from injuries and at the time of surgery.

3. *Is it an acquired or inherited disorder?*

Patients with inherited bleeding disorders can present anytime from birth until old age. Patients with mild hemophilia or von Willebrand disease may not have worrisome bleeding until their first trauma or surgery. Therefore, the presence of an abnormal aPTT in an older patient should *not* be ignored because "they are too old to have hemophilia." Classic hemophilia A and B (factors VIII and IX deficiency) are sex linked so it is important to ask about bleeding in brothers, cousins, and uncles. Von Willebrand disease is autosomal dominant but may have variable penetrance. Acquired bleeding disorders will often present suddenly with severe bleeding and newly abnormal coagulation tests. Often these patients have other illnesses, but autoimmune coagulation diseases can suddenly strike any previously healthy person.

4. *What tests do I need to perform and how do I interpret them?*

A patient with a suggestive history of bleeding should have a PT, aPTT, platelet count, and bleeding time (or PFA-100) performed. The following patterns are most often seen (Table 3.2):

- *Elevated aPTT only*: Factors VIII, IX, and XI deficiencies are associated with an increased aPTT and bleeding. Factor VIII

Table 3.2 Most common test results and likely (not exhaustive!) diagnoses

Elevated PT only: chronic liver disease, mild vitamin K deficiency

Elevated aPTT only:
  Not bleeding: lupus inhibitor, factor XII deficiency
  Bleeding: heparin contamination (if drawn through catheter – factor VIII deficiency or inhibitor, factor IX deficiency

Both PT and aPTT elevated: warfarin or heparin effect, severe liver disease, DIC
Abnormal bleeding time: aspirin, Cox-1 inhibitors, von Willebrand disease, platelet function defects, uremia, liver disease

and IX deficiency will present as classic "hemophilia." Factor XI deficiency has more variable bleeding tendencies and often is associated with post-surgical bleeding. Acquired factor inhibitors will present often with a sudden onset of bleeding. Factor XII and contact protein deficiencies do not have associated bleeding. Patients with lupus inhibitors rarely bleed. Some patients with antiphosopholipid antibodies will have bleeding if they have associated prothrombin deficiency. The laboratory clue is that they will also have an elevated PT.

- *Elevated PT only*: Only an isolated factor VII deficiency will present with an elevated PT. One only requires a factor VII level of 5–10% for adequate hemostasis, so most modest elevations (less than an INR of 3) will not lead to bleeding.

- *Elevated PT and aPTT*: The rare factors X, V, and II deficiencies have both an elevated PT and aPTT. More common etiologies are multiple deficiencies due to liver disease, vitamin K deficiency, or disseminated intravascular coagulation. Lupus inhibitors with associated antiprothrombin antibodies can also present with both tests elevated.

- *Decreased platelet counts*: See Chap. 7 for a discussion on thrombocytopenia.

- *Increased bleeding time/PFA-100*: It is seen either with von Willebrand disease or platelet function disorders. An elevated aPTT is seen only rarely in von Willebrand disease when the factor VIII level is below 30%.

Table 3.3 Additional tests to order in bleeding patients with normal screening tests

Plasma fibrinogen
Thrombin time
Reptilase time
Euglobulin clot lysis time
Factor XIII Level
Plasminogen activator inhibitor-1 level
Alpha$_2$-antiplasmin level

Patients who ingest aspirin or nonsteroidal antiinflammatory agents may have a prolonged bleeding time. Prolonged bleeding times are routinely seen in liver and renal disease. The prolonged bleeding times present in liver and renal disease patients are of little prognostic value for risk of bleeding.

Rare patients may have a normal PT, aPTT, platelet count, and bleeding time but have a bleeding diathesis. In these patients, one should check (Table 3.3):

- Plasma fibrinogen to rule out dysfibrinogenemia
- Euglobulin clot lysis time to rule out fibrinolysis
- Factor XIII level
- Plasminogen activator inhibitor-1 level
- Alpha$_2$ antiplasmin level

Suggested Reading

Harrison LB, Nash MJ, Fitzmaurice D, Thachil J. Investigating easy bruising in an adult. BMJ. 2017;356:j251.

Moenen FCJI, Nelemans PJ, Schols SEM, Schouten HC, Henskens YMC, Beckers EAM. The diagnostic accuracy of bleeding assessment tools for the identification of patients with mild bleeding disorders: a systematic review. Haemophilia. 2018;24(4):525–35.

Neutze D, Roque J. Clinical evaluation of bleeding and bruising in primary care. Am Fam Physician. 2016;93(4):279–86.

Hemophilia

4

Thomas G. DeLoughery

Introduction

Hemophilia A and B are X-linked bleeding disorders caused by factor VIII (FVIII) and factor IX (FIX) deficiency, respectively. Hemophilia A has a 1:5000 incidence among boys and comprises 80% of hemophilia cases, and hemophilia B makes up the remaining 20%. Patients with severe disease require ongoing care to manage bleeding complications and associated comorbidities. Patients with less severe disease will still need FVIII or FIX replacement and special care at times of trauma or surgical procedures. Some patients with mild disease may not present until adulthood and may minimize bleeding symptoms, considering them to be normal.

Pathophysiology and Classification

Normally, after initiation of coagulation, the tissue factor-VIIa complex activates factor IX. Factor IX, along with its co-factor VIII, then activates factor X. Patients with hemophilia bleed due to a lack of factor VIII or IX. Tissue factor-

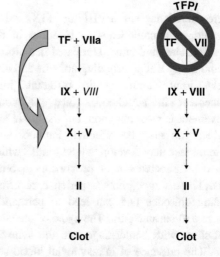

Fig. 4.1 Normal coagulation showing the role of TF+VIIa in activating both factors X and IX. When TAFI suppresses TF+VIIa, continued coagulation is dependent on IXa and its co-factor VIII

VIIa can directly activate factor X, but this reaction is soon quenched by formation of tissue factor pathway inhibitor making further thrombin generation dependent on factors VIII and IX (Fig. 4.1).

Classification is based on clinical severity of disease which generally correlates the level of factor deficiency. Severe disease is defined as less than 1% factor activity (<1 IU/dL), moderate disease 1–5% factor activity, and mild disease 5–40% factor activity. Patients with severe disease often have unprovoked bleeding. Those with

T. G. DeLoughery (✉)
Division of Hematology/Medical Oncology, Department of Medicine, Pathology, and Pediatrics, Oregon Health & Sciences University, Portland, OR, USA
e-mail: delought@ohsu.edu

© Springer Nature Switzerland AG 2019
T. G. DeLoughery (ed.), *Hemostasis and Thrombosis*, https://doi.org/10.1007/978-3-030-19330-0_4

moderate disease tend to bleed with trauma. However, previous hemarthroses (joint bleeds) or hemarthropathy (joint damage from previous bleeding) can increase the tendency towards bleeding. Individuals with mild disease often bleed only with severe trauma, surgery, or dental procedures. Measurement of baseline factor levels can help predict bleeding propensity.

Clinical Presentation and Symptoms

Hemarthrosis

Severe deficiency in FVIII or FIX, when untreated, classically leads to bleeding in the joints, muscles, and brain. Untreated hemarthroses commonly lead to crippling arthritis and ultimately joint failure with resultant joint replacement in adulthood. Knee or elbow involvement is most common, but the ankle and shoulder can also be affected. Patients with severe disease may develop "target joints" which tend to be affected out of proportion to other joints. These target joints experience recurrent bleeding episodes that can lead to permanent damage and chronic pain. The cycle of bleeding often starts with hemorrhage into the synovial space. The presence of intrasynovial blood sets up an inflammatory reaction leading to pain, warmth, and swelling. Subsequently, the synovium hypertrophies and develops increased vascularity; these new vessels are more friable which leads to more bleeding, creating a vicious cycle that ultimately leads to joint destruction.

In younger patients such as toddlers, the only sign of joint bleeding may be irritability and refusal to use a joint. Older children and adults will often describe a "tingling" in the joint, heralding the bleed. Patients with mild hemophilia may not associate their symptoms with a joint bleed and instead simply complain of frequent "sprained" ankles.

Hemarthroses cause underlying joint damage and make hemophiliac joints more prone to developing septic arthritis with a 15–40X greater risk than the general population. Initial presentation of a septic joint can be similar to that of a bleed. There can be mild warmth and severe pain, but septic joints will not improve with factor therapy and will continue to worsen. Patients with *Staphylococcus aureus* infection will typically have high fevers and elevated white counts at presentation.

Intramuscular Hematomas

Bleeding can occur in any muscle group. Iliopsoas muscle hematomas can be particularly devastating and life-threatening. Muscle bleeds in any limb can be complicated by compartment syndrome and may require surgical decompression if they progress despite factor replacement.

Iliopsoas hematomas may lead to compartment syndrome from blood tracking down the psoas muscle to cause compression of the femoral nerve with resulting paralysis of the quadriceps muscle group. Patients can present with thigh, hip, or groin pain and abdominal pain. A particular sign is hip flexion and lateral rotation due to paresthesia in the distribution of the femoral nerve.

Cerebral Hemorrhage

Cerebral hemorrhages are not uncommon in severely affected patients and are the leading cause of hemorrhagic death, especially in older patients. The bleeding may be due to minor trauma or may occur spontaneously. Patients classically present complaining of the worst headache of their lives. For patients presenting with signs suggestive of intracranial hemorrhage, factor should be given before imaging.

Diagnosis

Because both the FVIII and FIX genes are encoded on the X chromosome, hemophilia is a sex-linked disease. Hemophilia should be considered in any male patient presenting with unexplained or excessive bleeding. Patients may have affected grandfathers, uncles, and cousins but usually not parents. However, mothers can be symptomatic carriers with variable bleeding symptoms. Up to 30% of patients with newly diagnosed hemophilia will not have a family history of hemophilia; these represent new mutations. Conversely, von Willebrand disease, the most commonly inherited coagulopathy, is rarely associated with hemarthrosis. Since most types are autosomal dominant, patients with von Willebrand disease will usually have an affected parent or female relative.

Patients with mild hemophilia may not be diagnosed until adulthood, when an episode of trauma, dental extraction, or surgically induced bleeding leads to the diagnosis. Past episodes of bleeding are often minimized or not recognized as being abnormal. Some with mild hemophilia will have only mildly elevated aPTT and can go on to have severe bleeding if this laboratory abnormality is not further evaluated.

Once hemophilia is suspected, the diagnostic approach is straightforward. Patients with an elevated aPTT should have FVIII, FIX and von Willebrand levels assayed. Patients with normal FVIII and FIX levels should be screened for other bleeding disorders (Chap. 6).

Therapy

In theory, the treatment of hemophilia is simple—replace the missing factor. Plasma-purified and recombinant factor replacement is available for both hemophilia A and B (Table 4.1). In practice, treatment needs to be tailored to the individual needs of each patient. In addition, the increasing use of novel products has made choosing the best therapy more challenging.

Hemophilia A (Factor VIII Deficiency)

A number of FVIII replacement products exist; these range from "medium purity products" to pure recombinant products. Since all products derived from plasma sources are treated to inactivate hepatitis and HIV viruses, "purity" refers to the presence of other proteins. Some recombinant FVIII (rFVIII) products require plasma proteins

Table 4.1 Replacement products

Factor VIII
Low purity
Cryoprecipitate
Immunoaffinity purified
Hemofil-M (Baxter)
Monarc-M (Baxter)
Monoclate-P (CSL Behring)
Intermediate purified containing von Willebrand factor
Alphanate SD (Grifols)
Koate-DVI (Talecris)
Humate-P (CSL Behring)
Wilate (Octapharma)
Recombinant
Advate (Baxter)
Helixate (Bayer)
Kogenate (Bayer)
Recombinate (Baxter)
Refacto (Pfizer)
Xyntha (Pfizer)
Factor IX
Low purity (prothrombin complex concentrates) (<50 IX units/mg)
Bebulin VH (Baxter)
Profilnine SD (Grifols)
Kcentra (CSL Behring)
Higher purity (> 160 units/mg)
MonoNine (CSL Behring)
Alphanine SD (Grifols)
Recombinant
BeneFIX (Genetics Institute)
Rixubis (Baxter)

during production that are removed during processing, such as Helixate FS or Refacto, while other rFVIII preparations, including Advate or Xyntha, are albumin-free and have virtually no risk of viral transmission. Only high purity products are used to treat factor deficient coagulopathies. Intermediate purity plasma-derived FVIII products can be used to treat von Willebrand disease as they contain von Willebrand factor. It should be noted that viral transmission has not been observed with any rFVIII or modern virally inactivated plasma isolated products.

Theoretically, 1 unit of FVIII per kg will increase factor activity by 2 IU/dL or 2% (Table 4.2):

$$\frac{(\text{desired FVIII concentration} - \text{current level}) \times \text{weight in kg}}{2}$$

Table 4.2 Calculation of replacement doses of factors VIII and IX

Replacement dose for factor VIII

$$\frac{(\text{desired Factor VIII concentration} - \text{current level}) \times \text{weight } (\text{kg})}{2}$$

Replacement dose for factor IX

(desired Factor IX concentration − current level) × weight (kg)

Continuous infusion of products

Factor VIII: bolus of 50 units/kg followed by a continuous infusion of 4 units/hour guided by levels

Factor IX: load with 100 units/kg and then use a continuous infusion of 4–5 units/hour guided by levels

In an emergency one can assume the current level is zero and use the formula:

$$\frac{(\text{desired level})}{2} \times \text{weight in kg}$$

However, factor utilization differs among patients. Under times of surgical stress, there may be increased factor consumption. Therefore, for all but the simplest procedures, therapy should be guided by factor VIII levels. Infusions should be repeated every 8–12 hours to achieve the desired level. Another method that is useful for achieving stable levels of factor VIII is continuous infusion of the product. The infusion should start with a bolus of 50 units/kg and then a continuous infusion of factor VIII at ~4 units/kg/hour with adjustments guided by factor levels.

In a patient who has received multiple infusions, the history may be used to guide treatment for simple bleeds. A "recovery" study should be conducted before major surgeries are performed. This consists of measuring factor VIII levels pre-infusion and then 30 minutes and again 4 hours after the infusion of 20–50 units/Kg of factor VIII. The recovery study allows for accurate assessment of the amount of factor VIII needed for replacement in a specific individual.

Desmopressin, which increases FVIII levels through mobilizing von Willebrand factor release from the blood vessel lining, can be useful for treating minor bleeds and procedures for patients with mild disease. These patients will have a substantial rise in their FVIII level with administration of desmopressin. The intravenous dose is 0.3 mcg/kg diluted in 50 mL normal saline infused over 20–30 minutes one-half hour before the procedure, with a maximal dose of 20 mcg. The same dose can also be administered subcutaneously with a maximal dosing volume of 1.5 mL. The dose for nasal desmopressin (Stimate) is 150 mcg (one nasal squirt) in patients under 50 kg and 300 mcg (two squirts) in patients over 50 kg. Factor levels should increase 30–60 minutes after dosing and remain elevated for 6–12 hours. Dosing can be repeated in 12–24 hours although tachyphylaxis will occur due to depletion of von Willebrand storage sites.

Hemophilia B (Factor IX Deficiency)

In the past, FIX deficiency was treated using fresh frozen plasma (FFP) or prothrombin complex concentrates (PCC) derived by absorbing plasma from the vitamin K-dependent proteins such that the final product contained not only FIX but also factors II, VII, and X. These products are associated with several potential complications and thus are no longer used in the treatment of FIX deficiency. With the advent of highly purified FIX concentrates and recombinant FIX (rFIX) such as AlphaNine SD and BeneFIX, treatment of hemorrhage from FIX deficiency is no longer associated with excessive activation of the coagulation pathway. One unit of FIX per kilogram will increase factor activity by 1 IU/dL or 1%.

Dosing for the highly purified concentrate is

(desired FIX concentration − current level) × weight in kg

Dosing for rFIX is

$$\left[\left(\text{desired FIX concentration} - \text{current level}\right)\times \text{weight in kg}\right]\times 1.2$$

Treatment with FIX is more unpredictable than with FVIII as infused FIX has a more variable half-life; however, it is generally twice that of FVIII. Infusions should be repeated every 12–24 hours to achieve the desired level. As with factor VIII infusions, peak and trough should be measured in patients undergoing extensive procedures. Continuous infusions of factor IX should be preceded by a 100 units/kg loading dose followed by a continuous rate of 4–5 units/kg/h adjusted based upon levels.

Prophylactic Factor Use

Treatment guidelines for bleeding episodes are discussed in the next section. The most effective treatment of hemophilia is prevention of bleeding and its associated debilitating complications. Prophylactic treatment regimens have been shown to significantly reduce the number of bleeding episodes and the amount of joint disease while increasing quality of life. Furthermore, the costs associated with increased factor use are offset by the costs of treatment for bleeding and its complications. Prophylaxis is recommended in all patients with severe FVIII deficiency as well in those with moderate FVIII deficiencies that have bleeding complications. There are several prophylactic regimens used; a common FVIII prophylactic regimen is 25 IU/Kg on Mondays and Wednesdays with 50 IU/Kg on Fridays with the goal of less than one bleed per year. It is important to verify that the trough factor levels are >1%. The dosing schedule is often modified to match activities and routines, with the overall goal of prophylaxis to allow persons with hemophilia to live active normal lives, including noncontact sports. To accommodate differences in individual bleeding tendencies and activity level, the prophylactic factor replacement dose is increased if there is breakthrough bleeding or if trough factor levels arc <1%.

Patients with FIX deficiency often have a less severe bleeding phenotype compared to patients with the same severity of FVIII deficiency.

Nevertheless, prophylaxis is often considered in patients with severe FIX deficiency or in any FIX deficiency with bleeding complications. Standard FIX prophylaxis starts at 100 IU/Kg twice a week with the same goals and guidelines as those with FVIII deficiency

Now available are factor VIII and IX molecules with longer half-lives. For factor VIII, this is done by either attaching a human immunoglobulin Fc domain to the factor VIII molecular or PEGylation. The modifications lengthen the half-life by 1.5–1.8-fold and are used by some patients as prophylactic therapy to prevent bleeds

For factor IX products, the prolongation of half-life is in the range of 3–5-fold with modified products, and these products are preferred for prophylaxis in factor IX deficient patients since patients will only need an infusion once a week or even less. Beside factors modified with PEGylation and addition of the Fc receptor, there is a factor with human albumin attached.

Emicizumab

Emicizumab is a novel product to treat hemophilia A. This bispecific antibody binds factor XIa and X simulating the function of factor VIII. This product has been shown to dramatically reduce bleeding in patients. When used as prophylaxis, this product dramatically reduced bleeding rates when compared to patients receiving factor VIII prophylaxis. The drug is dosed by giving a loading dose of 3 mg/kg for 4 weeks and then either 1.5 mg/kg weekly, 3 mg/kg every other week, or 6 mg/kg every month. One drawback of this agent is that, for acute bleeds, patients will need factor VIII supplementation. The presence of emicizumab will interfere with all coagulation tests, including basic tests such as the aPTT, and will result in falsely high factor VIII levels. True factor VIII levels can only be determined by performing a chromogenic VIII level using bovine reactions which is only a reference lab procedure.

Thrombotic microangiopathy has been reported in patients who were receiving emicizumab and were treated with greater than 100 units/kg/24 h of activated prothrombin complex concentrates.

Guidelines for Specific Types of Bleeds (Table 4.3)

Hemarthrosis is managed by raising the factor VIII (or IX in hemophilia B) level to 100% acutely. Patients should initially rest and use ice on the joint, then gradually try to use it to prevent freezing of the joint. Hemarthroses can often be managed with 2–3 doses of factor replacement. FVIII is generally given every 12–24 hours, while FIX is given every 24–48 hours. In addition, for those patients not on prophylactic treatment (see above) a short course of multiple infusions to raise factor levels to ~50% may be useful for treating recurrent bleeds. Painful joints that do not respond to factor replacement may benefit from a short course of prednisone (60–80 mg/day for 3 days, then 40 mg/day for 2 days) once a septic joint is ruled out. If joint aspiration is necessary, factor levels should be at least 50% prior to aspiration. Infusions should continue until the pain stops.

Hematomas tend to respond to a target factor level of 80–100%. Large bleeds or those affecting vital structures will require more aggressive therapy (levels of 100%) or even drainage for limb-threatening bleeds. In patients with hemorrhage into limb compartments, close monitoring of neurologic function is essential, and infusions should be continued until the swelling resolves. If there is impending development of a compartment syndrome, fasciotomy may be necessary to preserve limb function.

For patients with *oral mucosal bleeding*, adjunctive therapy with antifibrinolytic agents is useful. Either epsilon aminocaproic acid (EACA) or tranexamic acid can be used. The dose of EACA is 100 mg/kg oral elixir slow swish and swallow followed by 50 mg/kg slow swish and swallow every 6 hours. Tranexamic acid is given 10–20 mg/kg orally every 8 hours. Often only a single dose of factor is required when antifibrinolytic therapy is used. Prior to most dental procedure, patients should receive 100% factor replacement. With procedures involving extractions, deep cleaning, or other procedures involving the gums, they should also receive either EACA 50 mg/kg slow swish and swallow every 6 hours or tranexamic acid 10–25 mg/kg PO BID. Individuals with factor deficiencies often

Table 4.3 General guidelines for factor replacement

Site of bleed	Hemostatic level	Hemophilia A	Hemophilia B
Joint	80–100% daily until resolved	40–50 units/kg daily	80 units/kg daily
Muscle	80–100%	25–40 units/kg per day until healed	50–60 units/kg daily
Oral	100%[a]	50 units/kg[a]	100 units/kg[a]
Nose	Initially 80–100%, then 30% until healing	40–50 units/kg, then 30–40 units per day	80–100 units/kg then 35–40 units every day
Gastrointestinal	Initially 100%, then 50% until healing	50 units/kg then 30–40 units/kg per day	100 units/kg then 30–40 units every day
Genitourinary	If conservative measures fail then give 30–50% until bleeding resolves	15–25 units/kg daily	30–50 units/kg every other day
Central nervous system	100% for 14 days	50 units/kg every 12 hours	100 units/kg every day
Surgery/trauma	80–120% until wound healing begins, then 50% until suture removed	50 units/kg then 40–50 units every 12 hours adjusted according to healing	100 units/kg then 50 units every day adjusted according to healing

Note: For severe or persistent minor bleeding, factor levels should be followed
[a]Antifibrinolytic agents are useful for oral bleeding

experience delayed oral bleeding after procedures (3–4 days after the procedure); thus, antifibrinolytic treatment should continue for 5–7 days.

Gastrointestinal bleeding should be treated with the initial goal of factor levels of 100%, and thereafter a trough level of 30% should be achieved until the lesion has healed. Patients with hemophilia will often have an underlying lesion as the source of their bleeding. Therefore, aggressive evaluation of the gastrointestinal tract is necessary after a bleeding episode.

Hematuria is a common complication in patients with hemophilia. Rare episodes of painless hematuria do not require investigation. Frequent, excessive hematuria, especially associated with other symptoms such as pain, requires aggressive evaluation to ensure there is not an underlying lesion present. Secondary to concerns for obstruction, hematuria is normally treated conservatively with rest and oral or intravenous hydration unless there is a drop in the hematocrit, pain, or bleeding lasting more than several consecutive days. When factor is used, a peak of 40–50% is targeted to control the bleed. Hydration is an important adjunct therapy. Antifibrinolytic therapy should not be used in this situation since this can lead to formation of insoluble thrombi in the ureters.

The presence of any *head trauma* in individuals with severe hemophilia, even with no significant bruising or swelling, should receive aggressive factor therapy. Any patient with hemophilia and a severe headache or new neurological signs should immediately receive factor replacement (aiming for 100% levels) *before* proceeding to an imaging study. In older patients, 50% of bleeds occur without a history of trauma.

Surgery in the Patient with Hemophilia

Surgical intervention requires close monitoring of the patient's factor levels. Close coordination among hematologist, surgeon, anesthesiologist, and nursing staff is paramount. Before any major procedure, a recovery study should be performed. One hour prior to surgery, the appropriate dose of factor should be administered to give a predicted level of 100–120% with a post-infusion level obtained to insure adequate factors levels for surgery. After surgery, a factor level should be obtained in the recovery room to guide the next dose. The trough should not fall below 70% for at least the first 48 hours after surgery. The trough level is gradually tapered but should be kept above 30% until full wound healing has occurred. For joint replacement, patients should have their levels increased to 50–80% before each physical therapy session to allow full participation in rehabilitation.

Inhibitors

Twenty five to 30% of patients with severe hemophilia A and ~3% of patients with hemophilia B develop antibodies or inhibitors to infused factors. Inhibitors generally present with decreased response to factor infusions. With FIX deficiency anaphylaxis can also occur, especially in the first 20 infusions of factor replacement. There are several predisposing factors for inhibitor development, including the type of gene mutation involved, age of the patient, and the number of factor infusions the patient has had. Inhibitor formation is most common in patients during their first 50 infusions. There is evidence that the type of factor replacement given—recombinant or plasma-derived—alters the risk for inhibitor development, with higher levels seen with recombinant factors seen in one clinical trial. An inhibitor should be suspected if a patient has poor bleeding control with factor use and has post-infusion factor levels that are significantly lower than predicted.

Inhibitor levels are measured in Bethesda units with 1 Bethesda unit (BU) defined as the amount of inhibitor that can neutralize 50% of factor VIII in a 50:50 plasma mix. Patents can have low (<5 BU)- or high (≥5 BU)-titer inhibitors which impacts the type of treatment that may be effective in bleeding episodes. With no recent exposure to factor, patients may have a significant reduction in their inhibitor titers that allows a "window" for use of factor VIII with severe hemorrhage. With re-exposure to factor the anti-body titer may rise dramatically. Therefore, inhibitor patients should not be exposed to any factor-containing product unless severe or life-threatening bleeding is present. Even with significant bleeding episodes, most inhibitor patients should be given a bypassing agent that treats the bleeding without exposing the patient to factor. Given the dynamic nature of inhibitors, the inhibitor titer should be followed over time.

Management of Factor Inhibitors

Therapy for patients with inhibitors can be challenging (Table 4.4). For low-titer inhibitors (<5 BU), the inhibitor may be overwhelmed with large doses of FVIII, but the inhibitor titer often increases after several days, rendering the continued use of factor ineffective. One strategy (Kasper) is to give 40 units VIII/kg plus 20 units/kg per BU of inhibitor. However, the mainstay treatment for patients with inhibitors is the use of bypassing agents. Bypassing agents act downstream in the coagulation cascade to induce the activation of thrombin and clotting without the need for FVIII or FIX. The two bypassing agents available are activated prothrombin complex concentrates (aPCC), with the name brand of FEIBA (factor eight inhibitor bypassing agent), and recombinant activated factor VII (rFVIIa), with the name brand of Novoseven.

Table 4.4 Therapy for inhibitors

Prothrombin complex concentrate
Dosing: 100 units/kg
Bebulin VH (Baxter)
Profilnine SD (Grifols)
Kcentra (CSL Behring)
Activated prothrombin complex concentrate
Dosing: 75 units/kg every 8 hours
FEIBA (Baxter)
Recombinant activated VII
Dosing: 90 mcg/kg every 2–3 hours
NovoSeven (Novo Nordisk)
Emicizumab
3 mg/kg for 4 weeks, then either
1.5 mg/kg weekly
3 mg/kg every other week
6 mg/kg every month

aPCC contains FII, FVII, FIX, FX, and small amounts of FVIII and helps induce thrombin production which is necessary for clot development. FEIBA dosing is 50–75 units/kg every 8–12 hours with a maximum dose of 200 units/kg. aPCC use can be complicated by thromboembolic events such as stroke, myocardial infarction, and DIC. As it contains FVIII, it can also induce an amnestic response.

Recombinant VIIa (rFVIIIa) can be used in both hemophilia A and B as well as Glanzmann thrombasthenia refractory to platelet transfusion. rFVIIa binds to exposed tissue factor and can directly activate factor X, thereby bypassing the FIX-FVIII step. Dosing is 90 mcg/kg every 2–3 hours. Three doses often suffice for joint bleeds, while prolonged administration (up to 10–14 days) is required for major surgery, muscle bleeds, or intercranial hemorrhage.

Emicizumab is being used more often in patients with inhibitors. As with patients without inhibitors, there was a dramatic reduction in bleeding rates with prophylactic use of Emicizumab, and many patients are now using this agent to prevent bleeding.

Immune tolerance induction (ITI) desensitization via frequent dosing of FVIII products, often requiring months to years, has been able to eliminate inhibitor levels in 60–80% of cases. Patients with maximal titers <200 BU, and titers <10 BU at ITI initiation, inhibitor duration <5 years, low-risk mutations (missense mutations rather than null or nonsense mutations), and younger age tend to do better. Successful treatment regimens range from 100 IU/kg three times a week to 50–200 IU/kg daily.

Immune suppression with agents such as corticosteroids, cyclophosphamide, mycophenolate, intravenous immunoglobulin, and rituximab has been attempted with variable success. There have been no randomized, controlled trials to assess treatment efficacy.

Plasmapheresis has been used in emergent situations to attempt to remove the inhibitor and replace it with donor plasma. However, there are several potential difficulties using this method, and it is generally not used as first-line therapy.

Future Therapy

Hemophilia is a popular target for gene therapy, as raising the factor levels only a few percent will drastically alter the bleeding phenotype. Trials are being performed with both adenovirus and retrovirus vectors to insert a normal gene into liver cells. Early results have been promising, but more work needs to be done to make this therapy widely available.

A monoclonal antibody against TFPI that in theory would increase prothrombotic activity is in clinical trials. Also in development is a process reducing antithrombin by interfering with its production by antisense technology. Both of these agents are in early trials and, if successful, hold the promise of another pathway to prevent bleeding in hemophilia patients.

Conclusions

This chapter provides a primer for the management of hemophilia. However, hemophilia is a chronic disease with complex complications that is best handled through the multidisciplinary approach available at hemophilia treatment centers (HTC). Even if a HTC is not nearby, patients would benefit from a consultation with a regional hemophilia center that can provide periodic input on prophylaxis, physical therapy, surgical, and social needs of the patient along with specialty testing that may not be readily available in the community.

Suggested Reading

Croteau SE. Evolving complexity in hemophilia management. Pediatr Clin N Am. 2018;65(3):407–25.

Dunn A. The long and short of it: using the new factor products. Hematology Am Soc Hematol Educ Program. 2015;2015:26–32.

Mahlangu J, Oldenburg J, Paz-Priel I, Negrier C, Niggli M, Mancuso ME, Schmitt C, Jiménez-Yuste V, Kempton C, Dhalluin C, Callaghan MU, Bujan W, Shima M, Adamkewicz JI, Asikanius E, Levy GG, Kruse-Jarres R. Emicizumab prophylaxis in patients who have hemophilia A without inhibitors. N Engl J Med. 2018;379(9):811–22.

Nogami K, Shima M. New therapies using nonfactor products for patients with hemophilia and inhibitors. Blood. 2019;133(5):399–406.

Srivastava A, Brewer AK, Mauser-Bunschoten EP, et al. Guidelines for the management of hemophilia. Haemophilia. 2013;19(1):e1–47.

Weyand AC, Pipe SW. New therapies for hemophilia. Blood. 2019;133(5):389–98.

Von Willebrand Disease

5

Thomas G. DeLoughery

Introduction

Von Willebrand disease (vWD) is the most common inherited bleeding disorder, affecting up to 1% of the population. Despite its relatively high prevalence, many features of the disease have remained controversial.

Pathogenesis and Classification

Von Willebrand factor (vWF) is critical for platelet interaction with damaged vasculature, aiding in platelet adhesion and aggregation. It is also involved in fibrin clot formation through its role as a carrier protein for factor VIII (Fig. 5.1). vWF circulates as a multimer that varies in molecular weight, with the highest multimers weighing up to 20,000,000 daltons. The larger molecular weight forms are the most effective at supporting the interaction between platelets and damaged endothelium. When vWF binds to damaged vessels (usually to exposed collagen), this alters the protein, creating a binding site for the platelet receptor Gp Ib. Thus, vWF is the "glue" between the platelet and damaged vessels. vWF is also the

carrier protein for factor VIII. Unless protected by vWF, the half-life of factor VIII is labile in the plasma due to inactivation by proteins C and S. vWD results from either decreased vWF levels or impaired vWF function.

Given the complexity of vWF, it makes sense that there are several forms of vWD (Table 5.1). *Type 1* is a quantitative defect and is the most common type of vWD, making up 65–80% of cases. It is caused by a reduction in normally functioning protein with most patients having between 5% and 40% of normal levels. Molecular studies have shown that different mutations in the von Willebrand gene cause decreased vWF levels due to mechanisms such as impaired intracellular transport, blocked transcription, and reduced half-life. In the *type 2* variants of vWF, there is a qualitative defect in which the protein's levels are unaffected, but the size and/or function is abnormal. *Type 2A* is the second most common subtype, making up 20–25% of cases, and is caused by decreased high molecular weight multimers of vWF, which are the most active form of the protein. *Type 2B* is a fascinating subtype in which there is a "gain-in-function" mutation allowing the vWF to bind to glycoprotein (GP) Ib even without collagen present. Therefore, the protein can bind to platelets even while freely circulating in the blood stream resulting in increased clearance and fewer numbers of the higher molecular weight forms. Mild thrombocytopenia is also present since the bound platelets are cleared with the sticky vWF. On the other hand, *type 2M* vWD

T. G. DeLoughery (✉)
Division of Hematology/Medical Oncology,
Department of Medicine, Pathology, and Pediatrics,
Oregon Health & Sciences University,
Portland, OR, USA
e-mail: delought@ohsu.edu

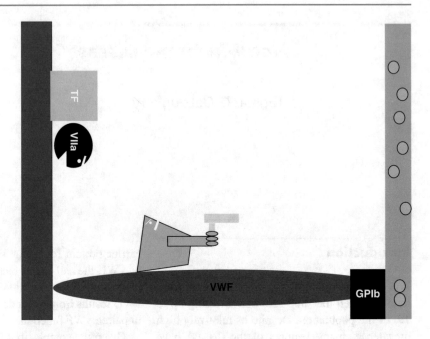

Fig. 5.1 The two roles of vWF—carrier of factor VIII and ligand for platelet adhesion

Table 5.1 Types of von Willebrand disease

Type 1: Low levels of all proteins with normal function

Type 2: Abnormal protein

   Type 2A: Abnormal protein leading to lower levels of high molecular weight multimers (HMWM)

   Type 2B: Abnormal protein with increased binding to GP Ib leading to lower levels of HMWM and increased platelet clearance

   Type 2N: Lack of factor VIII binding site leading to low factor VIII levels

   Type 2M: Abnormal protein with decreased binding to GP Ib but normal HMWM

Type 3: No vWF or factor VIII present

Pseudo-vWD: Abnormal Gp Ib with increased vWF affinity leading to lower levels of HMWM

ing vWF and factor VIII; this results in a severe phenotype that clinically mimics hemophilia. In fact, these patients will often present with severe bleeding, mucosal bleeding from impaired platelet function without the vWF, and soft tissue and joint hemorrhage from factor VIII deficiency. Finally, in "platelet-type" or "pseudo"-vWD, the platelet receptor has the "gain-of-function mutation" that acts like type 2B with reduced numbers of platelets and amounts of high molecular weight multimers.

Signs and Symptoms

is caused by the reduced affinity of vWF to GP 1b, thus reducing the activity of the factor without changing the size of multimers. Finally, *type 2 Normandy (2N)* is often mistaken for classic hemophilia because the vWF is unable to bind factor VIII, leading to low factor VIII levels (usually 5–15% but normal vWF levels). Unlike the sex-linked inheritance of classic hemophilia, the inheritance of Normandy type, as with other vWD subtypes, is autosomal dominant; males and females will be equally affected. *Type 3* vWD is rare (1:1,000,000) and is caused by a homozygous defect with no or very low levels of circulat-

Patients with vWD have "platelet-type" mucocutaneous bleeding. They will often have severe nosebleeds and large bruises. Patients will come to clinical attention due to bleeding with minor surgeries such as tonsillectomies. Women can suffer from heavy menses. In fact, in some series, up to one-third of women who present with the complaint of heavy menses will be found to have vWD. Unlike in classic hemophilia, joint bleeding is rare, except with type 3 or 2N patients. Patients often have a history of frequent bleeding as a child but with lessening of symptoms as adulthood is reached. Unless specifically questioned, patients often will not be aware of a significant bleeding history. Unexpected surgical bleeding can occur as the presenting problem in adulthood.

Testing

Testing for vWD can be challenging for several reasons. The plasma levels of vW protein in some patients can vary significantly, from abnormally low to just in the lower range of normal. Stress, such as trauma, can transiently elevate levels, and levels also tend to increase with increasing age. Finally, estrogens can greatly increase protein levels. Thus, knowing the patient's circumstances at the time of testing is important. Patients with histories suggesting platelet-type bleeding may require repeat testing to verify the diagnosis. Since vWF levels vary with the menstrual cycle, menstruating women should have levels checked between days 5 through 7 of their cycle.

The bleeding time or PFA-100 can screen patients with a history of bleeding for vWD. However, in patients with variable protein levels, these test results can also be normal when the levels are in the normal range. Therefore, a normal bleeding time in a patient with a good history for platelet- type bleeding does not eliminate the possibility of vWD.

Four tests are required to diagnose vWD (Tables 5.2 and 5.3). The tests are:

- Factor VIII activity
- von Willebrand antigen
- von Willebrand activity (sometimes called ristocetin cofactor activity [vWFR:Co])
- von Willebrand multimer analysis

Factor VIII activity is directly proportional to the amount of vWF that is present and its ability to carry factor VIII. The level of vWF antigen is an actual measurement of the protein. Von Willebrand activity can be measured in several ways. The classic test is ristocetin cofactor activity. Ristocetin is an antibiotic that was withdrawn from the market due to associated thrombocytopenia. Ristocetin causes binding of vWF to platelets. Ristocetin cofactor activity (vWFR:Co) serves as a rough measure of "von Willebrand activity." Newer assays can detect exposure of the active site that is correlated with activity. Multimer analysis shows the size distribution of von Willebrand protein multimers and helps with subtype differentiation.

vWD should be suspected if factor VIII and von Willebrand antigen and activity are below normal or if the vWF activity is significantly lower than vWF antigen regardless of the actual level of vWF activity. Since levels can vary, testing should be repeated if the initial panel is normal in those with high suspicion for vWD. Currently, levels below 30% are considered diagnostic for vWD. Patients with levels of 30–50% are labeled "bleeding with low von Willebrand factor."

Type 1 patients have uniform reductions in all three tests and normal crossed-immunoelectrophoresis. If the vWF activity/vWF antigen ratio is <0.6, a type 2 variant should be considered. A FVIII/vWF antigen ratio of

Table 5.3 Testing for von Willebrand disease

| Factor VIII level |
| von Willebrand antigen |
| von Willebrand activity |
| Multimer analysis |

Table 5.2 von Willebrand disease subtype laboratory results

	vWF:Ag	vWF: activity	Factor VIII	Multimer	RIPA
Type 1	↓	↓	↓	Normal multimer pattern	↓
Type 2A	Normal	↓	Normal or ↓	↓ HMW multimers	No response or ↓
Type 2B	Normal	↓	Normal or ↓	↓ HMW multimers	↑↑
Type 2N	Normal	Normal	↓↓	Normal multimer pattern	Normal
Type 2M	↓	↓↓	↓	Normal multimer pattern	↓↓
Type 3	<5%	<10%	<10%	Not visible	Absent

<0.7 should be concerning for hemophilia or vWD type 2N.

Patients lacking high-weight protein multimers need to be differentiated between types 2A, 2B, or pseudo-vWD. The ristocetin-induced platelet aggregation test (RIPA) can help differentiate among these types. Type 2B and the platelet type will show *increased* aggregation with addition of small amounts of ristocetin because of the "gain in function" affinity for GP 1b, while type 2A will have decreased or no activity. Unfortunately, RIPA is a point of care test not available at most institutions. However, since many of these defects are limited to certain areas of the vWF, molecular studies can be helpful in determining the different type 2 subtypes. Thus, if there is suspicion for type 2 vWD, peripheral blood can be sent out for exon 28 sequencing to certified facilities.

vWD 2N should be suspected in women who have low factor VIII levels, in cases when the inheritance appears to be autosomal dominant, or when the patient does not respond to factor VIII replacement. Diagnosis is established by performing a vWF-factor VIII binding study which is commercially available. The best diagnostic approach to 2M patients remains unsettled as there is still no consensus on how to perform and report testing; however, most cases will show the vWF activity/vWF antigen ratio is <0.6 with a normal multimer pattern on crossed-immunoelectrophoresis (Table 5.2). Direct sequencing of the vWF gene is being more commonly performed to help with exact diagnosis.

Therapy

Several therapies are available for vWD (Tables 5.4 and 5.5). Desmopressin or DDAVP causes release of stored vWF from storage pools (mainly from the endothelium). The majority of type 1 patients respond to desmopressin with vWF levels adequate to achieve hemostasis. Some type 2A patients may also respond. Desmopressin is usually avoided in type 2B and in platelet-type vWD. The fear is that such treatment will cause thrombocytopenia due to

Table 5.4 Therapy of von Willebrand disease

Intravenous desmopressin 0.3 ug/kg can be repeated daily
Intranasal desmopressin 300 ug (150 ug/nostril)
Humate-P or Alphanate
Levels below 30%: 40–50 IU/kg followed by 20 IU/kg every 12 hours
Levels above 30%: 20–40 IU/kg every day
Vonicog alfa (rVWF)
Minor/moderate bleed or surgery: 40–60 IU/kg
Major bleeding or surgery: 80 IU/kg
First dose to be given with factor VIII concentrates

Type 1	Desmopressin
Type 2A	Desmopressin (only effective in 10%), Humate-P or Alphanate
Type 2B	Humate-P, Alphanate, or Vonicog alfa
Type 2N	Desmopressin
Type 2M	Humate-P, Alphanate, or Vonicog alfa
Type 3	Humate-P, Alphanate, or Vonicog alfa
Platelet-Type	Platelets+(Humate-P, Alphanate, or Vonicog alfa), rVIIa

Table 5.5 Procedures

Desmopressin-responsive vWD: Infuse 0.3 ug/kg to end 45 minutes before procedure. May repeat every 24 hours. For major procedures, follow factor VIII levels with plan to keep troughs over 80%
Desmopressin unresponsive vWD
Humate-P or Alphanate to achieve peak over 120% and troughs of 80%:
Levels below 30%: 40–50 IU/kg followed by 20 IU/kg every 12 hours
Levels above 30%: 20–40 IU/kg every day
Vonicog alfa (rVWF) to achieve peak over 120%
Minor/moderate bleed or surgery: 40–60 IU/kg—trough >50%
Major bleeding or surgery: 80 IU/kg—trough >30%
First dose to be given with factor VIII concentrate

increased binding of vWF to the platelet, which in turn can cause increased platelet aggregation and platelet clearance. The dose of desmopressin for types 1 and 2A is 0.3 mcg/kg IV over 20–30 minutes with a maximal dose of 20 mcg. vWF levels should increase by 3–5× within 30–60 minutes and this increase should last 6–12 hours. Desmopressin is also available in a brand-name nasal spray which can be used before minor procedures. The dose for nasal desmopressin (Stimate) is one nasal squirt in patients under 50 kg and two squirts (one for each nostril) in patients over 50 kg. Stimate should be specified on the prescription because generic desmopressin is dosed inadequately for vWD. Tachyphylaxis can occur with repeated doses given every 24 hours due to exhaustion of endothelial stores. One significant side effect of desmopressin is retention of free water because it is a synthetic analog of antidiuretic hormone. In patients unable to control their water intake or in those receiving IV fluids, care must be taken not to induce hyponatremia which can cause significant morbidity and even death.

Several vWF containing plasma concentrates are available, including Humate-P and Alphanate. Infusion of the concentrates is associated with shortening of the bleeding time and normalization of multimer patterns. Ideally, the dosing is based on a patient's vWFR:Co. Factor concentrate is dosed either by factor VIII units or by von Willebrand units, both of which are listed on the vials. Suggested dosing for major bleeding or surgery is an intravenous bolus of 40 IU/kg (all dosing in *vWF* units) followed by 20 IU/kg every 12 hours for 3 days and then 20 IU/kg every day for 3–5 days. For patients with milder disease, 20–40 IU/kg every day may be effective. A recombinant product is now available—rVWF (vonicog alfa). Given that factor VIII levels can be very low, for urgent use a loading dose of factor VIII needs to be given with this product. Dosing is 40–60 IU/kg for mild to moderate bleeding and 80 IU/kg for major bleeding. Future doses are given every 12–24 hours—adjusted to have a trough level of 50% for 72 hours after surgery and then 30%. For urgent surgery or severe bleeding, a loading dose of factor VIII should also be given as per formulas in Chap. 4.

It is unclear what laboratory test best predicts hemostatic effect with infusion. A practical way to follow therapy is to follow vWFR:Co and aim for peak levels of more than 100% and troughs of more than 40%. Obviously, the dosing should be adjusted depending on the factor levels. In patients with type 3 vWD or those with very low factor VIII, factor VIII levels should be checked to ensure levels are adequate for hemostasis.

Cryoprecipitate contains a variable amount of vWF and can be used in emergencies until a more predictable source like Humate-P is available. Dosing is 10 units every 12 hours.

Therapy by vWD Subtype

Desmopressin is the mainstay of therapy for type 1 patients. However, all patients should be tested to confirm response by obtaining labs immediately before and 60 minutes after giving desmopressin (0.3 mcg/kg by IV or using the intranasal formulation). For minor procedures, desmopressin can be given once and then repeated daily in patients undergoing major surgeries. vWFR:Co levels should be followed in patients undergoing major procedures to ensure adequate hemostasis. For dental work, the addition of antifibrinolytic therapy such as Amicar (50 mg/kg QID) or tranexamic acid (10–20 mg/kg PO BID) is useful.

Ten percent of type 2 patients respond to desmopressin, so these patients should be tested for a response. Type 2A patients who do respond to desmopressin tend not to respond with as high of an absolute rise in factor or as long of a duration of response as type 1 patients. Patients without a response to desmopressin should receive a vWF-containing plasma concentrate, such as Humate-P or Alphanate or rVWF. Type 2 patients with menorrhagia tend to respond well to oral contraceptive pills or levonorgestrel-releasing intrauterine devices.

Therapy of type 2B is a vWF-containing plasma concentrate (Humate-P or Alphanate) or rVWF. Desmopressin may induce thrombocytopenia and worsen the bleeding diathesis since the abnormal vWF has a higher affinity for platelets and results in greater platelet clearance.

Type 2N patients often respond to desmopressin. For non-responders or major surgery, Humate-P, Alphanate, or rVWF can be used.

Type 2M patients require Humate-P or Alphanate.

Therapy of type 3 patients requires a vWF-containing plasma concentrate which also supplies the missing factor VIII or therapy with rVWF and supplemental factor VIII for the first dose. Many of these patients characteristically have "hemophiliac-type" bleeding and will require aggressive factor replacement. Ultimately many of these patents will require joint replacements due to hemarthroses.

Therapy of platelet-type vWD is challenging. If indicated, platelets and vWF-containing plasma concentrate need to be given concomitantly. A typical dose is 20 units of platelets followed by the appropriate dose of Humate-P. These patients represent a major management challenge and should only have procedures performed if absolutely necessary. In patients with refractory bleeding, recombinant factor VIIa may be useful.

Pregnancy

Levels of vWF increase dramatically with pregnancy. The vast majority of patients with type 1 vWD will normalize their levels with pregnancy and not require any therapy at the time of delivery. A von Willebrand panel at 32 weeks should be performed to ensure normal levels. Types other than type 1 may require therapy at the time

of delivery. It is desirable to avoid desmopressin or factor replacement until after the cord is clamped. Patient with severe non-type 1 vWD may have excessive postpartum bleeding and should receive aggressive therapy after delivery.

Suggested Reading

Castaman G, Goodeve A, Eikenboom J. Principles of care for the diagnosis and treatment of von Willebrand disease. Haematologica. 2013;98(5):667–74.

Kruse-Jarres R, Johnsen JM. How i treat type 2B von Willebrand disease. Blood. 2018;131(12):1292–13.

Leebeek FWG, Susen S. Von Willebrand disease: clinical conundrums. Haemophilia. 2018;24(Suppl 6):37–43.

Ng CJ, Di Paola J. Von Willebrand disease: diagnostic strategies and treatment options. Pediatr Clin N Am. 2018;65(3):527–41.

Peyvandi F, Mamaev A, Wang JD, Stasyshyn O, Timofeeva M, Curry N, Cid AR, Yee TT, Kavakli K, Castaman G, Sytkowski A. Phase 3 study of recombinant von Willebrand factor in patients with severe von Willebrand disease who are undergoing elective surgery. J Thromb Haemost. 2019;17(1):52–62.

von Lillicrap D. Willebrand disease: advances in pathogenetic understanding, diagnosis, and therapy. Blood. 2013;122(23):3735–40.

Other Inherited Bleeding Disorders

6

Thomas G. DeLoughery

Platelet Defects

Introduction

Inherited platelet defects fall into two general categories: congenital defects in platelet function and inherited thrombocytopenic disorders. These syndromes cause varying degrees of platelet-type bleeding ranging from minor to severe. In addition, several are associated with an increased risk of developing leukemia (Table 6.1).

Defective Platelet Function

Most patients with inherited disorders of platelet function have normal platelet counts. These patients present with signs of platelet-type bleeding such as nosebleeds and easy bruisability. Patients tend to be only mildly symptomatic and may have excessive bleeding with trauma and surgery. Although many patients on evaluation will be identified with specific defects of platelet

Table 6.1 Inherited defects of platelet function

Platelet function disorders with normal platelet numbers
Collagen aggregation defects (inheritance pattern varies)
Glanzmann thrombasthenia (AR)
Dense granule deficiency (autosomal recessive, AR)
Secretion defect (inheritance varies)
Thrombocytopenia (large platelets)
Alport's syndrome (autosomal dominant, AD)
Autosomal dominant thrombocytopenia (AD)
Bernard-Soulier (AR) syndrome
MYH 9 defects
Fechtner syndrome (AD)
Gray platelet syndrome (AD)
May-Hegglin anomaly (AD)
Montreal giant platelet syndrome (AD)
Thrombocytopenia (normal-sized platelets)
Chediak–Higashi syndrome (AR)
Thrombocytopenia with absent radius (TAR) (AR)
Factor V Quebec (AD)
Thrombocytopenia (small platelets)
Wiskott-Aldrich syndrome (X-linked)

aggregation, some patients will have a history of bleeding and a prolonged bleeding time or platelet function assay (PFA) closure time but no identifiable defects.

Diagnosis is made by prolonged bleeding or PFA closure time in the presence of a suggestive history. Platelet aggregation studies or flow cytometry for missing proteins can be useful in identifying specific defects such as Glanzmann thrombasthenia or Bernard-Soulier syndrome.

T. G. DeLoughery (✉)
Division of Hematology/Medical Oncology,
Department of Medicine, Pathology, and Pediatrics,
Oregon Health & Sciences University,
Portland, OR, USA
e-mail: delought@ohsu.edu

© Springer Nature Switzerland AG 2019
T. G. DeLoughery (ed.), *Hemostasis and Thrombosis*,
https://doi.org/10.1007/978-3-030-19330-0_6

Electron microscopy can identify abnormal platelet morphology. Increasingly, molecular testing is being used to identify specific defects. Panels using new generation sequencing technology can screen a large number (50–90) for mutations. Studies indicate that up to 50% or more of patients with previously undiagnosed bleeding disorders will have mutations found using this technology.

No specific therapy exists for these disorders. Many patients respond to desmopressin, and any patient identified with a platelet bleeding disorder should receive a trial of desmopressin to see if the PFA shortens. Platelets should be given for severe bleeding. All platelet products should be leukoreduced to prevent platelet alloimmunization. There is some data showing that recombinant factor VIIa is useful for patients with Glanzmann thrombasthenia who have severe bleeding or need major procedures. Antifibrinolytics such as tranexamic acid 1000 mg IV or 1300 mg oral tid can be useful for oral procedures or minor surgeries. Patients with RUNX1, ETV6, and ANKRD26 mutations have a higher risk for leukemia and need to have their blood counts monitored.

Congenital Thrombocytopenia

Congenital thrombocytopenia may be associated with a number of diseases. Most patients have only mild thrombocytopenia in the 50,000–100,000 uL range with varying degrees of bleeding.

Diagnosis can be easy if the thrombocytopenia is part of a well-defined syndrome. Some patients with milder disorders may be labeled as having "mild immune thrombocytopenia." A careful review of the family history or review of family members' blood counts will reveal the inherited nature of the thrombocytopenia.

Patients with mild thrombocytopenia and no symptoms do not require any therapy. Symptomatic patients often respond to desmopressin. Severely affected patients will require platelet transfusions.

Named Platelet Disorders

Platelet Function Disorders with Normal Platelet Numbers

Collagen aggregation defects (inheritance pattern varies): Patients have an isolated defect in aggregation to collagen.

Dense granule deficiency (autosomal recessive, AR): Platelets have no storage pools of ADP and serotonin. Patients may demonstrate reduced platelet aggregation, especially in response to epinephrine and collagen. Electron microscopy will reveal the abnormal platelet structure. Flow cytometry can detect the lack of granules due to lack of uptake of fluorescent dye by the affected platelets.

Glanzmann thrombasthenia (AR) is a severe bleeding disorder in which the platelets lack GP IIb/IIIa. Patients can have life-threatening bleeding from the time of birth. Platelet aggregation testing will demonstrate complete lack of aggregation to all agonists except ristocetin. Flow cytometry will detect the lack of either CD61 or CD41. In severely affected children, bone marrow transplantation can be curative.

Secretion defect (varies): It encompasses a large number of disorders, including cyclooxygenase deficiency and defects in mobilizing calcium.

Thrombocytopenia (Large Platelets)

Autosomal dominant thrombocytopenia (AD) is manifested by mild thrombocytopenia, larger (in some kindreds, normal size) platelets, and a mild bleeding diathesis. Some families have a markedly higher incidence of leukemias due to defects in RUNX1. In addition, patients who are carriers of Bernard-Soulier syndrome may have thrombocytopenia with large platelets on the blood smear and can be shown to have decreased expression of CD42.

Bernard-Soulier (AR) syndrome is a defect in platelet GP Ib. Platelet aggregation shows decreased response to ristocetin, and flow cytometry shows loss of CD42.

Gray platelet syndrome (AD) platelets have no alpha granules, giving the platelet a characteristic gray appearance on the peripheral smear. Some patients develop myelofibrosis later in life. Platelet aggregation is abnormal in response to ADP, collagen, and thrombin.

MHY9 defects (AD) are a group of syndromes due to mutations in the myosin heavy chain genes. The platelet defect is a thrombocytopenia with normal platelet function in most (but not all!) patients. Rare patients have been reported to have prolonged bleeding times/PFA that have responded to an infusion of desmopressin. A diagnostic clue is Döhle bodies in the leukocytes. Patients may also have nerve deafness, renal disease, and cataracts. Former names of these defect syndromes are Alport's, Fechner, and May-Hegglin syndromes.

Montreal giant platelet syndrome (AD) has large platelets and mild bleeding. Platelets show abnormal aggregation to ristocetin, ADP, and collagen.

Thrombocytopenia (Normal-Sized Platelets)

Chediak-Higashi syndrome (AR): Patients have albinism, recurrent infections, and inclusion bodies in leukocytes and macrophages. Platelets show abnormal aggregation in response to epinephrine and collagen.

Thrombocytopenia with absent radius (TAR) (AR): Patients have reduced number of bone marrow megakaryocytes. This syndrome may be a variant of Fanconi's anemia.

Quebec platelet disorders (AD): Patients have delayed bleeding after injury due to excessive fibrinolysis from release of excess fibrinolytic enzymes from the platelet. Platelet aggregation testing shows defects in aggregation to epinephrine and sometimes to ADP and collagen. Patients will have markedly elevated FDP but normal D-dimers on testing. Given this mechanism, antifibrinolytics are useful in treatment of bleeding in these patients.

Thrombocytopenia (Small Platelets)

Wiskott-Aldrich syndrome (X-linked): Patients have an immunodeficiency and severe eczema.

Platelets show abnormal aggregation to ADP, collagen, and thrombin.

Less Common Coagulation Disorder

Patients with classic hemophilia greatly outnumber those with these defects. Common features are variable bleeding and autosomal inheritance. Most of these patients are treated with plasma infusions with some important exceptions (Table 6.2).

Alpha₂-antiplasmin deficiency is rare, with patients showing umbilical stump bleeding, spontaneous joint and muscle bleeding, and excessive bleeding after trauma or surgery. The euglobulin clot lysis time may be normal, and diagnosis is made by measuring alpha₂-antiplasmin levels. One odd finding is a greater tendency for bleeding with increasing age. Therapy is with antifibrinolytic therapy.

Plasminogen activator inhibitor-1 deficiency presents in a similar fashion to alpha₂-antiplasmin deficiency. The euglobulin clot lysis time is more reliably shortened in these patients. Treatment is also with antifibrinolytic therapy.

Hypofibrinogenemic patients have a mild bleeding tendency. Total lack of fibrinogen (afibrinogenemia) has been reported with patients having a severe hemorrhagic disposition similar to classic hemophilia. Women have a higher risk of miscarriages and may benefit from prophylaxis. One unique feature is a propensity for spontaneous splenic rupture. Cryoprecipitate contains fibrinogen and is used for replacement. Recommended dosage is one bag for every 5–7 kg of body weight. For prolonged replacement, this initial dose can be followed by one bag of cryoprecipitate/15 kg body weight daily. One should aim for trough levels of 100 mg/dl. Fibrinogen concentrates (both recombinant and plasma derived) are now available and are dosed at desired rise in fibrinogen level/1.7 times weight in kilograms.

Dysfibrinogenemias have a variety of presentations ranging from asymptomatic (~50%), bleeding (~30%), to thrombosis (~20%). The PT-INR and aPTT are normal unless the fibrinogen activity is below 80 mg/dl. The thrombin

Table 6.2 Rare factor deficiencies

Factor	Normal plasma concentration (mg/dl)	Level needed for hemostasis	Half-life (hours)	Therapy
I	200–400	100 mg/dl	120	Cryoprecipitate
II	10	25%	50–80	Plasma
V	1	20–25%	24	Plasma, platelets
VII	0.05	15%	6	Plasma, RVIIA
VIII	0.01	100%	12	Concentrate, desmopressin
IX	0.3	100%	24	Concentrate
X	1	10–20%	25–60	Plasma, estrogens
XI	0.5	40–60%	40–80	Plasma
XIII	1–2	1–3%	150	Plasma
Alpha$_2$-antiplasmin	5–7	30% (?)	48	Antifibrinolytic agents
Plasminogen activator 1	0.005			Antifibrinolytic agents

time is usually prolonged, but cases of dysfibrinogenemias exist where the thrombin time is shortened. Specific assays of fibrinogen activity will show low levels. In dysfibrinogenemia, the fibrinogen antigen will be markedly elevated above activity levels and this discrepancy is the most valuable diagnostic clue. Therapy is with cryoprecipitate concentrates with dosage the same as for hypofibrinogenemia.

Prothrombin deficiency has markedly elevated PT-INR and aPTT with the PT-INR elevated to a greater degree. Patients often bleed soon after birth but tend not to get hemarthrosis. Bleeding patients should be treated with plasma to achieve a prothrombin level of 10–15% for minor bleeding and 20–40% for major bleeding or surgery. Given the long half-life of prothrombin, repeated transfusion may not be necessary for isolated bleeding episodes. For more aggressive therapy, one can use prothrombin concentrates such as prothrombin complex concentrates with loading dose of 20 units/kg and daily infusion of 5 units/kg adjusted to desired levels.

Factor V deficiency: Patients have a mild to moderate bleeding disorder. Levels of factor V tend not be greatly predictive of bleeding. PT-INR and aPTT are prolonged. One should always obtain a factor VIII level, due to the rare syndrome of combined factor V and VIII deficiency. Bleeding patients are treated with plasma to achieve a factor V level of 20–25%. Plasma is dosed as an initial infusion of 20 ml/kg followed by 5 ml/kg every 12 hours to achieve a trough of 25%. Platelets also contain factor V, and platelet transfusions may be useful in severe bleeding.

Factor VII deficiency is associated with severe bleeding, including a high frequency of intracranial hemorrhage. Oddly, some patients with very low levels do not manifest bleeding, and excessive thrombosis has been reported. Patients have an isolated PT-INR elevation. Therapy is with plasma to achieve a level of 15%. Factor VII has a short half-life so plasma must be infused frequently. Recombinant VIIa dosed at 15–30 ug/kg is also useful in these patients. In these patients, one can simply monitor the PT-INR with a goal of achieving a normal value. Due to the short half-life of factor VII, frequent dosing may be necessary.

Factor X deficiency is associated with severe bleeding including hemarthrosis and intracranial bleeding. The PT-INR and aPTT are prolonged. In bleeding patients, 15–20 ml/kg of plasma should be infused to achieve a factor X level of 15–20%. Prothrombin complex concentrates contain factor X and may be useful for severe bleeding. Loading dose is 20–30 units/kg and daily dosing is 10–15 units/kg. Factor X levels do rise with estrogens and this may be useful in symptomatic women. There is also a factor X concentrate that can be used for major procedures or severe bleeding. The dosing for bleeding is 25 units/kg every 24 hours until cessation of bleeding. For surgery, a factor X level of 70–90% prior to surgery should be aimed for and dosing is by this formula:

$$Body\ weight\ (Kg) \times (desired\ factor \times level\ increase) \times 0.5 = dose\ to\ be\ given$$

Factor XI deficiency has the most variation in bleeding tendencies of any factor deficiency, and the bleeding tendency is not closely associated with factor XI levels. The disease is most commonly found in the Ashkenazi Jewish population. Patients who are symptomatic tend to have a mild-to-moderate bleeding disorder with an isolated elevated aPTT. Patients tend to bleed after surgical procedures and after dental surgery. Some heterozygotes may also exhibit mild bleeding. The family and personal history of bleeding tends to be more reliable than factor levels.

Patients can be treated with plasma, but high levels (40–60%) are needed for hemostasis. Given that the half-life of factor XI is long, one can infuse a "loading dose" of 15 ml/kg plasma and then follow this with 3–6 ml/kg every 12 hours, with goal levels being 45% for major surgery and 30% for minor procedures. Given the volumes of plasma involved, there is increasing interest in the use of rVIIa, especially for trauma and major surgery, at low doses such as 15–30 ug/kg. Some patients may also respond to desmopressin. Increasingly antifibrinolytic agents such as tranexamic acid have shown good results in preventing procedural bleeding.

Factor XII deficiency: Homozygotes have unmeasurable aPTT. This factor deficiency is not associated with any excessive bleeding. In fact, a mild tendency toward thrombosis has been claimed. Deficiency of prekallikrein and high-molecular-weight kininogen present in a similar fashion with no excessive bleeding.

Factor XIII deficiency: Patients have a high incidence of intracranial hemorrhage and umbilical stump hemorrhage. Women may also suffer from frequent spontaneous abortions. Since factor XIII deficiency does not prolong the PT-INR or aPTT, specific factor levels must be done. Only low levels of XIII (1–3%) are needed for hemostasis, and this can be accomplished by prophylactic cryoprecipitate infusions 1 unit/10 kg every 3–4 weeks or by use of one of the recombinant factor XIII products.

Suggested Reading

Hsieh L, Nugent D. Rare factor deficiencies. Curr Opin Hematol. 2012;19(5):380–4.

Lee A, Poon MC. Inherited platelet functional disorders: general principles and practical aspects of management. Transfus Apher Sci. 2018;57(4):494–501.

Lentaigne C, Freson K, Laffan MA, Turro E, Ouwehand WH, BRIDGE-BPD Consortium and the ThromboGenomics Consortium. Inherited platelet disorders: toward DNA-based diagnosis. Blood. 2016;127(23):2814–23.

Menegatti M, Peyvandi F. Treatment of rare factor deficiencies other than hemophilia. Blood. 2019;133(5):415–24. https://doi.org/10.1182/blood-2018-06-820738. Epub 2018 Dec 17.

Noris P, Pecci A. Hereditary thrombocytopenias: a growing list of disorders. Hematology Am Soc Hematol Educ Program. 2017;2017(1):385–99.

Nurden AT, Nurden P. Inherited disorders of platelet function: selected updates. J Thromb Haemost. 2015;13(Suppl 1):S2–9.

Othman M. Rare bleeding disorders: genetic, laboratory, clinical, and molecular aspects. Semin Thromb Hemost. 2013;39(6):575–8.

Acquired Bleeding Disorders

7

Thomas G. DeLoughery

The most common bleeding disorders in older patients are acquired bleeding disorders. The most frequently occurring are immune thrombocytopenia, liver and renal disease, and DIC; these are discussed in other chapters. This chapter reviews other causes of acquired bleeding disorders.

Thrombocytopenia

Thrombocytopenia is a relatively common finding in hospitalized patients. For example, thrombocytopenia is very common in the critical care population, with platelet counts below 100,000/uL found in 25–40% of such patients. Finding the etiology is frustrating, as multiple factors may be producing the thrombocytopenia. A rational approach is to consider the differential from a mechanistic point of view. Thus, defects in platelet production, increased platelet sequestration, or increased platelet destruction (immune or nonimmune) can lead to thrombocytopenia.

The initial assessment of the patient should focus on whether the patient is bleeding or having thrombosis, the underlying disorder, current medications, and (if available) past medical history.

The mode of presentation can be an important clue to the etiology of the thrombocytopenia. Patients who present only with severe thrombocytopenia (<10,000/uL) and no other systemic signs or symptoms (outside of bleeding) and a normal blood smear most often will have either idiopathic or drug-induced immune thrombocytopenia.

If the patient is in the hospital, the reason for hospitalization is an important indicator in the evaluation of thrombocytopenia (Table 7.1). Thrombocytopenia may be a diagnostic clue for infection, TTP, or sepsis in patients who present with multiorgan system failure. In hospitalized patients with new-onset thrombocytopenia, this may be a manifestation of heparin-induced thrombocytopenia (HIT), may be drug-induced, or might be a harbinger of sepsis.

The patient who presents with moderate thrombocytopenia (50–100,000/uL range) can be a diagnostic problem. Despite the modest degree of thrombocytopenia, counts in this range are commonly seen in TTP and HIT. Patients with hypersplenism will have counts in this range. Often the nonspecific thrombocytopenia that occurs in postsurgical and critically ill patients will also be in this range. It is frequently difficult to specifically identify the etiology of modest thrombocytopenia.

T. G. DeLoughery (✉)
Division of Hematology/Medical Oncology,
Department of Medicine, Pathology, and Pediatrics,
Oregon Health & Sciences University,
Portland, OR, USA
e-mail: delought@ohsu.edu

© Springer Nature Switzerland AG 2019
T. G. DeLoughery (ed.), *Hemostasis and Thrombosis*,
https://doi.org/10.1007/978-3-030-19330-0_7

Table 7.1 Diagnostic clues to acquired bleeding disorders

Clinical setting	Differential diagnosis
Cardiac surgery	Cardiopulmonary bypass, HIT, dilutional thrombocytopenia
Interventional cardiac procedure	Abciximab or other IIb/IIIa blockers, HIT
Sepsis syndrome	DIC, ehrlichiosis, sepsis, hemophagocytosis syndrome, drug-induced, misdiagnosed TTP, mechanical ventilation, pulmonary artery catheters
Pulmonary failure	DIC, *Hantavirus* pulmonary syndrome, mechanical ventilation, pulmonary artery catheters
Mental status changes/seizures	TTP, ehrlichiosis
Renal failure	TTP, dengue, HIT, DIC
Cardiac failure	HIT, drug-induced, pulmonary artery catheter
Postsurgery	Dilutional, drug-induced, HIT
Acute liver failure	Splenic sequestration, HIT, drug-induced, DIC

Table 7.2 Initial approach to thrombocytopenia

1. Obtain detailed history – especially any and all drug exposures
2. Assess for lymphadenopathy and hepatosplenomegaly
3. Review blood smear
4. Check liver function and renal function
5. Check LDH

Table 7.3 Differential diagnosis of isolated thrombocytopenia

Production defects
   Amegakaryocytic thrombocytopenia
   Carbamazepine
   Alcohol
Sequestration
Immune destruction
   Idiopathic
   Drug-induced
   HIV
   Sepsis
   Posttransfusion purpura
   Heparin-induced thrombocytopenia
Nonimmune destruction
   Thrombotic microangiopathies
   Microangiopathic hemolytic anemia
   DIC

Diagnostic Approach (Table 7.2)

Medication is a common cause of thrombocytopenia. Patients should be carefully questioned about over-the-counter medicine or "natural" remedies. Hospitalized patients need their medication sheets reviewed with all the medicines the patient has received noted.

Examination of the blood smear can quickly reveal whether pseudothrombocytopenia is present and it can verify the degree of thrombocytopenia. The smear should be carefully reviewed for presence of schistocytes. An evaluation for DIC should be performed. Laboratory assessment of liver and renal function should also be reviewed. A markedly elevated level of LDH out of proportion to other liver function abnormalities is often seen in TTP and *Hantavirus* pulmonary syndrome. In TTP, fractionation of the LDH reveals elevation of all isoenzymes consistent with multiorgan damage. If there is any suspicion of HIT, a HIT assay should be immediately obtained.

Etiologies of Thrombocytopenia (Table 7.3)

Decreased Production

So-called acquired amegakaryocytic thrombocytopenia is relatively rare. Most marrow disorders that lead to thrombocytopenia will cause other cell lines to be affected. The leading cause of isolated thrombocytopenia due to marrow problems is heavy (more than one-fifth per day) use of alcohol that leads to a megakaryocytic maturation defect. Clinically the platelets are small (MPV low). The count remains depressed for 3–5 days after alcohol is stopped but then rapidly rises with a "rebound" thrombocytosis. Thiazides and carbamazepine may also be associated with reduced platelet production. Late-stage HIV patients may have prolonged thrombocytopenia due to pyrimethamine and other medicines.

Rare patients with autoimmune amegakaryocytic thrombocytopenia may present with severe thrombocytopenia but do not respond to steroids or immunoglobulin. On marrow biopsy they have diminished to absent megakaryocytes. The etiology is due to suppressor T-cells repressing megakaryocyte production. Therapy is with cyclosporine or anti-thymocyte globulin. Thrombopoietic agonists such as eltrombopag or romiplostim are being used to treat this more recently.

In elderly patients, mild thrombocytopenia may be the first indicator of a myelodysplastic syndrome. Patients with myelodysplasia usually have an elevated MCV even if anemia is absent. Advanced molecular diagnostic techniques such as next-generation sequencing can be helpful.

Small platelets are a diagnostic clue to marrow production defects. A history of alcohol or carbamazepine use is also helpful to establish the diagnosis. Often bone marrow examination with cytogenetics is required to document the reduction in megakaryocyte number or to search for evidence of myelodysplasia. If available, the platelet reticulocyte count may be helpful if it is low.

Sequestration

Splenomegaly due to any cause can lead to thrombocytopenia. Usually the platelet count is above 50,000/uL. The splenomegaly from increased venous pressures seen with congestive heart failure and respiratory failure may account for the mild thrombocytopenia seen in these disorders. Although the splenomegaly seen with liver disease is often blamed for a concomitant thrombocytopenia, this can also be due to lack of thrombopoietin synthesis or to immune destruction.

Most patients do not require treatment; however, some patients may need higher counts for surgery. Platelet growth factors – eltrombopag, avatrombopag, or lusutrombopag – can be used to raise the count. These agents need to be started 1–2 weeks before the procedure.

Increased Destruction: Immune

Immune destruction is the most common cause of thrombocytopenia. Often these patients will have low platelet counts (<20,000/uL) but large platelets. Contrary to popular belief, these patients will respond to platelet transfusion, but the half-life of the transfused platelet is dramatically shortened (see below). Causes include:

- *Immune Thrombocytopenia (ITP)*: Discussed at length in Chap. 11. ITP is a classic autoimmune disorder of young women. Usually it presents in an otherwise healthy person with the onset of increased bruising and petechiae. ITP is a diagnosis of exclusion. Treatment is evolving but initial therapy is steroids, with splenectomy for steroid failures. Severe thrombocytopenia with bleeding can be treated with immunoglobulin or anti-D.
- *Sepsis*: An almost universal finding in patients with sepsis syndrome is thrombocytopenia. Classically this has been ascribed to DIC or nonspecific immune-mediated platelet destruction. One mechanism is cytokine-driven hemophagocytosis of platelets. The patients with hemophagocytosis have higher rates of multiple organ system failure and higher mortality rates. Inflammatory cytokines, especially M-CSF, are thought responsible for inducing the hemophagocytosis. Since there is no specific therapy for the thrombocytopenia, therapy is supportive.

Three infectious agents, *Ehrlichia*, *Hantavirus*, and leptospirosis, are associated with multisystem illness and thrombocytopenia. Both human granulocytic *Ehrlichia* and human monocytic *Ehrlichia* present with moderate thrombocytopenia and lymphopenia. Review of the peripheral smear in *Ehrlichia* may reveal the organism in the neutrophils or monocytes. *Hantavirus* presents with respiratory failure and thrombocytopenia. The findings of hemoconcentration, thrombocytopenia, left-shifted white blood counts, and greater than 10% circulating immunoblasts are almost diagnostic of *Hantavirus* in the clinical setting of respiratory failure. Leptospirosis presents with fevers and headache – conjunctival injection can be a diagnostic clue. Laboratories show a left shift in the white count and elevated liver function tests.

Table 7.4 Most common drugs implicated in drug-induced thrombocytopenia

Anti-GP IIb/IIIa agents
　Abciximab
　Eptifibatide
　Tirofiban
Antimicrobials
　Amphotericin B
　Aztreonam
　Daptomycin
　Flucloxacillin
　Linezolid
　Piperacillin
　Rifampin
　Sulfisoxazole
　Trimethoprim-sulfamethoxazole
　Vancomycin
Antiseizure
　Carbamazepine
　Phenytoin
　Valproic acid
H2-blockers
　Cimetidine
　Ranitidine
Nonsteroidal antiinflammatory agents
　Aceclofenac
　Ibuprofen
　Naproxen
Other drugs
　Acetaminophen
　Amiodarone
　Haloperidol
　Heparin
　Hydrochlorothiazide
　Oxaliplatin
　Quinidine
　Quinine
　Simvastatin
　Tacrolimus

Drugs: Many of the drugs used in modern medicine have been associated with thrombocytopenia (Table 7.4). The most common drugs implicated in thrombocytopenia include heparin, antibiotics (sulfa drugs, beta-lactams), quinidine, and nonsteroidal antiinflammatory agents. However, the list of drugs implicated in drug-induced thrombocytopenia is extensive, and any drug started within the last 3 months must be considered suspect.

Drug-induced thrombocytopenia is severe and sudden in onset. Usually the thrombocytopenia resolves when the drug is cleared from the body.

Quinidine thrombocytopenia is associated with an HUS-like syndrome as described in Chap. 12.

Therapy consists of stopping the drugs. Patients with very low platelet counts often will not respond to steroids and immunoglobulin infusions.

Severe thrombocytopenia has been reported in 0.5–2% of patients receiving specific GP IIb/IIIa inhibitors. The mechanism of thrombocytopenia is unknown but is speculated to be related to conformational changes in GP IIb/IIIa induced by binding of the inhibitors. Experience with abciximab has shown that infusion of immunoglobulin is not helpful. Platelet transfusions result in a prompt rise in platelet count until the drug is cleared from the patient.

Posttransfusion Purpura: Patients with this rare disease will have the explosive onset of severe thrombocytopenia 1–2 weeks after receiving blood products. PTP occurs in patients who lack common platelet antigens such as PL_{A1}. For unknown reasons, exposure to the antigens from the transfusion leads to rapid destruction of the patient's own platelets. Unlike most immune thrombocytopenias, bleeding may be severe in PTP. The diagnostic clue is thrombocytopenia in a patient who has recently received a red cell or platelet blood product. Treatment consists of steroids. Immunoglobulin is useful in severe cases. Rare patients may require plasmapheresis. The patient's thrombocytopenia will resolve in a few months. If patients with a history of PTP require further transfusions, the red cells should be washed, and only PL_{A1} negative platelets should be given.

Heparin-Induced Thrombocytopenia (HIT): Heparin can induce a unique form of immune thrombocytopenia. Unfortunately, some of these patients will then develop severe thrombosis. HIT is discussed in more detail in Chap. 22.

Increased Destruction: Nonimmune DIC – Discussed in Chap. 8.

Thrombotic Microangiopathies – Discussed in Chap. 12.

Dysfunctional Platelets

Subtle testing of platelet function has revealed that acquired abnormalities in function are extremely common, but the clinical significance of these abnormalities is controversial. Of the many agents and diseases which result in impaired platelet performance, only the few reviewed below appear to be of clinical significance.

Drugs: Multiple drugs have been shown to inhibit platelet function, but clinical bleeding has only been associated with a few. Antiplatelets such as aspirin have been shown to be associated with a higher risk of bleeding in clinical trials. Ketorolac (Toradol) has also been associated with significant clinical bleeding. This is especially true with combined use of ketorolac and heparin.

Acquired platelet dysfunction was first seen with carbenicillin therapy but has been reported with multiple antibiotics, especially early anti-pseudomonas penicillins. Infusions of therapeutic doses of ticarcillin and carbenicillin into normal volunteers will reproducibly raise the bleeding time by the third or fourth day of drug administration. In some patients this prolongation of the bleeding time will persist for up to 2 weeks. The newer anti-pseudomonal antibiotics do not appear to have significant antiplatelet effects.

Myeloma: Increased bleeding times indicative of platelet dysfunction have been described in patients suffering from myeloma. Abnormal platelet function, including decreased aggregation, decreased adhesion, and procoagulant activity, has been described. This may be due to the abnormal protein coating the platelet. A severe and potentially fatal bleeding diathesis due to a paraprotein with affinity for platelet glycoprotein IIIa has been reported. These platelet function defects decline with treatment of the myeloma.

Cardiopulmonary Bypass. As discussed in Chap. 10, the complex milieu of cardiopulmonary bypass may cause multiple and profound changes at all levels of hemostasis. Along with thrombocytopenia, some patients will have profound platelet dysfunction. Patients with post-pump thrombocytopenia may require multiple platelet transfusions to stop microvascular bleeding, and raising the platelet count above 100,000/uL may be required to compensate for the platelet function defect.

Diagnosis and Therapy: Classically patients with inhibition of platelet function will have "platelet-type" bleeding: bruising, diffuse muco-sal oozing, and epistaxis. The diagnosis of platelet inhibition is a clinical one based on the patient's underlying illnesses and the medications that they are receiving. The bleeding time or PFA-100 time is only modestly useful. A normal bleeding time rules out platelet dysfunction as a cause of bleeding, and a prolonged one is suggestive of a platelet defect. However, an abnormal bleeding time has never been shown to be predictive of bleeding in any situation. The clinical history of prior bleeding is a better predictor of future hemorrhagic complications.

Appropriate treatment of severe bleeding believed due to abnormal platelet function is platelet transfusion. Desmopressin may augment platelet function in a number of disorders. However, desmopressin has been associated with thrombosis in older patients and should be used cautiously. Raising the hematocrit to more than 30% by transfusion or by use of erythropoietin will also improve hemostasis in uremia and perhaps in other disorders. Cryoprecipitate will shorten the bleeding time in uremia and liver failure.

Acquired Coagulation Factor Deficiency

Acquired defects of hemostasis may first present with either prolongation of routine coagulation laboratory values or with a serious bleeding diathesis. Frequently DIC and liver disease present with both PT and aPTT elevated. If there is no evidence of either disorder, then further testing is needed. A 50:50 mix that corrects establishes the presence of factor deficiency. One that does not correct (even with added phospholipids) suggests a specific factor inhibitor.

The first step in evaluation is to obtain a prothrombin time (PT) and an activated partial thromboplastin time (aPTT). One should ensure the sample is obtained from a peripheral vein. Samples drawn through heparin-locked catheters, even with elaborate manipulation to prevent contamination, can result in falsely elevated results. Three patterns of defects may be seen (Table 7.5). Isolated elevations of the PT are indicative of an isolated factor VII deficiency. Isolated elevations

Table 7.5 Four causes of elevated aPTT and response to 50:50 mix

1. Factor deficiency – corrects
2. Antiphospholipid antibodies – does not fully correct
3. Factor inhibitors – corrects at time 0 but then prolongs
4. Heparin, direct anticoagulants – does not correct (usually obvious from history)

Table 7.6 Interpretations of elevated PT and/or aPTT

PT only
Factor VII deficiency
  Congenital
  Acquired
    Vitamin K deficiency
    Liver disease
Factor VII inhibitor
Rarely in patients with modest decreases of factor V or X
PTT only
Contact factor XI, IX, VIII deficiency
Contact factor XI, IX, VIII specific factor inhibitor
Heparin contamination
Antiphospholipid antibodies
Both
Factor X, V, or II deficiency
Factor X, V, II inhibitor
Improper anticoagulant ratio (hematocrits >60 or <15)
High doses of heparin (elevation of aPTT greater relative to PT)
Large warfarin effect (elevation of PT greater relative to aPTT)
Low fibrinogen (<80 mg/dl)

of the aPTT are typically due to heparin contamination; lupus inhibitors; isolated defects of VIII, IX, and XI; or the contact pathway. Mixing studies can provide information to narrow the list of possible diagnoses. Prolongation of both the PT and aPTT suggests multiple defects or deficiency of factors II, V, or X. Marked prolongation of the PT and aPTT can also be seen with low levels of fibrinogen (< 50 mg/dl) (Table 7.6).

Patients with hematocrits of greater than 60% may have spurious elevations of the PT and aPTT due to improper plasma/anticoagulant ratio in the sample tube. Further coagulation tests are ordered based on the PT and aPTT to define the defect better if the reason for the coagulation deficiency is not apparent by the history (i.e., severe liver disease).

Vitamin K Deficiency

Vitamin K is critical in the synthesis of coagulation factors II, VI, IX, and X, protein C, protein S, and protein Z. Patients obtain vitamin K from food sources and from metabolism of intestinal flora. Vitamin K is used as a cofactor in gammacarboxylation of the vitamin K-dependent proteins. The gammacarboxylation involves oxidation of vitamin K. Vitamin K is recycled in a step blocked by warfarin. Despite being a fat-soluble vitamin, body stores of vitamin K are low and the daily requirement is 1 ug/kg/day.

Vitamin K deficiency can present dramatically. Once the body stores of vitamin K are depleted, production of the vitamin K-dependent proteins ceases, and the INR will increase rapidly to extreme levels. This can be seen in patients with poor nutrition who have a mildly prolonged INR going into surgery and several days postoperatively have an INR of 50.

The diagnosis is suspected when there is a history of prolonged antibiotic use or malnourishment. One must also suspect vitamin K deficiency in a previously healthy patient who presents with an elevated INR that corrects with 50:50 mix. This is a common presentation of accidental or surreptitious warfarin or rat poison ingestion.

Treatment of vitamin K deficiency is by replacement of vitamin K. Most patients will respond rapidly to 10 mg orally. For a more rapid response, 5–10 mg may be given intravenously over at least 60 minutes. However, anaphylaxis has been reported with rapid infusion of vitamin K. Alternatively, plasma can be used for the bleeding patient. At least 3–4 units (15 ml/kg) of plasma may be needed until the administered vitamin K takes effect. For life-threatening bleeding, 25–50 units of prothrombin complex concentrates can be given.

Antibiotics

Antibiotics can affect vitamin K metabolism in two ways. Most antibiotics with activity against anaerobes can sterilize the gut, eliminating microbial production of vitamin K. Certain cephalosporins that contain the N-methylthiotetrazole (NMTT) group can inhibit vitamin K epoxide reductase. This prevents the normal recycling of vitamin K. The most commonly implicated antibiotics are cefamandole, cefoperazone, cefotetan, cefmenoxime, and cefmetazole. NMTT is released from the antibiotic and circulated with a half-life of 24–36 hours. The NMTT metabolite can accumulate in patients with renal failure. The use of prophylactic vitamin K (10 mg orally/day) with these antibiotics has dramatically reduced the incidence of vitamin K deficiency. Prophylactic vitamin K should be considered for every patient on these antibiotics.

Malnutrition

Since vitamin K stores are labile, patients with poor nutritional status are liable to become vitamin K-deficient. This is especially true if a patient has biliary problems or is on drugs that interfere with vitamin K metabolism. Aggressive use of nutritional supplements and parental nutrition has greatly reduced malnutrition-related vitamin K deficiency.

Rat Poison/"Superwarfarin"

Warfarin used to be the rodenticide in commercially available rat poisons. But then certain rats (by anecdote from New York City) became resistant to warfarin. Now rat poison contains brodifacoum as the main rodenticide. Brodifacoum binds and irreversibly inhibits vitamin K recycling. Furthermore, it is highly fat-soluble and has a long half-life. Patients who ingest rat poison present with an elevated PT-INR that is only transiently responsive to fresh frozen plasma or to small doses of vitamin K. Diagnosis is established by measuring brodifacoum levels. High doses of vitamin K, 25–50 mg three times per day, may be required for months to treat brodifacoum ingestion. While in the past most cases were deliberate attempts to poison oneself or others, more recently cases are being identified as being due to adulterated recreation drugs such as synthetic cannabinoids.

Specific Acquired Factor Deficiencies

Alpha$_2$ antiplasmin deficiency most commonly occurs in DIC and acute promyelocytic leukemia. As discussed in Chap. 27, rare patients with excessive bleeding and low levels of alpha$_2$ antiplasmin may benefit from antifibrinolytic therapy. Rare cases of acquired alpha$_2$ antiplasmin deficiency associated with severe bleeding have been reported in amyloidosis.

Plasminogen activator inhibitor-1 deficiency has infrequently been reported in amyloidoses. Diagnosis is by finding a long euglobulin clot lysis time and very low levels of PAI-1.

Hypofibrinogenemia is most commonly seen in liver diseases, following thrombolytic therapy, in dilutional coagulopathies from massive transfusions, and in severe DIC. Patients commonly exhibit bleeding with fibrinogen levels lower than 100 mg/dl. Since the formation of the fibrin clot is the endpoint of the PT and PTT, patients with low fibrinogen levels will have artifactually elevated PT and aPTTs. Therapy is with cryoprecipitate, with an expected increase in plasma fibrinogen of at least 100 mg/dl after 10 bags.

Dysfibrinogenemias are most often seen in liver disease. Patients with hepatoma may also have dysfibrinogenemia. It is assumed that the liver dysfunction results in abnormal glycosylation of the fibrinogen which results in a dysfunctional molecule. The presence of an abnormal fibrinogen is established by an abnormal thrombin time, elevated levels of FDPs with normal D-dimers, and a discrepancy between fibrinogen activity and antigen. Most patients do not require specific therapy.

Prothrombin deficiency occurs in two clinical situations: antiphospholipid antibody disease and with topical thrombin therapy discussed in detail below under factor V deficiency.

Approximately 5% of patients with lupus inhibitors will have antibodies that react with prothrombin. The antibodies do not react with the active site but lead to increased consumption of the molecule. Rarely this may result in bleeding.

Patients with antiphospholipid antibodies may have elevated prothrombin times for two reasons. One is that antiphospholipid antibody cross-reacts with the prothrombin time. The other cause is due to antiprothrombin antibodies. The 50:50 mix will only correct with the antiprothrombin antibodies. Remember that these antibodies are not inhibitors but lead to increased factor degradation and factor deficiency.

Therapy for antiprothrombin antibodies is with steroids. A reasonable dose is prednisone 60 mg every day. Prothrombin can be provided by factor infusions, but the half-life will be short due to increased consumption. Most patients respond promptly to steroids.

Factor V deficiency　Factor V inhibitors can be seen in patients after the use of topical thrombin. Several weeks after surgery, the patient will develop antibodies to bovine thrombin. Many patients will also develop an antibody to the bovine factor V that is often also present in the bovine thrombin. This antibody will readily cross-react with human factor V. Rarely, antibodies to human thrombin will also be seen.

Patients may present with severe bleeding or with an inhibitor detected on routine laboratory screening. The thrombin time is always prolonged as it is performed using bovine thrombin. If factor V antibodies are present, the PT and aPTT will also be prolonged, and they will behave as an inhibitor in the 50:50 mix. Due to presence of the inhibitor, Factor V levels are reduced.

Many patients with factor V antibody do not bleed. One reason may be that platelet factor V, inside the platelet alpha granule, is protected from circulating antibodies. For the bleeding patient, therapy with plasma and platelets may be used. The antibodies will disappear in several weeks. With the advent of better purification methods and recombinant technology, the incidence of this has markedly decreased.

Acquired factor V deficiency has also been reported with myeloproliferative syndromes. These patients demonstrate a reduced half-life of factor V with plasma transfusion.

Factor VII deficiency　is usually seen with vitamin K deficiency or with liver disease. Factor VII has the shortest half-life of the vitamin K-dependent proteins, and its levels fall first as vitamin K supplies fall. Rare inhibitors of factor VII have been reported. For unclear reasons, levels of factor VII fall in severe illness and may lead to prolongation of the INR.

Factor VIII deficiency　due to specific factor antibodies is the most common acquired factor deficiency. This can be seen in hemophilia (discussed in Chap. 4), autoimmune disease, older patients, and postpartum.

Patients with acquired factor VIII inhibitors present with diffuse bleeding. Unlike in classic hemophilia, these patients will have bruises covering large areas of their body. Patients can bleed from any site, but the gastrointestinal tract is most common. Postpartum factor VIII inhibitors can appear several weeks after delivery.

Patients will have elevated aPTTs that behave like an inhibitor on the 50:50 mix (no correction). Factor levels show a low factor VIII. Sometimes testing results are indeterminate between a specific factor VIII inhibitor and lupus inhibitor. Levels of factor VIII will "increase" with dilution of the test plasma in patients with a lupus inhibitor but not with true factor VIII inhibitors. Also, it is rare for patients with lupus inhibitors to have significant bleeding. The strength of the factor VIII inhibitor is reported in "Bethesda units." Due to the complex kinetics, these levels in acquired factor VIII inhibitors are often difficult to measure and interpret.

Therapy is twofold, aimed at correcting the hemostatic defect and at driving away the inhibitor. The specific therapy to correct the hemostatic defect is reviewed in detail in Chap. 4.

For very low-level inhibitors (<5 BU), treatment is directed toward trying to overpower the inhibitor.

For higher-level inhibitors, activated pro-thrombin complex concentrate at a dose of 75 units/kg twice/day can be used. Especially in older patients, the use of these products may be complicated by thrombosis. Due to these concerns, recombinant VIIa has become more frequently used for inhibitor patients. For bleeding patients, the dosing of rVIIa is 90 ug/kg repeated every 2–3 hours until the bleeding has stopped. For patients who require surgery or have life-threatening bleeding, the rVIIa should be "weaned" by decreasing the dose to every 6 hours for several days after 2–3 days of successful every 2–3-hour therapy.

Most patients with acquired factor VIII inhibitor antibodies will not fully inhibit porcine FVIII. Recombinant porcine factor VIII (Obizur) is now available and should be used for major bleeding episodes or if procedures need to be performed. The dosing starts at 200 units/kg with frequent checks of factor VIII levels to determine subsequent dosing based on keeping trough levels above 50–100%.

Patients with factor VIII inhibitors should receive immunosuppression to eliminate the inhibitor. Up to one-third of patients may transiently respond to immunoglobulin (1 g/kg per day for 2 days). Given the high rate of morbidity, aggressive immunosuppression should be started with prednisone 60 mg/day plus oral cyclophosphamide 100 mg/day. This should be continued until factor levels increase and the inhibitor titer decreases. Increasingly it is being reported that patients respond to rituximab therapy (375 mg/m^2/week × 4 or 1000 mg × 2 separated by 14 days), and early use of this agent needs to be considered.

Factor IX deficiency rarely occurs as an acquired antibody. Therapy for bleeding is with rVIIa. Immunosuppression is also indicated.

Factor X deficiency Multiple case reports describe factor X deficiency in amyloidosis. The amyloid appears to bind the factor X. Acquired deficiency of factor X appears to be more common in patients with splenic involvement by amyloid. Patients have responded to anti-

myeloma therapy. In patients with massive splenomegaly, splenectomy has been associated with improved factor X levels. In younger patients, bone marrow transplant may be an option.

Factor XI deficiency due to inhibitors can be seen in patients with autoimmune disease – especially lupus. These are rarely associated with bleeding.

Factor XIII deficiency is rarely seen with drugs such as isoniazid, phenytoin, or procainamide or in inflammatory bowel disease. Patients can have severe bleeding with normal coagulation parameters but low factor XIII levels. As with other acquired inhibitors, patients respond to immunosuppression.

Acquired Von Willebrand Disease

Acquired von Willebrand disease (VWD) has been reported to occur in lymphomas, myeloproliferative syndromes, myeloma, and monoclonal gammopathies and with the use of certain drugs. Acquired deficiency of von Willebrand proteins (VWF) can occur by several mechanisms. One is by protein absorption to the surface of the malignant cell. Malignant cells in lymphomas, myelomas, and Wilms tumors can express GP Ib. Another mechanism is by antibody binding to the protein.

Patients on mechanical support such as ventricular assist devices or ECMO will develop acquired VWD that will persist until the device is removed. Acquired VWD has also been reported with severe aortic stenosis and mitral regurgitation.

The most common drug-induced etiology is administration of hydroxyethyl starch. Bleeding is seen, especially with prolonged use of these agents or with the use of more than 1.5 l/day. Decreased levels of both VWF and factor VIII are seen, but many patients will have a type 2 defect with selective loss of higher weight VWF multimers. Levels rise after the agent is stopped, but some patients may require factor replacement if severe bleeding is present. Rarely, acquired VWD has been reported with valproic acid and ciprofloxacin.

Patients with acquired VWD can present with type 1 (decreased protein) or type 2 (abnormal multimers) disease. The diagnosis is suggested by lack of personal or family history of a bleeding diathesis. Levels of factor VIII, ristocetin cofactor activity, and von Willebrand antigen are decreased. Platelet levels of VWF are normal, suggesting depletion of circulating VWF from the plasma. Crossed immunoelectrophoresis is used to differentiate type 1 from type 2 disease.

Desmopressin is effective in many patients with acquired type 1 and type 2 disease. Consistent with the antibody-mediated destruction, the magnitude and duration of desmopressin effect is often reduced in acquired VWD. In some patients it is not effective. Recent reports indicate that high-dose immunoglobulin is also effective in reversing acquired VWD. For bleeding patients, high doses of Humate-P is indicated with frequent monitoring of factor VIII levels. For patients with very intense inhibitors, rVIIa may prove useful. If present, treatment of the hematologic neoplasm is also effective.

In patients with acquired VWD due to devices such as ECMO, the VWD will resolve rapidly when the patient is no longer using the device. Infusion of VWD is often ineffective as it will be rapidly degraded. Similar with valvular disease, repair or replacement of the valve is the most effective treatment.

Suggested Reading

Alberio L. My patient is thrombocytopenic! Is (s)he? Why? And what shall I do? A practical approach to thrombocytopenia. Hamostaseologie. 2013;33(2):83–94.

Al-Nouri ZL, George JN. Drug-induced thrombocytopenia: an updated systematic review, 2012. Drug Saf. 2012;35(8):693–4.

Charlebois J, Rivard GÉ, St-Louis J. Management of acquired von Willebrand syndrome. Transfus Apher Sci. 2018;57(6):721–3. https://doi.org/10.1016/j.transci.2018.10.012. Epub 2018 Oct 30.

Coppola A, Favaloro EJ, Tufano A, Di Minno MN, Cerbone AM, Franchini M. Acquired inhibitors of coagulation factors: part I-acquired hemophilia A. Semin Thromb Hemost. 2012;38(5):433–46.

Feinstein DL, Akpa BS, Ayee MA, Boullerne AI, Braun D, Brodsky SV, Gidalevitz D, Hauck Z, Kalinin S, Kowal K, Kuzmenko I, Lis K, Marangoni N, Martynowycz MW, Rubinstein I, van Breemen R, Ware K, Weinberg G. The emerging threat of superwarfarins: history, detection, mechanisms, and countermeasures. Ann N Y Acad Sci. 2016;1374(1):111–22.

Franchini M, Lippi G, Favaloro EJ. Acquired inhibitors of coagulation factors: part II. Semin Thromb Hemost. 2012;38(5):447–53.

Kruse-Jarres R, Kempton CL, Baudo F, Collins PW, Knoebl P, Leissinger CA, Tiede A, Kessler CM. Acquired hemophilia A: updated review of evidence and treatment guidance. Am J Hematol. 2017;92(7):695–705. https://doi.org/10.1002/ajh.24777. Epub 2017 Jun 5.

Loo AS, Gerzenshtein L, Ison MG. Antimicrobial drug-induced thrombocytopenia: a review of the literature. Semin Thromb Hemost. 2012;38(8):818–29.

Mitta A, Curtis BR, Reese JA, George JN. Drug-induced thrombocytopenia: 2019 Update of clinical and laboratory data. Am J Hematol. 2019;94(3):E76–8.

Scharf RE. Drugs that affect platelet function. Semin Thromb Hemost. 2012;38(8):865–83.

Tiede A, Rand JH, Budde U, Ganser A, Federici AB. How I treat the acquired von Willebrand syndrome. Blood. 2011;117(25):6777–85.

Disseminated Intravascular Coagulation

8

Thomas G. DeLoughery

Disseminated intravascular coagulation (DIC) may be seen in patients with a variety of disease states. DIC can present with a spectrum of findings ranging from asymptomatic abnormal laboratory findings to florid bleeding or thrombosis. DIC is always a consequence of another pathologic process and represents the final common pathway of coagulation dysregulation.

Pathogenesis

DIC is the clinical manifestation of inappropriate thrombin (IIa) activation (Table 8.1). Inappropriate thrombin activation can be due to causes such as sepsis, obstetric disasters, and others. The activation of thrombin leads to (1) conversion of fibrinogen to fibrin, (2) activation of platelets (and their consumption), (3) activation of factors V and VIII, (4) activation of protein C (and degradation of factors Va and VIIIa), (5) activation of endothelial cells, and (6) activation of fibrinolysis:

Table 8.1 Consequences of excessive thrombin generation

1. Conversion of fibrinogen to fibrin → thrombosis and depletion of fibrinogen
2. Activation of platelets → thrombocytopenia
3. Activation of factors V, VIII, XI, XIII → thrombosis and depletion of coagulation factors
4. Activation of protein C → depletion of factors V and VIII and eventually protein C
5. Activation of endothelial cells → expression of tissue factor
6. Activation of fibrinolysis → lysis of thrombi and depletion of fibrinogen

1. *Conversion of fibrinogen to fibrin* leads to formation of fibrin monomers and excessive thrombus formation. In most patients these thrombi are rapidly dissolved by excessive fibrinolysis. In certain clinical situations, especially cancer, excessive thrombosis will occur. In cancer patients this is most often a deep venous thrombosis. Rare patients, especially those with pancreatic or lung cancer, may have severe DIC with multiple arterial and venous thromboses. Non-bacterial thrombotic endocarditis can also be seen in these patients.
2. *Activation of platelets (and their consumption)*. Thrombin is the most potent physiologic activator of platelets, and so in DIC there is increased activation of platelets. These activated platelets are consumed with resultant thrombocytopenia. Platelet dysfunction is

T. G. DeLoughery (✉)
Division of Hematology/Medical Oncology, Department of Medicine, Pathology, and Pediatrics, Oregon Health & Sciences University, Portland, OR, USA
e-mail: delought@ohsu.edu

© Springer Nature Switzerland AG 2019
T. G. DeLoughery (ed.), *Hemostasis and Thrombosis*,
https://doi.org/10.1007/978-3-030-19330-0_8

55

also present. Platelets that have been activated and have released their contents but still circulate are known as "exhausted" platelets which can no longer function to support coagulation. The fibrin degradation products in DIC can also bind to GP IIb/IIIa and inhibit further platelet aggregation.

3. *Activation of factors V, VIII, XI, and XIII.* Activation of these factors can promote thrombosis and they are then rapidly cleared by antithrombin. This can lead to depletion of all the prothrombotic clotting factors and antithrombin. This can lead to both thrombosis and bleeding.

4. *Activation of protein C* further promotes degradation of factors Va and VIIIa as well as decreasing protein C levels.

5. *Activation of endothelial cells*, especially in the skin, may lead to thrombosis and in certain patients – especially those with meningococcemia – purpura fulminans. Endothelial damage will downregulate thrombomodulin which prevents activation of protein C and leads to further reductions in levels of activated protein C.

6. *Activation of fibrinolysis* leads to breakdown of fibrin monomers, formation of fibrin thrombi, and increased circulating fibrinogen. In most patients with DIC, the fibrinolytic response is brisk. This is why most patients with DIC present with bleeding and prolonged clotting times.

Etiology

In essence, anything that leads to an overproduction of thrombin can cause DIC. This overproduction of thrombin can result from an immense number of clinical situations (Table 8.2). A few of the more common ones are discussed below.

Infection can lead to DIC via several pathways. Endotoxin produced by gram-negative bacteria results in expression of tissue factor by both endothelial cells and monocytes. Certain organisms such as *Rickettsia* and viruses of the herpes family can directly infect

Table 8.2 Etiologies of DIC

Adenocarcinomas
Amniotic fluid embolism
Burns
Intravascular hemolysis
Infections
Leukemia
Penetrating brain injury
Placental abruption
Retained fetal death in utero
Shock
Snake bites
Trauma

endothelial cells, resulting in tissue factor expression. The hypotension produced by sepsis can lead to tissue ischemia and tissue factor expression.

Cancers, primarily adenocarcinomas, can result in DIC. Highly vascular tumor cells are known to express tissue factor. In addition, some tumor cells can express a direct activator of factor X ("cancer procoagulant"). In acute promyelocytic leukemia and to a lesser degree in other leukemias, tissue factor and other enzymes lead to thrombin generation. Patients with DIC in leukemia present with fulminant bleeding syndromes. For mysterious reasons, many patients with DIC due to cancer present with thrombosis. This may be due to the inflammatory state which accompanies cancer or it may be a unique part of cancer biology.

DIC due to *obstetrical* causes is rare but can be deadly. Fulminant DIC is a hallmark of amniotic fluid embolism. A fetus retained after dying in utero can lead to DIC within a week due to exposure of maternal plasma to macerated fetal products.

Patients with severe *trauma* often have DIC. Their coagulation defects are due to tissue trauma and may be complicated by hypothermia and dilution due to resuscitation with crystalloid fluids. Some have postulated a unique type of coagulopathy – acute coagulopathy of trauma – that is due to excessive activation of protein C leading to decreases in factors V and VIII. In addition, there is excessive fibrinolysis due to activated protein C binding plasminogen activator inhibitor – 1.

Clinical Presentation (Table 8.3)

Patients can present in one of four ways with DIC:

1. *Asymptomatic*. Patients can present with laboratory evidence of DIC but no clinical problems. This is often seen in sepsis and in cancer. However, with further progression of the underlying disease, these patients may rapidly become symptomatic.
2. *Bleeding*. Most patients with DIC bleed. The bleeding is due to a combination of factor depletion, platelet dysfunction, thrombocytopenia, and excessive fibrinolysis. These patients may present with diffuse bleeding from IV sites, surgical wounds, etc.
3. *Thrombosis*. Despite general activation of the coagulation process, thrombosis is unusual in most patients with DIC. The exceptions include cancer patients, trauma patients, and certain obstetrical patients. Most often the thrombosis is venous, but arterial thrombosis can also be seen.
4. *Purpura Fulminans*. DIC in association with symmetric limb ecchymosis and necrosis of the skin is seen in two situations. One, primary purpura fulminans, is most often seen after a viral infection. In these patients, the purpura fulminans starts with a painful red area on an extremity that rapidly progresses to a black ischemic area. In this situation, acquired deficiency of protein S is often found. These patients will have laboratory evidence of DIC.

Secondary purpura fulminans is most often associated with meningococcemia but can be seen in any patient with overwhelming infection. Post-splenectomy sepsis syndrome patients are also at risk. Patients present with signs of sepsis; the skin lesions often involve the extremities and may lead to amputations.

Diagnosis

There is no one test that will diagnose DIC; one must match the test to the clinical situation (Table 8.4).

Screening Tests The PT-INR and aPTT are usually elevated in severe DIC but may be normal or shortened in chronic forms. One may also see a shortened aPTT in severe acute DIC due to large amounts of activated II and factor X "bypassing" the contact pathway. aPTTs as short as 10 seconds have been seen in acute DIC. The platelet count is usually reduced but may be normal in chronic DIC. Serum fibrinogen is decreased in acute DIC but again may be in the "normal" range in chronic DIC.

"Specific Tests" These are tests which allow one to deduce that abnormally high concentrations of IIa are present:

- *Ethanol Gel and Protamine Test*: Both of these older tests detect circulating fibrin monomers. Circulating fibrin monomers are seen when IIa acts on fibrinogen. Usually the monomer polymerizes with the fibrin clot, but when there is too much IIa, these monomers can circulate. Detection of circulating fibrin monomer means there is too much IIa and DIC is present.

Table 8.3 Clinical presentations of DIC

Asymptomatic – laboratory abnormalities only
Severe bleeding – especially from sites of minor trauma such as IV sites
Thrombosis
Purpura fulminans
Severe DIC
Microvascular thrombosis with area of skin ischemia/necrosis

Table 8.4 Testing for DIC

PT-INR, aPTT, fibrinogen level: non-specific
Protamine sulfate: detects circulating fibrin monomers. Specific but not sensitive
Ethanol gel: detects circulating fibrin monomers. Sensitive but not specific
Fibrin(ogen) degradation products
D-dimers (fibrin degradation product)

- *Fibrin Degradation Products (FDPs)*: Plasmin acts on the fibrin/fibrinogen molecule to cleave the molecule in specific places. The resulting degradation product levels will be elevated in situations of increased fibrin/fibrinogen destruction (DIC, fibrinolysis). The FDPs are typically mildly elevated in renal and liver disease due to reduced clearance.
- *D-Dimers*: When fibrin monomers bind to form a thrombus, factor XIII acts to bind their "D" domains together. This bond is resistant to plasmin and thus this degradation fragment is known as the "D-dimer." High levels of D-dimer indicate that (1) IIa has acted on fibrinogen to form a fibrin monomer that bonded to another fibrin monomer and (2) this thrombus was lysed by plasmin.

Other tests that are sometimes helpful:

- *Thrombin time (TT)*: This test is performed by adding IIa to plasma. Thrombin times are elevated in (1) DIC (FDPs interfere with polymerization), (2) the presence of low fibrinogen levels, (3) dysfibrinogenemia, and (4) the presence of heparin (very sensitive).
- *Reptilase time*: This is the same as thrombin time but is performed with a snake venom that is insensitive to heparin. Reptilase time is elevated in the same conditions as the thrombin time with the exception of the presence of heparin. Thrombin time and reptilase time are most useful in evaluation of dysfibrinogenemia.
- $F_{1.2}$: $F_{1.2}$ is a small peptide cleaved off when prothrombin is activated to thrombin. Thus high levels of $F_{1.2}$ are found in DIC but may also be seen in other thrombotic disorders. This test is of limited clinical value.
- *Antithrombin levels* are decreased in DIC and can help with diagnosis of difficult cases. Levels can also be low in acute venous thrombosis and severe liver disease.

Therapy The best way to treat DIC is to treat the underlying disease state. However, one must replace factors if depletion occurs and bleeding

Table 8.5 Therapy of DIC

Follow PT-INR, aPTT, platelets, and fibrinogen
Protime >INR 2.0 *and* aPTT abnormal – infuse 2–4 units of FFP
Platelets <50–75,000/uL – give 6 platelet concentrates
Fibrinogen <150 mg/dl – give 10 units of cryoprecipitate
Heparin – give only if the patient is having thrombosis

ensues (Table 8.5). General guidelines for replacement are:

- Protime >INR 2.0 *and* aPTT abnormal – infuse 2–4 units of FFP.
- Platelets <50,000/uL – give 1 unit of platelet concentrate or one plateletpheresis unit/10 kg body weight.
- Fibrinogen <150 mg/dl – give 10 units of cryoprecipitate.
- Heparin – give only if the patient is having thrombosis.

Plasma replacement is needed to correct multiple factor deficiencies. Past concern about "feeding the fire" is not clinically valid. One should strive to bring the aPTT down to less than 1.5 times normal if possible. Keeping the fibrinogen level over 100 mg/dl is also important.

As mentioned above, platelets are both low and dysfunctional in DIC. Accordingly, the goal for platelet levels over 50,000/uL is needed to compensate.

Heparin therapy is reserved for the patient with thrombosis. Its use in acute promyelocytic leukemia patients is still controversial. Due to the derangements of coagulation factors, one should follow heparin levels or use low molecular weight heparin instead of following the aPTT. Reliance on the aPTT to follow heparin therapy may lead to over- or undertreatment of patients.

Therapy for purpura fulminans is controversial. Primary purpura fulminans, especially that seen with post-varicella autoimmune protein S deficiency, has responded to plasma infusion titrated to keep the protein S level more than 25.

Anecdotes suggest a response to immune globulin (1 mg/kg × 2 days) or steroids in these patients. Heparin has been reported to control the DIC and extent of necrosis. A reasonable starting dose in these patients is 5–8 units/kg/h.

Very sick patients with secondary purpura fulminans have been treated with plasma drips, plasmapheresis, and continuous plasma ultrafiltration. Heparin therapy alone has not been shown to improve survival. Much attention has been given to replacement of natural anticoagulants such as protein C and antithrombin III as therapy for purpura fulminans. Multiple randomized trials have shown negative results for the use of antithrombin III. Trials using protein C concentrates have shown more promise in controlling the coagulopathy of purpura fulminans and improving outcomes in sepsis, especially in patients who also have DIC.

Suggested Reading

Chalmers E, Cooper P, Forman K, Grimley C, Khair K, Minford A, Morgan M, Mumford AD. Purpura fulminans: recognition, diagnosis and management. Arch Dis Child. 2011;96(11):1066–71.

Colling ME, Bendapudi PK. Purpura fulminans: mechanism and management of dysregulated hemostasis. Transfus Med Rev. 2018;32(2):69–76. https://doi.org/10.1016/j.tmrv.2017.10.001. Epub 2017 Oct 16.

Gando S, Levi M, Toh CH. Disseminated intravascular coagulation. Nat Rev Dis Primers. 2016;2:16037. https://doi.org/10.1038/nrdp.2016.37.

Giordano S, Spiezia L, Campello E, Simioni P. The current understanding of trauma-induced coagulopathy (TIC): a focused review on pathophysiology. Intern Emerg Med. 2017;12(7):981–91.

Levi M, Scully M. How i treat disseminated intravascular coagulation. Blood. 2018;131(8):845–54.

Scully M, Levi M. How we manage haemostasis during sepsis. Br J Haematol. 2019;185(2):209–18.

Liver and Renal Disease

9

Thomas G. DeLoughery

Liver Disease

While it has been accepted for years that patients with liver disease are at risk of bleeding, there has been a more recent realization that, for most patients, this hazard has been overstated and that paradoxically, thrombosis may also be a risk. Most bleeding in liver disease patients is due to mechanical reasons such as a ruptured varix rather than an underlying coagulopathy. In addition, classic tests of coagulation fail in many patients to fully assess their hemostatic capacity.

Pathogenesis of Defects

Patients with severe liver disease have multiple coagulation defects that can put them at risk of bleeding (Table 9.1). These defects are due to:

1. *Decreased coagulation factor synthesis –* Nearly all the major coagulation factors and their inhibitors are synthesized in the liver. The exceptions are factor VIII and von Willebrand factor. Most factor VIII is synthe-

Table 9.1 Coagulation defects in liver disease

Bleeding
Decreased synthesis of coagulation factors
Increased consumption of coagulation factors
Thrombocytopenia
Platelet function defects
Increased fibrinolysis
Prothrombotic
Decreased synthesis of natural anticoagulants

sized in the liver, but in liver failure the plasma levels are often elevated due to release from endothelial stores.

2. *Thrombocytopenia –* It used to be thought that the hypersplenism which often accompanies liver disease resulted in platelet sequestration. However, it is now appreciated that the liver is the main site of thrombopoietin production and that platelet production is reduced in liver disease. This explains why splenectomy or shunting procedures often do not improve platelet counts in patients with liver disease. Additionally, patients with hepatitis C appear to have a higher risk of immune thrombocytopenia and may have very low platelet counts.

3. *Platelet dysfunction –* This is due to a number of causes. The reduced clearance of fibrin degradation products and plasmin will lead to platelet dysfunction. Fibrin degradation products can bind and inhibit GP IIb/IIIa. Plasmin will degrade platelet receptors. Also found in patients with liver disease is an ill-characterized

T. G. DeLoughery (✉)
Division of Hematology/Medical Oncology,
Department of Medicine, Pathology, and Pediatrics,
Oregon Health & Sciences University,
Portland, OR, USA
e-mail: delought@ohsu.edu

© Springer Nature Switzerland AG 2019
T. G. DeLoughery (ed.), *Hemostasis and Thrombosis*,
https://doi.org/10.1007/978-3-030-19330-0_9

increase in the bleeding time. It has been speculated that the increase in nitric oxide levels found with liver disease may result in platelet inhibition. Often the bleeding time is prolonged but the patient has no evidence of increased bleeding. In evaluation of the prolonged bleeding time, one must carefully ask about excessive bleeding with minor trauma. Again, bleeding history is more predictive of future bleeds than is bleeding time.

4. *Increased factor consumption* – Patients with liver disease appear to have an increased consumption of clotting factors. This is due to delayed clearance of activated enzymes leading to increased coagulation. These patients are also more prone to minor and major bleeds leading to greater consumption of factors.

5. *Primary fibrinolysis* – Liver disease is the most common cause of primary fibrinolysis. This occurs due to a decrease in hepatic production of fibrinolytic inhibitors and delayed clearance of plasmin. There are also data showing that levels of TAFI (thrombin activatable fibrinolysis inhibitor) are low in patients with liver disease. Evidence of enhanced fibrinolysis can be found in 30% of patients with end-stage liver disease. Fibrinolysis is evaluated by measuring the euglobulin clot lysis time. Values of less than 60 minutes (normal being more than 60) indicate a fibrinolytic state. Bleeding seen with fibrinolysis is diffuse bleeding from multiple sites or persistent oozing from surgical sites or minor wounds.

However these "anticoagulant" defects can be balanced by "procoagulant" propensities. Levels of natural anticoagulants – protein C, protein S, and antithrombin – are decreased also due to lack of synthesis. Detailed measurement of coagulation potential such as the thrombin generation assay or thromboelastography demonstrates preserved coagulation in patients with liver disease despite abnormal screening tests of hemostasis. In addition, liver disease patients are at increased risk of thrombosis – both due to a greater number of hospital stays and illness but perhaps also, in some patients, the loss of anticoagulants tips them toward hypercoagulability.

Evaluation and Treatment of Coagulation Defects in Liver Disease

It is important to remember that, despite abnormal laboratory studies, the most common cause of bleeding in liver disease is a mechanical defect (hole in vessel). Thus, evaluation in patients with severe bleeding should be aimed at identifying sites of bleeding. Many patients will have dramatic gastrointestinal bleeding due to bleeding varices or gastric ulcers. In these situations replacement of coagulation factors provides an "adjunctive therapy" role to definitive therapy. Except for certain coagulation defects (thrombocytopenia, fibrinolysis), corrections of mild-to-moderate coagulation defects in the severely bleeding patient are not important, and correction of severe coagulation defects is impossible.

An initial screen of the bleeding patient should consist of the hematocrit, platelet count, INR/aPTT, fibrinogen, D-dimer, and euglobulin clot lysis time (Table 9.2). Since DIC can commonly complicate liver disease, evaluation for DIC should be done on unstable patients with liver disease.

In the rapidly bleeding patient, the "magic five" (HCT, INR, aPTT, platelets, fibrinogen) should be checked every few hours to guide therapy (Table 9.3). Ideally, therapeutic goals should be:

- Protime >INR 2.0 *and* aPTT abnormal: give 2 units of FFP.
- Platelets <50,000: give 6 platelet concentrates or one plateletpheresis unit.
- Fibrinogen <150 mg/dl: give 10 units of cryoprecipitate.
- Hematocrit <21%: give packed red cells.

Table 9.2 Evaluation of the bleeding patient with liver disease

aPTT
D-dimer
Euglobulin clot lysis time (if available)
Fibrinogen level
INR
Platelet count
Thromboelastography (if available)

Table 9.3 Therapy of coagulation defects associated with bleeding in liver disease

Protime >INR 2.0 *and* aPTT abnormal: FFP

Platelets <50–75k: platelet concentrates

Fibrinogen <150 mg/dl: 10 units of cryoprecipitate

Hematocrit <21%: packed red cells

Antifibrinolytics

Epsilon-aminocaproic acid (EACA):

    IV bolus – 4–5 g given over 1 hour followed by a continuous infusion of 1 g per hour for 8 hours

    Oral dosing – 4 g every 4 hours

Tranexamic acid:

    IV – 1000 mg IV bolus followed by 1000 mg IV every 6–8 hours

    Oral dosing – 1300 mg every 6–8 hours

Thromboelastography (TEG) is being used more frequently to assess coagulation defects in liver disease. Studies have suggested this is a more accurate reflection of coagulation than standard testing, and its use may more accurately guide blood product replacement.

However, it is often difficult to lower the PT-INR in patients with severe liver disease due to the short half-life of factor VII and the minimal changes one achieves with FFP (increase of 5% per unit of FFP for all clotting factors). Consequently, therapy should not be aimed at complete correction of abnormal laboratory values. Overzealous attempts to totally correct the INR to <2–3 are unproductive and will result in volume overload. Also, an increased plasma volume may increase portal pressures, thereby increasing the risk of more bleeding. Keeping the platelet count above 50,000/uL and the fibrinogen greater than 150 mg/dl is more important than correction of the protime.

Abnormal fibrinolysis is an often overlooked cause of bleeding in patients with liver disease. Bleeding in these patients tends to be characterized by diffuse oozing from minor trauma. Often these patients are futilely treated with massive amounts of fresh frozen plasma before the fibrinolytic defect is discovered. Diagnosis is made by demonstrating a shortened euglobulin clot lysis time or by excess fibrinolysis on the TEG. If these tests are not available, increased fibrinolysis should be suspected in any patients with prolonged bleeding. In the patient who is bleeding from fibrinolysis, a trial of antifibrinolytic therapy is warranted (Table 9.3). The patient should be screened for DIC and significant urinary tract bleeding.

A current area of research is the use of prothrombin complex concentrates (PCC) to treat severe coagulopathies in patients with liver disease. Older PCC were associated with increased risk of thrombosis, but the newer products that contain both pro- and anticoagulant vitamin K-dependent proteins appear to be safer.

Preparation for Surgery

Patients with liver disease often require surgical procedures. Pre-surgical laboratory screening should consist of the hematocrit, platelet count, INR/aPTT, fibrinogen, D-dimer, and euglobulin clot lysis time. Patients with compensated fibrinolysis may rapidly defibrinate during surgical procedures. Before surgery, the platelet count should be increased to over 50,000/uL and the fibrinogen to over 150 mg/dl. Plasma can be used to lower the INR/aPTT but often only a minimal reduction will result. In patients with severe disease, it is not feasible to try to lower the INR below 2.0. Recall that an isolated elevation of the INR is indicative of factor VII deficiency and is not associated with increased risk of bleeding. If available, thromboelastography can provide better information about the patient's hemostatic status. The patient should be carefully monitored during the procedure and platelets and fibrinogen aggressively replaced.

Liver Transplantation

The advent of liver transplantation has significantly impacted the survival of patients with severe liver disease. Patients may require astonishing amounts of blood during the procedure. Totals of more than 100 units of red cells and plasma are not unusual in these patients. Before liver transplant is considered, baseline coagulation status should be determined. However, baseline coagulation defects are not predictive of bleeding with surgery. Certain operative features are more predictive of bleeding. Patients who have had previous abdominal surgery often require extensive dissection of adhesions and will require aggressive blood product support. A long anhepatic time will require frequent checks of coagulation status and monitoring of replacement products. One should anticipate that, when the clamps are released to allow blood flow to the new liver, a "burst" of fibrinolysis will occur. In some patients a heparin-like inhibitor is also released. The coagulopathies that occur during this period are the most challenging. In patients with very severe bleeding, one should check the euglobulin clot lysis time. Severe fibrinolysis should be treated with antifibrinolytic therapy until the patient is stable. If the new liver "takes," the coagulation defects will rapidly resolve.

Uremia

Patients with renal disease can have both a bleeding and a thrombotic diathesis. The thrombotic complications of renal disease are discussed in acquired hypercoagulable states (Chap. 18). Uremic patients may have spontaneous bleeding or may be at risk for bleeding with procedures.

Before the advent of renal replacement therapy, bleeding was a common complication of uremia. Life-threatening bleeding is uncommon, but dialysis patients have a high incidence of gastrointestinal bleeding and subdural hematomas. Patients with end-stage renal disease have a high incidence of underlying gastrointestinal lesions such as angiodysplasia and gastritis which may bleed.

Pathogenesis

The defect in uremia appears to be a platelet function defect. The bleeding time and PFA 100 are usually prolonged. Von Willebrand factor levels are always normal or supranormal. Abnormalities of both platelet adhesion and aggregation are seen. The old glass bead retention test that measured platelet adhesion to glass beads is prolonged in uremic patients. Platelet aggregation studies reveal defects in aggregation with ADP and epinephrine. One determinant of the prolonged bleeding time is the hematocrit level. Patients with hematocrits below 30% have markedly prolonged bleeding times. It is speculated that with low hematocrits, the red cells flow laminarly and are not able to "push" platelets into the vessel wall. Blood coagulation factors appear not to be affected, and unless other problems are present, the INR/aPTT are not prolonged.

Evaluation

Uremic patients who are bleeding should have INR/aPTT and platelet count performed. Patients with uremia are prone to vitamin K deficiency, so assessment of the prothrombin time is important. The half-life of both unfractionated and low molecular weight heparin is prolonged in renal failure. Patients will receive a bolus of heparin with dialysis, and the rare patient will have a prolonged anticoagulant effect. Low molecular weight heparins are cleared in the kidneys, and if the dose is not adjusted, levels can increase to supranormal levels. Bleeding times are prolonged in renal disease. Unfortunately there is little correlation between prolongation of the bleeding time and actual bleeding, especially with procedures.

Therapy (Table 9.4)

Patients who are severely uremic and bleeding may respond to aggressive dialysis. If the patient is having life-threatening bleeding, the use of heparin anticoagulants should be avoided.

Infusion of cryoprecipitate has been shown to correct the bleeding defect. The mechanism of action is unknown. Ten units every 12 hours will usually correct the bleeding time. Too aggressive use of cryoprecipitate will raise the plasma fibrinogen to very high levels that, theoretically, could promote thrombosis. Also, the effect of cryoprecipitate is not consistent and may fail to halt uremic bleeding.

Table 9.4   Therapy for uremic bleeding

Acute
Aggressive dialysis
Cryoprecipitate 10 units
Desmopressin 0.3 ug/kg
If hematocrit under 30%, red cell transfusions
Long term
Estrogen 0.6 mg/kg for 5 days
Erythropoietin to raise hematocrit over 30%

Desmopressin has been shown to be effective in uremic patients and results in a shorter bleeding time for at least 4 hours. The reason DDAVP works in uremia is unknown. Since levels of factor VIII and von Willebrand protein are already elevated in uremia, elevation of these proteins does not appear to be a mechanism. It has been speculated that DDAVP effect is either via a platelet aggregation promoting effect or via increasing the level of functional von Willebrand protein.

Infusion of conjugated estrogens will shorten the bleeding time. The dose is 0.6 mg/kg/day intravenously for 5 days. The exact mechanism is unknown, but improved vascular integrity has been proposed. One advantage of estrogens is that the effect appears to be long-lasting and can persist for 2 weeks after infusion

Raising the hematocrit above 30% will shorten the bleeding time. This can be done either acutely by transfusion or chronically with the use of erythropoietin. It is speculated that increasing the red cell mass will increase platelet-vessel wall interactions. For purposes of hemostasis, the target hematocrit with the use of erythropoietin should be greater than 30%.

Suggested Reading

Hedges SJ, Dehoney SB, Hooper JS, Amanzadeh J, Busti AJ. Evidence-based treatment recommendations for uremic bleeding. Nat Clin Pract Nephrol. 2007;3(3):138–53.

Lisman T, Porte RJ. Pathogenesis, prevention, and management of bleeding and thrombosis in patients with liver diseases. Res Pract Thromb Haemost. 2017;1(2):150–61.

Loffredo L, Pastori D, Farcomeni A, Violi F. Effects of anticoagulants in patients with cirrhosis and portal vein thrombosis: a systematic review and meta-analysis. Gastroenterology. 2017;153(2):480–7.

Pavord S, Myers B. Bleeding and thrombotic complications of kidney disease. Blood Rev. 2011;25(6):271–8.

Cardiac Bypass and Ventricular Assist Devices/ECMO

10

Thomas G. DeLoughery

Introduction

More than 100,000 patients undergo cardiopulmonary bypass surgery each year. Coronary bypass surgery may be complicated by blood loss and sometimes a severe bleeding diathesis. Patients presenting for cardiac surgery may have preexisting bleeding defects or may develop severe defects during or after surgery. Also, over the past decade, more patients are having ventricular assist devices implanted either as a bridge to cardiac transplant or permanently as "destination therapy." Similar hemostasis issues are seen with the use of ECMO (extracorporeal membrane oxygenation).

Preoperative Coagulation Defects

Anticoagulation. Many patients who present for surgery are already anticoagulated, most often for the underlying heart disease (Table 10.1). If needed, rapid reversal (4–6 hours) of warfarin can be achieved with the use of vitamin K, given as 5 mg over 1 hour by slow intravenous infusion.

Table 10.1 Management of the patient on anticoagulation

Warfarin
Elective procedures
1. Stop warfarin 5 days before procedure
2. Start enoxaparin 1 mg/kg every 12 hours
3. Give last dose evening before surgery and hold morning dose
4. Check PT-INR/aPTT morning of surgery
Emergency procedures
1. Stop warfarin
2. Give 5 mg slow intravenous push of vitamin K if INR greater than 2.0
3. If INR still elevated before surgery, use 2–4 units of FFP as pump prime, or give 25–50 units/kg of prothrombin complex concentrates
Direct oral anticoagulant
Apixaban: Hold 48 hours
Dabigatran: Hold 48hours–72 hours if significant renal disease
Edoxaban: Hold 48 hours
Rivaroxaban: Hold 48 hours

Alternatively, fresh frozen plasma can be used to prime the cardiac bypass machine, or prothrombin complex concentrates given. If clinically feasible, patients should stop warfarin 1 week before the procedure. For the rare patient that requires bridging, the last dose of low molecular weight heparin should be given the morning before surgery.

Congenital heart disease patients may have several potential coagulation defects. Patients with cyanotic heart disease and high hematocrits will have spurious elevation of the INR/PTT due

T. G. DeLoughery (✉)
Division of Hematology/Medical Oncology,
Department of Medicine, Pathology, and Pediatrics,
Oregon Health & Sciences University,
Portland, OR, USA
e-mail: delought@ohsu.edu

© Springer Nature Switzerland AG 2019
T. G. DeLoughery (ed.), *Hemostasis and Thrombosis*,
https://doi.org/10.1007/978-3-030-19330-0_10

to alteration of the plasma/anticoagulant ratio. This occurs with hematocrits of more than 60%. The coagulation laboratory needs to be notified before testing is done. The laboratory can prepare a special tube with the proper amount of anticoagulant for the patient's hematocrit.

Many patients with congenital heart disease have a bleeding diathesis which is associated with a prolonged bleeding time but no obvious platelet abnormalities. The etiology of this defect is unknown, but rare patients may have severe bleeding with surgery or other procedures. If patients are responsive to desmopressin, this agent can be given preoperatively.

Patients with severe pulmonary hypertension can develop acquired type 2A von Willebrand disease. This may be due to destruction of the high molecular weight multimers by the damaged pulmonary endothelium. The affected patients can also have marked thrombocytopenia and a severe bleeding diathesis. Patients with pulmonary hypertension and bleeding should undergo a phlebotomy to lower the hematocrit to less than 65%. This reduction in hematocrit can increase the platelet count and ease the severity of the von Willebrand disease.

Cardiopulmonary Bypass

Cardiac bypass results in very complex and still poorly defined defects in all aspects of hemostasis (Table 10.2).

The flowing of blood over artificial surfaces results in activation of the contact coagulation system, leading to factor XI activation and kinin activation. The activation of the contact pathway is also a potent activator of the fibrinolytic system. The relevance of contact pathway activation has

Table 10.2 Coagulation defects associated with cardiopulmonary bypass surgery

1. Activation of contact pathway
2. Activation of fibrinolysis
3. Activation of tissue factor pathway
4. Activation of platelets
5. Platelet function defects

recently been challenged due to the persistence of coagulation defects in patients with deficiencies of the contact pathway undergoing bypass.

The tissue factor pathway is also activated during bypass. Monocyte activation is observed with the expression of tissue factor. The inflammatory response to surgery and bypass may also lead to expression of endothelial cell tissue factor. This expression of tissue factor results in persistent thrombin generation during the surgery, despite the large amounts of heparin given during bypass.

Platelets can be activated by contact with the artificial surfaces in the bypass machine. Excessive activation of platelets depletes their granules, leading to the circulation of "spent platelets." Platelet function is also inhibited by loss of the key receptors, GP Ib and IIb/IIIa. This is due in part to cleavage of platelet GP IIb/IIIa by activated proteolytic enzymes and in part to binding of the receptor GP Ib to the artificial surface.

Finally, there is activation of the fibrinolytic system. Fibrinolytic activation is via both the contact pathway and by release of endothelial tPA due to the stress of surgery and hypothermia.

Large amounts of heparin are used for the bypass machine to prevent thrombosis of the filters. Levels of heparin can reach as high as 5 units/ml with anti-Xa levels of 3–7 IU/ml. These large doses need to be reversed at the end of surgery to prevent bleeding. Since protamine has a shorter half-life than heparin, patients rarely may experience "heparin rebound." High doses of protamine can lead to coagulation defects or the inhibition of platelet function.

The magnitude of the bleeding diathesis is related to surgery length and long "pump runs." Complex dissections, such as those needed during lung transplants or repeat cardiac surgeries, also lead to additional bleeding.

Prevention and Therapy

Prophylactic use of platelets or plasma prior to surgery has been shown to be ineffective except in a few select cases. Patients with preexisting thrombocytopenia or platelet dysfunction may benefit from preoperative platelet transfusions to improve platelet function.

The use of desmopressin remains controversial. Initial studies indicated that it could reduce bleeding in cardiac bypass surgery. More recent studies have not confirmed these early trials. In patients with significant blood loss, perioperative use of desmopressin may help reduce bleeding.

Bypass surgery produces nonspecific activation of many enzymes, especially those of the fibrinolytic system. Therefore, the use of inhibitors of the fibrinolytic system has been advocated. Aprotinin was the most studied but was removed from the market due to thrombotic complications. Both tranexamic acid and epsilon aminocaproic acid are widely used to conserve blood during surgery. A recent trial showed high-dose tranexamic acid (50 mg/kg) did reduce need for blood products without increasing the risk of thrombosis.

Approach to the Bleeding Bypass Patient (Table 10.3)

If the patient is still in the operating suite and starts to have microvascular bleeding, one should check a full panel of coagulation testing including the platelet count, INR, PTT, and fibrinogen. Patients who have had multiple transfusions of cell-saver blood or of packed red cells may have dilutional coagulation defects that need to be replaced with heparin and cryoprecipitate. In the bleeding patient still on bypass, an infusion of desmopressin is indicated. Given a platelet defect, if the INR/aPTT are in the normal range and the patient is still bleeding, transfusion of platelets is indicated, even with platelet counts over 100,000 uL.

If bleeding occurs in the postoperative setting, coagulation tests should be run and surgical hemostasis achieved. Again, attention should be paid to the INR/PTT and fibrinogen level. Often patients will respond to empiric transfusions of platelets. In the immediate postoperative state, a thrombin time should be checked to ensure the patient is not having heparin rebound.

Table 10.3 Approach to bleeding cardiac surgery patient

Bleeding and still in operating room
1. Check PT-INR, aPTT, fibrinogen, and platelet count
2. Replace any deficits
3. If still bleeding, administer desmopressin 0.3 Ug/kg
4. If still bleeding, administer one platelet transfusion
5. If still bleeding, check euglobulin clot lysis time and, if prolonged, administer antifibrinolytic agent

Bleeding postoperatively
1. Assess surgical sites
2. Check PT-INR, aPTT, fibrinogen, and platelet count
3. Replace any deficits
4. If still bleeding, check thrombin time – if elevated give 50 mg protamine
5. If still bleeding, administer one platelet transfusion
6. If still bleeding, check euglobulin clot lysis time and if prolonged administer antifibrinolytic agent
7. If still bleeding and INR is elevated, give 1000 units of prothrombin complex concentrates
8. If still bleeding, either 30 ug/kg of rVIIa or 2000 units of activated prothrombin complex concentrates

For bleeding refractory to these maneuvers, a variety of therapies have been proposed. There is more frequent use of low-dose prothrombin complex concentrates 1000 units if the INR remains elevated. If bleeding continues, low-dose rVIIa 30 ug/kg can be tried. Some groups have used low-dose activated PCC 2000 units for recalcitrant bleeding.

Ventricular Assist Devices (VADs)

VADs are frequently being used either as a "bridge" to transplantation or as long-term cardiac support. Early devices required aggressive anticoagulation and resulted in high rates of both bleeding and thrombosis. Newer devices use continuous flow and appear to be less thrombogenic but still require anticoagulation. A combination of aspirin 81 mg/day and warfarin targeted to INR 1.5–2.5 is used. Pump thrombosis may occur most commonly in the first 6 months and is heralded by an increase in LDH – perhaps reflecting red cells disrupted by pump turbulence created by the thrombus. Thrombosis is treated either by transplantation, device replacement, or thrombolytic therapy. With long-term use of VADs, increased bleeding can been seen. The pump leads to loss of high molecular weight von Willebrand multimers, leading to a type 2A acquired von Willebrand disease (vWD). Also, patients with continuous flow pumps are prone to developing gastrointestinal arterial venous malformations. The combination of loss of von Willebrand factor, aspirin, and AVMs can lead to gastrointestinal bleeding. Also, patients with VADs who need surgery may have massive surgical bleeding.

The diagnosis of acquired vWD can be difficult as levels of von Willebrand protein and activity tend to be elevated; factor VIII levels and activity may be elevated as well. The platelet function assay is markedly elevated which is a diagnostic clue, and an abnormal multimer assay is diagnostic. Therapy of bleeding is difficult as infused Humate-P can often be ineffective as the infused vWD is rapidly degraded. Lowering INR goal can lead to less bleeding but will increase the risk of stroke.

Extracorporeal Membrane Oxygenation (ECMO)

ECMO is increasingly used in both children and adults with respiratory failure. It is essential an "artificial lung" that can oxygenate the blood to provide support when the lungs – even with maximal ventilatory support – cannot support the person. Like with VADs, there can be complex coagulopathies with ECMO. Acquired vWD also occurs very rapidly with onset of going on ECMO and resolves quickly when it is removed. Anticoagulation is required during ECMO, but much controversy remains over the best way to monitor – ACT, aPTT, heparin levels (anti-Xa), or thromboelastography. Platelet consumption is also common, and transfusion is frequently required to keep the count about 50,000/uL. Heparin resistance is common both due to the marked inflammatory state these sick patients will have and consumption of antithrombin.

Many protocols recommend monitoring antithrombin levels and replacement if below 60–70%, but again there is little consistency among ECMO centers about this. An alternative for patients with heparin resistance and especially those with heparin-induced thrombocytopenia is using the direct thrombin inhibitor bivalirudin (usually dosing is 0.1–0.2 mg/kg/h titrated to ACT).

Special Situations

Heparin-induced thrombocytopenia (HIT) is common in patients being considered for cardiac surgery. Since anticoagulation is necessary to undergo bypass, the presence of HIT can be a challenge. One strategy is to wait until the titer of the HIT antibody has decreased enough to be undetectable. This clearance of the HIT antibody may take a few weeks. When the platelet aggregation assay or serotonin release assay is negative, the patient can be re-exposed to heparin for the few hours needed for surgery. This window of opportunity can be used for bypass. If surgery is needed more urgently, then heparin alternatives are needed. Most experience is with argatroban and bivalirudin (Table 10.4). Argatroban has been reported to be effective in patients with HIT needing bypass surgery. One recommended dosing strategy is a bolus of 0.1 mg/kg followed by an infusion of 5–10 ug/kg/min to keep the activated clotting time (ACT) between 300 and 400 seconds. Most experience with bivalirudin dosing has been with a 1 mg/kg bolus and infusion at 1.75–2.5 mg/kg/h to keep the ACT >300 seconds.

Table 10.4 Alternative anticoagulation agents for patients with HIT

Argatroban
Bolus 0.1 ug/kg
Infusion of 5–10 ug/kg/min to keep ACT between 300 and 400 seconds
Bivalirudin
Bolus: 1 mg/kg bolus with a 50 mg bolus added to the priming
Infusion of 1.75–2.5 mg/kg/hour to keep ACT >250

"*Redos*": Patients who present for a repeat cardiac surgery are at high risk for significant bleeding. These patients require complex dissections of tissue planes and will have greater blood loss. They will have longer "pump runs" and a higher incidence of bypass-induced coagulation defects. All of these patients should receive antifibrinolytic therapy to help prevent blood loss.

Suggested Reading

Baumann Kreuziger LM, Kim B, Wieselthaler GM. Antithrombotic therapy for left ventricular assist devices in adults: a systematic review. J Thromb Haemost. 2015;13(6):946–55.

Davidson S. State of the art – how i manage coagulopathy in cardiac surgery patients. Br J Haematol. 2014;164(6):779–89.

Doyle AJ, Hunt BJ. Current understanding of how extracorporeal membrane oxygenators activate haemostasis and other blood components. Front Med (Lausanne). 2018;5:352.

Muslem R, Caliskan K, Leebeek FWG. Acquired coagulopathy in patients with left ventricular assist devices. J Thromb Haemost. 2018;16(3):429–40.

Myles PS, Smith JA, Forbes A, Silbert B, Jayarajah M, Painter T, Cooper DJ, Marasco S, McNeil J, Bussières JS, McGuinness S, Byrne K, Chan MT, Landoni G, Wallace S, ATACAS Investigators of the ANZCA Clinical Trials Network. Tranexamic acid in patients undergoing coronary-artery surgery. N Engl J Med. 2017;376(2):136–48.

Raffini L. Anticoagulation with VADs and ECMO: walking the tightrope. Hematology Am Soc Hematol Educ Program. 2017;2017(1):674–80. https://doi.org/10.1182/asheducation-2017.1.674.

Ranucci M. Hemostatic and thrombotic issues in cardiac surgery. Semin Thromb Hemost. 2015;41(1):84–90.

Immune Thrombocytopenia

11

Thomas G. DeLoughery

Introduction

Immune thrombocytopenia (ITP) is a common condition affecting about 1 in 20,000. This review will go over the presentation of ITP, the diagnosis, and then treatment options. Finally, ITP in specific clinical situations will be reviewed.

Pathogenesis and Epidemiology

ITP is due to autoantibodies binding to platelet surface proteins, most often to the platelet receptor GP IIb/IIIa. These antibody-coated platelets then bind to Fc receptors in macrophages and are removed from circulation. The initiating event in ITP is unknown. It is speculated that the patient responds to a viral or bacterial infection by creating antibodies which cross-react with the platelet receptors. Continued exposure to platelets perpetuates the immune response. ITP that occurs in childhood appears to be an acute response to viral infection and usually resolves. ITP in adults may occur in any age group but is seen especially in young women.

Although it had been thought that most adults who presented with ITP went on to have a chronic course, more recent studies have shown that 30–50% of patients may be "cured" with steroids. In addition, it often appears that even if patients have modest residual thrombocytopenia, as long as their counts are over 30,000/uL, no therapy is required.

Symptoms

Presentation can range from an asymptomatic patient with low platelets found on a routine blood count to massive bleeding. Typically, patients first present with petechiae – small bruises 1 mm in size – on the shins. True petechiae are only seen in severe thrombocytopenia. Patients will also notice frequent bruising as well as bleeding from the gums. Patients with very low platelet counts will notice "wet purpura" – blood-filled bullae – in the oral cavity. Life-threatening bleeding is a very unusual presenting sign unless other problems (trauma, ulcers) are present. The physical examination is only remarkable for stigmata of bleeding such as petechiae. The presence of splenomegaly or lymphadenopathy weighs strongly against a diagnosis of ITP.

T. G. DeLoughery (✉)
Division of Hematology/Medical Oncology, Department of Medicine, Pathology, and Pediatrics, Oregon Health & Sciences University, Portland, OR, USA
e-mail: delought@ohsu.edu

© Springer Nature Switzerland AG 2019
T. G. DeLoughery (ed.), *Hemostasis and Thrombosis*,
https://doi.org/10.1007/978-3-030-19330-0_11

Diagnosis

Extremely low platelet counts with a normal blood smear in an otherwise healthy patient is diagnostic of ITP. One should question the patient carefully about drug exposure (see drug-induced thrombocytopenia), especially about over-the-counter medicines, "natural" remedies, or recreational drugs.

There is no laboratory test that "rules in" ITP; rather, it is a diagnosis of exclusion. The blood smear should be carefully examined for evidence of microangiopathic hemolytic anemias (schistocytes), bone marrow disease (blasts, teardrop cells), or any other evidence of a primary bone marrow disease. In ITP, the platelets may be larger than normal, but finding some platelets the size of red cells should raise the issue of congenital thrombocytopenia. One should exclude pseudo-thrombocytopenia, which is the clumping of platelets due to a reaction to the EDTA anticoagulant in the tube and is clinically harmless.

Antiplatelet antibody assays appear to be specific but not sensitive and may be useful when the diagnosis is difficult to make. In a patient without a history of autoimmune disease or symptoms, empiric testing for autoimmune disease is not recommended. Patients who present with ITP should be tested for both HIV and hepatitis C. These are the most common viral causes of secondary ITP, and both have prognostic and treatment implications.

The role of bone marrow examination is controversial. Patients with a classic presentation of ITP (young woman, normal blood smear) do not require a bone marrow exam before therapy is initiated. Patients who do not respond to initial therapy or who have other blood abnormalities should have a bone marrow aspiration. The rare entity of amegakaryocytic thrombocytopenia can present with a similar clinical picture to ITP but will not respond to steroids. Bone marrow aspiration reveals the absence of megakaryocytes in this entity. It is rare, however, that another hematological disease is diagnosed in patients with a classic clinical presentation of ITP.

Measurement of thrombopoietin and reticulated platelets may provide clues to diagnosis.

Patients with ITP paradoxically have normal or only mildly elevated thrombopoietin levels. The finding of a significantly elevated thrombopoietin level should lead to questioning of the diagnosis. One can also measure "reticulated platelets" (also called immature platelet fraction) which are analogous to the red cell reticulocytes. Patients with ITP (or any platelet destructive disorder) will have high levels of reticulated platelets. These tests are not recommended for routine testing but may be helpful in difficult cases.

Therapy

Therapy in ITP should be guided by the patient's signs of bleeding and not by slavish adherence to measuring numbers; patients tend to tolerate their thrombocytopenia well. It is unusual to have life-threatening bleeding with platelet counts over 5000/uL in the absence of mechanical lesions. Rare patients will have antibodies that interfere with the function of the platelet; these patients can have profound bleeding with only modestly lowered platelet counts. A suggested cutoff for treating newly diagnosed patients is 20,000/uL but needs to be guided by the clinical presentation.

Initial Therapy (Table 11.1)

The primary therapy of ITP is glucocorticoids – either prednisone or dexamethasone. A widely used alternative to prednisone 1 mg/kg/day is dexamethasone 40 mg/day for 4 days. This induces a more rapid rise in the platelet count

Table 11.1 Acute therapy of ITP

Dexamethasone 40 mg/day × 4 days; repeat 3–4 times

For bleeding patients or counts below 5–10,000/uL

  Immunoglobulin 1 g/kg IV repeat in 24 hours or
  Anti-d (WinRho) 75 ug/kg once

Refractory patients

  Immunoglobulin 1 g/kg continuous infusion over 24 hours and

  Continuous infusion platelets (one plateletpheresis unit/6 hours or one platelet concentrate/hour)

with several studies suggesting high response and remission rates. An aggressive approach such as 4-day cycle every 14 days times 3 or 4 has been used in studies with high response rates.

For rapid induction of a response, there are two options. Intravenous immunoglobulin (IVIG) at 1 g/kg once or intravenous anti-D antibody at 50–75 ug/kg as a single dose can induce a response in over 80% of patients in 24–48 hours. IVIG has several drawbacks including risks of aseptic meningitis and of inducing thrombosis. The use of anti-D is limited to Rh-positive patients who have not had a splenectomy. It should not be used in patients who are Coombs positive for fear of provoking more hemolysis. Rarely, anti-D has been reported to cause a severe hemolytic DIC syndrome which has led to restrictions in use and recommendations that patients be observed for 8 hours after infusion with frequent monitoring for hemoglobinuria.

For patients who are severely thrombocytopenic and do not respond to initial therapy, one option is a continuous infusion of platelets (one unit over 6 hours) and IVIG 1 g/kg for 24 hours to raise the platelet count.

Patients with severe thrombocytopenia who relapse after steroids have several options for further management as discussed below. Some patients may only require several courses of repeated doses of anti-D or IVIG to transiently increase the platelet count, with resultant higher counts lasting for many months. Patients who do not respond to initial ITP therapies have multiple options. These can be divided into several broad groups – curative therapies, thrombopoietin agonists, and anecdotal therapies.

Chronic Therapies (Table 11.2)

Splenectomy

In patients with severe thrombocytopenia who do not respond or who relapse with tapering of prednisone, splenectomy should be strongly considered. Splenectomy will induce a good response in 60–70% of patients and is durable in most patients. Splenectomy carries a short-term surgical risk and the lifelong risk of increased suscep-

Table 11.2 Therapeutic options in patients who don't respond to splenectomy

Rituximab 375 mg/m^2 weekly × 4 or 1000 mg × 2 14 days apart
TPO-mimetics
Eltrombopag starting at 50 mg daily, can increase to 75 mg/daily if suboptimal response
Romiplostim started at 3 ug/kg weekly, may increase by 1 ug/kg amount weekly if response suboptimal to maximal dose of 10 ug/kg
Fostamatinib starting at 100 mg BID, increasing to 150 mg BID if needed
Azathioprine 125 mg/day
Cyclophosphamide 1 g/m^2 repeated every 28 days
Danazol 200 mg/qid +/− azathioprine
Mycophenolate 1000 mg BID
Vincristine 1.4 mg/m^2 IV weekly

tibility to overwhelming sepsis as discussed below. However, the absolute magnitude of these risks is low and is often lower than that of continued prednisone therapy or of continued cytotoxic therapy.

Timing of splenectomy depends on the patient's presentation. Most patients should be given a 6-month trial of steroids or other therapies before proceeding to splenectomy. However, patients who persist with severe thrombocytopenia despite initial therapies or who are suffering intolerable side effects from therapy should be considered sooner for splenectomy.

The risk of overwhelming sepsis varies by indications for splenectomy but appears to be about 1% or less. The use of pneumococcal vaccine and recognition of this syndrome have helped lessen the risk. Asplenic patients need to be counseled about the risk of overwhelming infections and should be vaccinated for pneumococcus, meningococcus, and Haemophilus influenzae and should wear an ID bracelet noting splenectomized state.

Rituximab

Rituximab has been shown to be very active in ITP. Most studies use the standard dose of 375 mg/m^2 weekly for 4 weeks, but many investigators are using the "immunosuppression" dose of 1000 mg given twice, on day 1 and day 14. The response time can vary; patients may demonstrate a rapid response or may take up to 12 weeks for their counts to go up – median time to response is 6 weeks. Overall the response rate of rituximab is about 60%, but only approximately 20% of patients overall will remain in long-term remission. Patients may respond by going back into remission with further doses of rituximab. There is no evidence yet that "maintenance" therapy or monitoring CD19/CD20 cells can help further the duration of remission.

Although not "chemotherapy," rituximab is not without risks. Many patients can get infusion reactions and these can be severe in 1–2% of patients. In a meta-analysis the fatal reaction rate was 2.9%. Patients with chronic hepatitis B infections can develop reactivation with rituximab. Finally, the very rare but devastating complication of progressive multifocal leukoencephalopathy has been reported.

Thrombopoietin (TPO)-Mimetics

Despite very low circulating platelet counts, levels of platelet growth factor thrombopoietin do not increase, which keeps platelet production low. Recently, two TPO-mimetics have been approved for use in patients with ITP.

Romiplostim
Romiplostim is a "peptibody" – a combination of a peptide that binds and stimulates the TPO receptor and an Fc domain to extend its half-life. It is administered in a weekly subcutaneous dose starting at 3 ug/kg. ITP patients demonstrate a response rate of 80–88% to romiplostim, with most patients having persistent responses.

The major side effect of romiplostim seen in clinical trials was marrow reticulin formation (marrow fibrosis) which occurred in ~ 5% of patients and appeared to reverse with cessation of the drug.

Eltrombopag
The other available TPO-mimetic is eltrombopag. This is an oral agent that stimulates the TPO receptor by binding the transmembrane domain and activating it. The drug is given orally starting at 50 mg/day (25 mg for patients of Asian ances-

try or those with liver disease) and can be escalated to 75 mg/day. The drug needs to be taken on an empty stomach. Eltrombopag also has been shown to be effective for chronic ITP with response rates similar to romiplostim. Eltrombopag shares with romiplostim the risk for marrow fibrosis. Its unique side effect is a 3–7% incidence of elevated liver function tests seen in clinical trials that did appear to resolve in most patients, but liver function tests need to be monitored in patients receiving eltrombopag.

Clinical Use of TPO-Mimetics
The clearest indication for use of TPO-mimetics is in patients who have failed several therapies and remain symptomatic or on intolerable doses of other medications such as prednisone. The clear benefits are their relatively safety and high rates of success. The main drawback is the need for continuing therapy as the platelets will return to baseline shortly after these agents are stopped. Right now there is no clear indication for one medication over the other.

Fostamatinib
This agent is a Syk (spleen tyrosine kinase) inhibitor. This kinase is active in macrophages and may play a role in the uptake of antibody-coated platelets. Clinical studies in patients refractory to multiple therapies showed a sustained response rate of ~ 20% with use of this agent. Median responses were seen as soon as 2 weeks. The side effects were diarrhea, nausea, neutropenia, and hypertension. The dose is 100 mg bid which can be escalated to 150 mg bid if patients do not have a platelet count over 50,000/ul by 4 weeks. If there is no response by 12 weeks, the drug should be stopped.

Other Options

In the literature, there are numerous options for treatment of ITP – most of these are anecdotal, enrolled small number of patients, and sometimes included patients with mild thrombocytopenia. These can be tried in patients who have failed standard therapies and have bleeding. The agents with the most data are:

- *Danazol* 200 mg four times daily is thought to downregulate the macrophage Fc receptor. The onset of action may be delayed, and a therapeutic trial of up to 4–6 months is advised. Danazol is very effective in antiphospholipid antibody syndrome with ITP and may be more effective in pre-menopausal women. Once a response is seen, danazol should be continued for 6 months, and then an attempt should be made to see if the agent can be weaned.
- *Vincristine* 1.4 mg/m^2 weekly has a low response rate, but if a response is going to occur, it will occur rapidly within 2 weeks. Thus, a prolonged trial of vincristine is not needed; if no platelet rise is seen in several weeks, the drug should be stopped.
- *Azathioprine* 150 mg po daily, like danazol, demonstrates a delayed response and requires several months to assess for response. Recently it has been reported that the related agent *mycophenolate* 1000 mg bid is also effective in ITP.
- *Cyclophosphamide* 1 gm/m^2 IV repeated every 28 days has been reported to have a high response rate of up to 40%. Although considered more "aggressive," this is a standard immunosuppressive dose and should be considered in patients with very low counts. Patients who have not responded to single-agent cyclophosphamide may respond to multi-agent chemotherapy with agents such as etoposide and vincristine plus cyclophosphamide.

A Practical Approach to the Refractory Patient

One approach is to divide patients into "bleeders" and "nonbleeders." Patients with bleeding have either very low platelet counts (under 5000/uL) or have had significant bleeding in the past. Non-bleeding patients have platelet counts above 5000/uL and no history of severe bleeding.

Patients who bleed and do not respond to splenectomy should first start with rituximab since it is not cytotoxic and is the only other "curative" therapy. Patients who are rituximab non-responders should then be tried on TPO-mimetics, and then, if TPO-mimetics don't work, fostamatinib. Patients who still do not respond and persist with severe disease with bleeding should receive aggressive therapy with immunosuppression. One approach to consider is bolus cyclophosphamide. If this is unsuccessful, then one can consider using a combination of azathioprine or mycophenolate plus danazol. Since it may take 4–6 months for this combination to work, these patients may need frequent IVIG therapy to maintain a safe platelet count.

Patients with persistent ITP but not significant bleeding ("nonbleeders") should be tried on danazol and other relatively "safe" agents. If this fails, rituximab or TPO-mimetics can be considered. Before one considers cytotoxic therapy, the risk of the therapy must be weighed against the risk of the thrombocytopenia. The mortality from ITP is fairly low (5%) and is restricted to patients with severe disease. Patients with only moderate thrombocytopenia and no bleeding are often better served with conservative management. There is little justification for the use of continuous steroid therapy in this group of patients given the long-term risks.

Special Situations

Surgery

Patients with ITP who need surgery either for splenectomy or for other reasons should have their platelet counts increased to a level above 20–30,000/uL before surgery. Most patients with ITP have increased platelet function and will not have excessive bleeding with these platelet counts. For patients with platelet counts below this level, an infusion of immunoglobulin or anti-D may rapidly increase the platelet counts. If the surgery is elective, short-term use of TPO agonists to raise the counts can also be considered.

Pregnancy

Up to 10% of pregnant women will develop low platelet counts during their pregnancy. The most common etiology is "gestational thrombocytopenia." This is an exaggeration of the low normal platelet count seen in pregnancy women. Counts may fall as low as 50,000/uL by the time of delivery. No therapy is required as the fetus is not affected and the mother does not have an increased risk of bleeding. Pregnancy complications such as HELLP syndrome and thrombotic microangiopathies also present with low platelet counts, but these can be diagnosed by history.

Women with ITP can either develop the disease during pregnancy or have a worsening of the symptoms during pregnancy. Counts often dramatically drop during the first trimester. Early management should be conservative with low doses of prednisone to keep the count above 10,000/uL. Immunoglobulin is also effective but there are rare reports of pulmonary edema. Rarely, patients who are refractory will require splenectomy, which may be safely performed in the second trimester. For delivery, the count should be greater than 30,000/uL, and for an epidural, platelet count should be greater than 50,000/uL.

Most controversy centers on management of the delivery. In the past it was feared that fetal thrombocytopenia could lead to intracranial hemorrhage, and Caesarean section was always recommended. It now appears that most cases of intracranial hemorrhage were due to alloimmune thrombocytopenia and not ITP. Furthermore, the nadir of the baby's platelet count is not at birth but several days after.

It appears the safest course is to proceed with a vaginal or C-section delivery determined by obstetrical indications and then immediately check the baby's platelet count. If the platelet count is low in the neonate, immunoglobulin will raise the count. Since the neonatal thrombocytopenia is due to passive transfer of maternal antibody, platelet destruction will abate in 4–6 weeks.

Pediatric Patients

There are several distinct differences in pediatric ITP syndromes. Most patients' ITP will resolve in weeks with only a minority of patients transforming into chronic ITP (5–10%). The rates of serious bleeding are lower, with rates of intracranial hemorrhage of 0.1–0.5% being seen. For most patients with no or mild bleeding, management is now largely expectant due to the perception that the risks of therapies are higher than that of bleeding. For patients with bleeding, use of IVIG, anti-D, or a short course of steroids can be used. Given the risk of overwhelming sepsis later in life, splenectomy is often deferred as long as possible. There is growing use of rituximab due to concerns of the use of agents such as cyclophosphamide or azathioprine in children. Studies are starting to appear about the use of TPO-mimetic in the pediatric population.

Evans Syndrome

Evans syndrome is defined at the combination of autoimmune hemolytic anemia (AIHA) and ITP. These cytopenias can present simultaneously or sequentially. Patients with Evans syndrome are thought to have a more severe disease process, to be more prone to bleeding, and to be more difficult to treat; the rarity of this syndrome makes this hard to quantify.

The classic clinical presentation of Evans syndrome is severe anemia and thrombocytopenia. Children with Evans syndrome often have complex immunodeficiencies such as autoimmune lymphoproliferative syndrome. In adults, Evans syndrome most often complicates other autoimmune diseases such as lupus. There are reports of Evans syndrome occurring as a complication of T-cell lymphomas. Often, the autoimmune disease can predate the lymphoma diagnosis by months or even years.

In theory, the diagnosis is straightforward: a Coombs-positive hemolytic anemia in the setting of a clinical diagnosis of immune thrombocytopenia. The blood smear will show spherocytes and a diminished platelet count. The presence of other abnormal red cell forms should raise the issue of an alternative diagnosis.

It is uncertain how vigorously one should search for other underlying diseases. Many patients will already have the diagnosis of an underlying autoimmune disease. The presence of lymphadenopathy should raise the concern of lymphoma.

Initial therapy is high-dose steroids (2 mg/kg/day). Intravenous immunoglobulin should be added if severe thrombocytopenia is present. Patients who cannot be weaned off prednisone or relapse after prednisone course is finished should be considered for splenectomy. However, these patients are at higher risk of relapsing. Increasingly, rituximab is being used with success. For patients who fail this, sirolimus starting at 2–3 mg/m^2/day, aiming for a trough of 4–15 ng/ml, has been reported to be effective.

Suggested Reading

Bussel J, Arnold DM, Grossbard E, Mayer J, Treliński J, Homenda W, Hellmann A, Windyga J, Sivcheva L, Khalafallah AA, Zaja F, Cooper N, Markovtsov V, Zayed H, Duliege AM. Fostamatinib for the treatment of adult persistent and chronic immune thrombocytopenia: results of two phase 3, randomized, placebo-controlled trials. Am J Hematol. 2018;93(7):921–30.

Bylsma LC, Fryzek JP, Cetin K, Callaghan F, Bezold C, Mehta B, Wasser JS. Systematic literature review of treatments used for adult immune thrombocytopenia in the second-line setting. Am J Hematol. 2019;94(1):118–32.

Cooper N. State of the art – how I manage immune thrombocytopenia. Br J Haematol. 2017 Apr;177(1):39–54.

Kelton JG, Vrbensky JR, Arnold DM. How do we diagnose immune thrombocytopenia in 2018? Hematology Am Soc Hematol Educ Program. 2018;2018(1):561–7.

Neunert CE, Cooper N. Evidence-based management of immune thrombocytopenia: ASH guideline update. Hematology Am Soc Hematol Educ Program. 2018;2018(1):568–75.

Thrombotic Microangiopathy (TTP/HUS)

12

Thomas G. DeLoughery

Introduction

The thrombotic microangiopathies (TMs) are a group of diseases which share the traits of microvascular occlusion, thrombocytopenia, and microangiopathic hemolytic anemia. Common to these diseases is a dramatic presentation and often fulminant illness. Although these diseases share some common characteristics, course and prognosis may vary.

Classification

Since the underlying pathophysiology and etiology of many of the TMs are unknown, any classification scheme is imprecise (Table 12.1). In addition, many of the signs and symptoms of TM overlap, especially thrombotic thrombocytopenic purpura (TTP) and hemolytic-uremic syndrome (HUS). However, several classic syndromes do stand out such as TTP and typical and atypical HUS. Pregnancy is associated with a unique TM, known as HELLP syndrome, which consists of hemolytic anemia, elevated liver function tests,

Table 12.1 Classification of thrombotic microangiopathies

TTP
Classic TTP
Relapsing TTP
Chronic TTP
HUS
Typical HUS
Atypical HUS
Pregnancy-related HUS
Pregnancy-related TTP
HELLP syndrome
Postpartum HUS
Therapy-related HUS
Calcineurin HUS
Stem cell transplant HUS
Drug-related HUS

and low platelets. The characteristic presentations of TTP and HUS may also occur during pregnancy and the postpartum period. Finally, some drugs are associated with HUS-like syndromes. This chapter will discuss TTP in detail and compare and contrast it with the other syndromes.

Classic Thrombotic Thrombocytopenic Purpura (TTP)

Clinical Presentation

Many patients with TTP will first have a prodrome of a flu-like or diarrheal illness. Patients

T. G. DeLoughery (✉)
Division of Hematology/Medical Oncology,
Department of Medicine, Pathology, and Pediatrics,
Oregon Health & Sciences University,
Portland, OR, USA
e-mail: delought@ohsu.edu

© Springer Nature Switzerland AG 2019
T. G. DeLoughery (ed.), *Hemostasis and Thrombosis*,
https://doi.org/10.1007/978-3-030-19330-0_12

Table 12.2 Thrombotic thrombocytopenic purpura pentad

Microangiopathic hemolytic anemia
Thrombocytopenia
Renal insufficiency
Fever
Mental status changes

can present with a variety of conditions ranging from general malaise to sudden death. The disease can strike at any age, though 20–40 years of age is most common. Women are affected more than men in a 2:1 ratio.

The classic reported pentad of fever, mental status changes, renal insufficiency, thrombocytopenia, and microangiopathic hemolytic anemia is seen in less than 50% of patients (Table 12.2). As described below, the pentad can range in severity from mild to severe.

Neurological

Neurological complaints range from mild confusion to a stroke-like syndrome. Most patients with TTP will have neurological complaints, although in mild cases these symptoms must be elicited by direct questioning. Patients complain of tiredness, confusion, and headaches. Seizures are common and may be recurrent. Patients can also develop transient focal neurological defects which may wax and wane over several hours. MRI can show reversible posterior leukoencephalopathy.

Hematologic

The diagnostic criteria for TTP and other TMs depend on the hematologic picture. By definition patients are thrombocytopenic. This is due to spontaneous aggregation of platelets and their deposition on damaged endothelial surfaces. The platelet count may range from 80,000/uL in mild cases of TTP to less than 1000/uL in severe cases. The median platelet count is 20,000/uL. In mild cases of TTP, the thrombocytopenia is mistakenly ascribed to other etiologies, and diagnosis is delayed. The platelet function is impaired due to continual platelet activation; this leads to the circulation of "spent platelets." Even though a seemingly adequate number of platelets are circulating, they are unable to support hemostasis. Thus, clinical bleeding is often present with platelet counts which are not dramatically decreased.

The hematocrit in TTP is low due to the hemolysis. Patients will have clinical testing consistent with hemolysis – high reticulocyte counts and LDH and indirect bilirubin with low haptoglobin. A direct antibody (Coombs) test will be negative. Review of the peripheral smear is diagnostic for microangiopathic hemolytic anemia. One should carefully examine the smear for red cell fragments. Critically ill patients may have rare schistocytes on a smear, but in TTP and other TMs, there is at least one red cell fragment per high-powered field. The presence of microangiopathic hemolytic anemia is the sine qua non for diagnosis of any TM. The LDH is strikingly elevated, often over two to four times normal. The source of the LDH is not only lysed red cells. On fractionation, LDH fractions 5 and 4 are increased, suggesting damage beyond just the red cells. The patient's coagulation status can be otherwise normal. Markers of DIC such as FDPs and D-dimers may be absent or present in only low titers (i.e., 1–2 ng/dl).

Renal

Patients with TTP present with renal insufficiency and, unlike with HUS, rarely have renal failure. The creatinine is usually only mildly to moderately elevated. Often the urinalysis will show hemoglobinuria and mild proteinuria.

Gastrointestinal

Patients can present with ileus and frank bowel necrosis from ischemia. Pancreatitis due to microvascular occlusion or small bowel infarction may also be seen.

Pulmonary

Although not classically described, patients may present with pulmonary infiltrates and respiratory insufficiency.

Cardiac

Patients will often have signs of cardiac ischemia and can have arrhythmias due to myocardial microinfarctions. Many patients who die of TTP will have sudden death, suggesting that cardiac ischemia/infarction may play a prominent role in fatal cases.

Pathogenesis

The etiology is now thought to be related to spontaneous platelet aggregation induced by von Willebrand factor. When von Willebrand factor is first synthesized, it is a very large polymer (ultra-large von Willebrand factor) that can cause spontaneous platelet aggregation without first binding to collagen. These ultra-large forms are reduced by a protease – ADAMTS13 – to less than 20 million daltons in molecular weight. Ultra-large von Willebrand multimers are found in patients with TTP, and most patients with the classic form of TTP have antibodies directed against ADAMTS13. This would fit with the observations that TTP occurs more often in young women, in patients suffering from lupus, can be recurrent, and may respond to immunosuppressant therapy. However, it appears that a minority of patients with classic TTP have normal levels of ADAMTS13, so other factors must be involved in stimulating platelet aggregation in these patients.

Differential Diagnosis

Given the variety of nonspecific symptoms associated with TTP, accurate diagnosis may be difficult. As mentioned, the classic pentad is present in less than 50% of patients. Patients seen initially are often given a variety of diagnoses ranging from alcohol withdrawal to septic shock syndrome. Since TTP may be seen in patients with lupus, confusion exists between the two diagnoses. One report indicates that 24% of patients dying with lupus cerebritis had pathologic evidence of TTP. TTP should always be considered, especially in young patients who develop a dramatic multisystem illness unexpectedly. TTP is a treatable disorder. It is essential to review the smear in any sick patient with even mild thrombocytopenia to look for schistocytes. Testing for ADAMTS13 is helpful, but treatment should not be delayed waiting on results. Very low (<5–10%) levels are diagnostic of TTP.

Therapy (Table 12.3)

Untreated TTP is rapidly fatal. Mortality in the pre-plasma era ranged from 95 to 100%. Present-day plasma exchange therapy is the cornerstone of TTP treatment and has reduced mortality to less than 20%. However, despite adequate therapy, patients often die either of refractory disease or suddenly during the early course of therapy.

Steroids in doses of 60 mg/day intravenously of prednisone are routinely given. This should be continued until the patient has fully recovered. Very mild cases of TTP (no neurologic symptoms) may be treated with prednisone alone with institution of plasma exchange at the slightest hint of disease progression.

Plasma infusion is beneficial, perhaps due to replenishing deficient ADMATS13. Plasma exchange has been shown to be superior to simple plasma infusion. This may be due to the ability of plasma exchange to deliver very large volumes of fresh frozen plasma. In patients who cannot be immediately exchanged, plasma infusions should be started at a dose of one unit every 4 hours.

Plasma exchange demonstrates a superior outcome compared to use of plasma transfusions. Patients with all but the mildest cases of TTP should receive 1.5 plasma-volume plasma exchanges for at least 5 days. Plasma exchange should be continued daily until the LDH has normalized. Patients should then be weaned off, starting with every-other-day exchange. If the platelet count falls or LDH rises, everyday exchange should be reinstated. Since the platelet count can be affected by a variety of external

Table 12.3 TTP: therapy

Prednisone 60–120 mg/day
1.5 plasma-volume plasma exchange, using plasma as replacement fluid
Rituximab 375 mg/m^2 if ADAMTS-13 inhibitors present
Caplacizumab 11 mg IV before the first exchange and then 11 mg sub-q for at least 30 days after the last exchange

influences, the LDH tends to be a more reliable marker of disease activity.

Platelet transfusions are contraindicated in patients with TTP. Transfusions of platelets sometimes lead to clinical deterioration of the patient. After platelet transfusion, patients with TTP can develop respiratory failure or seizures. Platelet transfusion should be limited to truly life-threatening situations such as intracranial hemorrhage. In most patients with TTP, there is very little justification for platelet transfusion. In severely thrombocytopenic patients, line placement for plasma exchange should be performed by an experienced person. This approach to line placement has been shown to be safe in patients with coagulation defects.

Rituximab is discussed below.

Caplacizumab is a monoclonal antibody fragment directed against von Willebrand factor that blocks its interaction with the platelet protein receptor Gp Ib. It is given as 11 mg IV day one before plasma exchange, then 11 mg subcutaneously after the first day's exchange, and then daily for at least 30 days after the last plasma exchange. If at that time ADAMTS-13 activity level is not above 10%, therapy should extended. Side effects are increased bleeding, mainly nosebleeds. Its use has been associated with shortening the time to normalization of platelet counts, need for plasma exchange, and frequency of relapses. There does appear to be a "rebound" increase in relapses when the drug is stopped, especially if the ADAMTS-13 levels are still low. Currently caplacizumab's place in therapy – as first line for all patients or just those with severe or refractory disease – is unknown.

Refractory Patients (Table 12.4)

Patients with TTP vary in their response to plasma exchange. Patients with refractory disease can present with two general patterns: the patient who slowly responds or who responds rapidly but continues to require daily plasma exchange or the patient who worsens while on exchange. In patients with refractory disease with

Table 12.4 Options to consider for refractory patients

Cryo-poor plasma
Twice daily 1 plasma-volume plasma exchange
Vincristine 1.4 mg/m² day 1 and then 1 mg days 4, 7, and 10
If not already started
Rituximab 375 mg/m² weekly × 4 therapy for refractory TTP
Caplacizumab 11 mg IV before the first exchange and then 11 mg sub-q for at least 30 days after the last exchange

ADAMTS-13 levels about 10%, an alternative diagnosis such as aHUS needs to be considered.

Slow responders often just require patience. Some patients will require several weeks of exchange before they recover. In patients with active but stable disease, anecdotal evidence exists regarding the effectiveness of infusion of vincristine (1.4 mg/m² IV, capped at 2 mg on day 1 and then 1 mg on days 4, 7, and 10) or rituximab 375 mg/m² weekly for 4 weeks. Patients should be evaluated for other causes of thrombocytopenia such as heparin-induced thrombocytopenia, folate deficiency, or thrombocytopenia due to other drugs such as antibiotics.

Patients who worsen while being treated are fortunately rare but present difficult challenges. In a patient with TTP who is worsening, one should ensure the patient does not have another syndrome such as vasculitis or infection. These processes may present with a microangiopathy and multisystem failure. One maneuver which may be helpful in the worsening patient is to increase exchange to one volume twice per day. Use of vincristine or rituximab may be indicated. Although splenectomy has been advocated, it is risky in the seriously ill patient with TTP. Splenectomy should only be considered as a desperate measure.

Prevention of Recurrences

Twenty to 30% of patients with spontaneous TTP will relapse. Most of these patients have been found to have antibodies directed against ADAMTS13. The use of rituximab in these patients appears to dramatically reduce the relapse rate.

Another group of patients who relapse appears to have congenital TTP. A surprising feature is that the first attack of TTP may not occur until adulthood. These patients will have very low (<5%) ADAMTS13 but no inhibiting antibody. Patients with congenital TTP will require plasma infusions (usually 2 units FFP every 2–4 weeks indefinitely) to prevent relapses. Recombinant ADAMTS13 is being developed and should be a benefit to these patients.

Role of Rituximab in TTP

The role of rituximab in treating TTP has become established as it clearly reduces the risk of relapse. The timing remains controversial; a prudent approach would be to use it in patients with inhibiting antibodies to ADAMTS13. A fairly recent recommendation is that patients in remission have their ADAMTS13 monitored and rituximab preemptively used if the levels fall below 10–20%. However, this is an evolving area of research.

Role of ADAMTS13 Levels

Blood should be sent immediately with start of plasma exchange for ADAMTS13 levels. Three patterns will be found:

- Very low levels (<10%), positive inhibitor: classic TTP, autoimmune; consider adding rituximab
- Very low levels (<10%), no inhibitor: congenital TTP, will need long-term plasma infusions to prevent relapses
- Not low levels (>10%), negative inhibitor: can be TTP, consider other diagnoses or atypical HUS

Hemolytic-Uremic Syndrome (HUS)

HUS was recognized as a separate syndrome in 1954. Classically, it is the triad of renal failure,

microangiopathic anemia, and thrombocytopenia. Two major forms are recognized, a "typical" form seen in young children with a prodrome of diarrhea and an "atypical" form.

Typical HUS

Typical HUS (also referred to as HUS D+) is typically seen in children under the age of 4 but can occur at any age. There is often a prodrome of infectious diarrhea, usually bloody. Patients come to medical attention due to symptoms of renal failure. In HUS, thrombocytopenia can be mild in the 50,000/uL range. Extrarenal involvement is common in typical HUS. Neurologic involvement may be seen in 40% of patients with seizure being the predominant feature. Elevated liver function tests are seen in 40% of patients, and 10% of patients will have pancreatitis. Patients with classic HUS will respond to conservative therapy and renal replacement therapy. Unfortunately, although most patients recover some renal function, many will have long-term renal damage. Currently, for most patients there is no role for plasma exchange even with severe disease. Patients should have their stool tested for Shiga toxin at presentation and cases reported to the health department as these cases may represent a widespread outbreak of enterohemorrhagic *Escherichia coli*.

Atypical HUS

Atypical HUS is an HUS not related to an infectious source. Many patients will present with spontaneous HUS and will have progressive disease leading to renal failure despite plasma exchange. The presence of severe hypertension can be a clinical clue. Many patients will be found to have defects in complement inhibition that lead to complement activation and renal damage. Renal transplant in some patients will result in recurrence of the HUS. The C5a blocker eculizumab is very effective in preserving and restoring renal function in these patients; it should be started as soon as the atypical HUS is

Table 12.5 Workup of TTP/HUS

Laboratories to obtain before plasma exchange
[a]ADAMTS13 activity and inhibitor
[a]Complement C3 level
If suspicious of aHUS
[a]Complement C3
[a]Complement factor B
[a]Complement factor H
[a]Complement factor I
[a]Membrane cofactor protein (MCP)

[a]Note: these are the most common – rarer – defects that have been reported, and up to 50% of patients with aHUS will not have a demonstrable defect even with the use of molecular panels.

recognized with a loading dose of 900 mg weekly times 4 weeks and then 1200 mg every other week. The role of testing for complement defects is controversial; many can be found only by genetic screening, and even those negative for defects will respond to treatment. A suggested workup is given in Table 12.5. Patients who respond to anti-complement therapy with stabilization of renal function may be able to stop therapy, but the relapse rate may be as high as 30%. If patients do stop anti-complement therapy, they need to be monitored closely for signs of relapse.

Pregnancy-Related TM

Pregnancy-Related TTP

TTP can occur anytime during pregnancy, often leading to diagnostic confusion due to the overlapping clinical presentation between TTP and HELLP syndrome. There does appear to be a unique presentation of TTP which occurs in the second trimester at 20–22 weeks. The fetus is uninvolved with no evidence of infarction or thrombocytopenia if the mother survives. The pregnancy appears to promote the TTP since the TTP will resolve with termination of the pregnancy and can recur with the next pregnancy. Therapy includes termination of the pregnancy or attempting to support the patient with plasma exchange until delivery. Up to 30% of patients will relapse with future pregnancies; this information must be weighed in planning future pregnancies.

HELLP Syndrome Weinstein introduced the acronym HELLP syndrome to describe a variant of preeclampsia. The acronym HELLP syndrome (*h*emolysis, *e*levated *l*iver tests, *l*ow *p*latelets) describes a variant of preeclampsia. Classically, HELLP syndrome occurs after 28 weeks of gestation in a patent suffering from preeclampsia. The preeclampsia need not be severe. The first sign is a drop in the platelet count followed by abnormal liver function tests. Signs of hemolysis are present with abundant schistocytes on the smear and a high LDH. HELLP can progress to liver failure and deaths have been reported due to hepatic rupture. Unlike TTP, fetal involvement is present in the HELLP syndrome with fetal thrombocytopenia reported in 30% of cases. In severe cases, elevated D-dimers consistent with DIC are also found. Delivery of the child will most often result in cessation of the HELLP syndrome, but refractory cases will require dexamethasone. Patients should be closely observed for 1–2 days after delivery as the hematologic picture can transiently worsen for up to 48 hours before improving. A severe variant of HELLP syndrome may be seen in patients with antiphospholipid antibody disease who present at 20–24 weeks with HELLP. These patients may have continuing thrombosis refractory to heparin and may require pregnancy termination to stop the process.

Postpartum HUS

An unusual complication of pregnancy is an HUS seen up to 28 days postpartum. This form of HUS is now recognized as a form of atypical HUS, and eculizumab therapy should be started once TTP is ruled out.

Therapy-Related HUS

Thrombotic microangiopathies (TMs) are seen commonly in patients receiving a number of therapies. These TMs can range from being an indication for adjustment of therapy to a rapidly fatal disorder.

Calcineurin Inhibitor HUS

The first case of TM associated with cyclosporine (CSA) was reported soon after its introduction. It is most often seen after a calcineurin inhibitor is started and should be considered with the appearance of a falling platelet count, falling hematocrit, and rising LDH. Some cases have been fatal. However, the TM often resolves with decreasing the dosage of the offending medicine or changing to another agent. The etiology appears to be direct endothelial or renal damage caused by these drugs. Thrombocytopenia and microangiopathy may only reflect vascular damage.

Stem Cell Transplant TM

TM can complicate both autologous and allogeneic stem cell transplants. The incidence ranges widely, depending on the criteria used to diagnose TM, but it is in the range of 15% for allogeneic and 5% for autologous stem cell transplants. Several types of TM are recognized in stem cell transplantation. One is "multi-organ fulminant" which occurs early (20–60 days after transplant), has multi-organ system involvement, and is often fatal. This has also been associated with severe CMV infection. Another type of TM is similar to calcineurin inhibitor HUS. A third type is the "conditioning" TM which occurs 6 months or more after total body irradiation and is associated with primary renal involvement. Finally, patients with systemic CMV infections will present with a TM syndrome related to vascular infection with CMV. The etiology of bone marrow transplant-related TTP seems different from that of "classic" TTP. Alterations of the von Willebrand factor cleaving protease have not been found in stem cell-related TM. This would seem to implicate therapy-related vascular damage.

The therapy of stem cell transplant TM is evolving. Patients should have their calcineurin inhibitor doses reduced. Although plasma exchange is often tried, patients with fulminant or conditioning TM often fail to respond. Increasingly, first-line therapy is with eculizumab as multiple case reports show improved outcomes with use of this agent. In patients with rising LDH and falling platelets who show signs of renal damage – proteinuria and hypertension – use of eculizumab should be considered. Measuring levels of sC5-9 can detect over-activation of complement. Many patients with stem cell TM will be found to have mutations in complement regulatory genes.

Drug-Related TM

TM was most commonly seen with the antineoplastic agent mitomycin C, with an incidence of 10% when a dose of more than 60 mg is used. The onset is slow, with the first sign being a falling platelet count months after therapy has been stopped. This is followed by a relentless course of renal failure and death. Now the most common antineoplastic drug causing TM is gemcitabine. As with mitomycin, the appearance of the TM syndrome with gemcitabine can be delayed and may be fatal. Severe hypertension often precedes the clinical appearance of the TM. The use of plasma exchange is not recommended as there is increasing data that a brief course of eculizumab may be helpful. VEGF inhibitors such as bevacizumab and sunitinib can also be associated with TM. Once the TM resolves, eculizumab can be stopped as the incidence of relapse appears to be very low. Since advanced cancer itself can be associated with a TTP-like syndrome, the thrombocytopenia and hemolysis may be due to the cancer and not the cancer treatment.

Although TMs have been reported with other antineoplastic drugs including carboplatin and gemcitabine, the newest drug class now featured in case reports are the thienopyridines: ticlopidine, clopidogrel, and prasugrel. The incidence of TTP with ticlopidine may be as high as 1:1600 with the incidence with clopidogrel much less – 0.0001% – but since it is widely prescribed, it is the second most common cause of drug-induced TM. Cases are also reported with the newest agent prasugrel; incidence is unknown. Almost all cases of clopidogrel- and prasugrel-induced TM occur within 2 weeks of starting the drug.

Unlike ticlopidine TM where very low levels of ADAMTS13 are found, levels are normal in clopidogrel- and prasugrel-induced TMs. All patients with thienopyridines TM should receive plasma exchange as it appears this is effective in controlling the process.

Suggested Reading

Chiasakul T, Cuker A. Clinical and laboratory diagnosis of TTP: an integrated approach. Hematology Am Soc Hematol Educ Program. 2018;2018(1):530–8.

Coppo P, Cuker A, George JN. Thrombotic thrombocytopenic purpura: toward targeted therapy and precision medicine. Res Pract Thromb Haemost. 2018;3(1):26–37.

Gupta M, Feinberg BB, Burwick RM. Thrombotic microangiopathies of pregnancy: differential diagnosis. Pregnancy Hypertens. 2018;12:29–34.

Olson SR, Lu E, Sulpizio E, Shatzel JJ, Rueda JF, DeLoughery TG. When to stop eculizumab in complement-mediated thrombotic microangiopathies. Am J Nephrol. 2018;48(2):96–107.

Raina R, Krishnappa V, Blaha T, Kann T, Hein W, Burke L, Bagga A. Atypical hemolytic-uremic syndrome: an update on pathophysiology, diagnosis, and treatment. Ther Apher Dial. 2019;23(1):4–21. https://doi.org/10.1111/1744-9987.12763. Epub 2018 Oct 29.

Shatzel JJ, Taylor JA. Syndromes of thrombotic microangiopathy. Med Clin North Am. 2017;101(2):395–415. https://doi.org/10.1016/j.mcna.2016.09.010. Epub 2016 Dec 27.

Weitz IC, Deloughery T. Effective treatment of chemotherapy induced atypical Haemolytic Uraemic Syndrome: a case series of 7 treated patients. Br J Haematol. 2018;183(1):136–9.

Non-blood Product Agents for Bleeding Disorders

Thomas G. DeLoughery

Several non-plasma-derived agents exist for therapy of bleeding disorders (Table 13.1). All of these agents share the common qualities of being relatively non-specific and having potential life-threatening complications.

Desmopressin

Desmopressin (DDAVP) is a synthetic analog of antidiuretic hormone. Administration of desmopressin in normal volunteers raises the levels of both factor VIII and von Willebrand proteins severalfold. In patients with mild factor VIII deficiency, desmopressin can raise levels 2–3 times. The factor VIII levels achieved may support hemostasis for minor surgeries and dental procedures. In von Willebrand disease, the response depends on the type of disease. Most type 1 patients and some type 2A will have a robust response to desmopressin. Type 2B and pseudo-von Willebrand patients may develop severe thrombocytopenia with desmopressin. Patients with factor XI deficiency have also been reported to occasionally respond to desmopressin.

T. G. DeLoughery (✉)
Division of Hematology/Medical Oncology,
Department of Medicine, Pathology, and Pediatrics,
Oregon Health & Sciences University,
Portland, OR, USA
e-mail: delought@ohsu.edu

The reason administration of desmopressin leads to this increase in factor VIII is unknown. Direct administration of desmopressin to endothelial cells does not result in von Willebrand protein release, implying the presence of a second messenger or some other indirect effect.

Desmopressin is also useful in patients with some congenital bleeding disorders. Patients with inherited platelet disorders may respond to desmopressin. Finally, approximately half of patients with bleeding and prolonged bleeding times but no identifiable defect will respond to desmopressin. Patients with uremia will also demonstrate shortening of the bleeding time with desmopressin. This may be due to a rise in newly released von Willebrand factor.

Patients with inherited bleeding disorders should be tested for their response to desmopressin. Patients with factor VIII deficiency should have factor VIII levels done before and 45 min after the infusion ends. Patients with von Willebrand disease should have a von Willebrand panel and a PFA-100 performed before and after. Patients with platelet dysfunction should just have PFA-100 performed.

Desmopressin is available in two forms. The intravenous form is dosed as 0.3 ug/kg mixed in normal saline and infused over 15–30 min. It takes 45 min after dosing to achieve full hemostatic effect. A nasal form of desmopressin (Stimate) is also available. Each squirt contains 150 ug of desmopressin. The dose for patients

Table 13.1 Non-blood product agents for bleeding disorders

Desmopressin
IV: 0.3 ug/kg over 30 min
Nasal: Over 50 kg – one squirt of 150 ug in each nostril
Under 50 kg – one squirt of 150 ug total
Aminocaproic acid
IV: 5 g bolus, then 500–1000 mg/h
Oral: 5 g bolus, then 2 g every 2 h
Tranexamic acid
IV: 10 mg/kg every 6–8 h, 1000 mg IV preoperatively
Trauma: 1 g load and 1 g over 8 h
Oral: 25 mg/kg every 6–8 h, 1300 mg TID
Conjugated estrogens
0.6 mg/kg IV for 5 days

over 50 kg is one squirt in each nostril, and for those under 50 kg, one squirt total. Patients who use Stimate should be instructed in its use to ensure proper application of the medicine. It is also essential that patients are actually prescribed Stimate and are not given generic desmopressin. The generic desmopressin is dosed for enuresis, not VWD, and contains a woefully inadequate dose (1.5 mg/ml vs 0.1 mg/ml).

Since desmopressin is an analog of antidiuretic hormone, water retention is the major side effect. For most patients with occasional use of the drug, this is not a problem. However, in surgical patients who are receiving intravenous free water and desmopressin, life-threatening hyponatremia may result. Surgical patients and other patients who cannot control their fluid intake should have serum sodium and urine output monitored.

Rare reports of patients with pre-existing vascular disease receiving desmopressin and then developing thrombosis exist. It is unclear what risk desmopressin poses to patients with underlying vascular disease.

Aminocaproic Acid and Tranexamic Acid

Aminocaproic acid and tranexamic acid function as antifibrinolytic agents by blocking the binding of plasmin to fibrinogen. These agents are useful in three situations. One is in the presence of excessive fibrinolysis. This most often occurs with liver disease but it may rarely complicate amyloidosis or rare congenital defects. Antifibrinolytic agents are also useful as adjunctive therapy for oral or dental procedures in patients with a bleeding diathesis. Finally, in patients with severe thrombocytopenia, the use of antifibrinolytic agents may reduce bleeding.

Thirdly, there has been increased interest in tranexamic acid use in trauma and surgical patients. The CRASH-2 trial demonstrated a reduction in mortality with early use (<3 h) of tranexamic acid in patients with significant hemorrhage. These findings are consistent with data from military hospitals. The WOMEN trial demonstrated that 1 g of tranexamic acid given to women with blood loss of more than 500 ml after vaginal delivery or 1000 ml after C-section has a risk reduction of death of 0.81 with no increased risk of thrombosis. There is also considerable data that prophylactic use of tranexamic acid before surgeries with high risk of blood loss (spine, orthopedic) is also effective at reducing bleeding. There are ongoing randomized trials of tranexamic acid in many different clinical situations.

Currently the use of tranexamic acid should be considered in:

- Trauma patients (within 3 h)
- Severe postpartum hemorrhage
- Total hip or knee arthroplasty
- Pre-procedure in patients with bleeding disorders
- Bleeding in patients with liver disease

The major hazard associated with these drugs is the fact that they strengthen thrombi and prevent lysis of thrombi. In areas of confined bleeding such as ureteral hemorrhage, use of antifibrinolytic agents may lead to obstruction. In the presence of DIC where fibrinolysis is a secondary process, the use of antifibrinolytic agents may induce severe thrombosis. Long-term use of aminocaproic acid has been associated with the development of a generalized myopathy.

The dose of aminocaproic acid is a bolus of 5 g given over 1 h followed by a continuous infusion of 1 g per hour. Oral regimens vary. One approach is to use a 5 g oral bolus and then give 2 g every 2 h immediately after an oral procedure for the first day, cutting back to 4 g every 4 h for the next 2 days.

The dosing for tranexamic acid is 10 mg/kg IV bolus followed either by 10 mg/kg IV every 6–8 h or 25 mg/kg every 6–8 h orally. Frequently a flat preoperative dose of 1000 mg is used in orthopedic surgery. The oral dosing of tranexamic acid makes it useful for oral surgery and other minor procedures. In the United States, a 1300 mg (two 650 mg pills) three times a day is approved for treatment of heavy periods. In patients on dialysis or several renal diseases, the dose should be cut in half.

Aprotinin

Aprotinin is a non-specific protease inhibitor which inhibits fibrinolytic enzymes as well as a variety of other enzymes. Aprotinin has been shown in cardiac surgery to reduce the use of blood products but has been removed from the market due to increased risk of thrombosis.

Conjugated Estrogens

High doses of conjugated estrogens have been reported to ameliorate bleeding in patients with uremia. The dosing is 0.6 mg/kg per day intravenous or orally for 5 days. The hemostatic effect of estrogens can last for 2 weeks. The reason estrogens are effective in slowing uremic bleeding is unknown.

Recombinant VIIa (rVIIa)

Although initially developed for use in hemophilia patients with inhibitors, there are more and more reports of the use of rVIIa for complex bleeding diatheses (Table 13.2). Most established use of this agent is for hemophilia patients with inhibitors, acquired factor inhibitors, factor VII

Table 13.2 Current uses of rVIIa

| Factor VIII inhibitors |
| Factor IX inhibitors |
| Factor XI deficiency |
| Factor VII deficiency |
| Glanzmann thrombasthenia |
| Severe liver disease |
| Reversal of fondaparinux |

and XI deficiencies, plus Glanzmann thrombasthenia. More controversial is its use for acquired coagulation defects in trauma patients, patients with liver disease, and patients' bleeding while being anticoagulated with novel anticoagulants such as dabigatran and warfarin overdoses. Much of this data exists in case series and isolated reports – the real value of rVIIa in these settings is unknown, and increasing data suggests this agent may be of no benefit beyond its role in patients with factor deficiencies or Glanzmann.

Suggested Reading

Desborough MJ, Oakland KA, Landoni G, Crivellari M, Doree C, Estcourt LJ, Stanworth SJ. Desmopressin for treatment of platelet dysfunction and reversal of antiplatelet agents: a systematic review and meta-analysis of randomized controlled trials. J Thromb Haemost. 2017;15(2):263–72.

Franchini M. The use of desmopressin as a hemostatic agent: a concise review. Am J Hematol. 2007;82(8):731–5.

Goldstein M, Feldmann C, Wulf H, Wiesmann T. Tranexamic Acid Prophylaxis in Hip and Knee Joint Replacement. Dtsch Arztebl Int. 2017;114(48):824–30.

Ker K, Edwards P, Perel P, Shakur H, Roberts I. Effect of tranexamic acid on surgical bleeding: systematic review and cumulative meta-analysis. BMJ. 2012;344:e3054. https://doi.org/10.1136/bmj.e3054.

Lamba G, Kaur H, Adapa S, Shah D, Malhotra BK, Rafiyath SM, Thakar K, Fernandez AC. Use of conjugated estrogens in life-threatening gastrointestinal bleeding in hemodialysis patients--a review. Clin Appl Thromb Hemost. 2013;19(3):334–7. https://doi.org/10.1177/1076029612437575. Epub 2012 Mar 12.

Ramirez RJ, Spinella PC, Bochicchio GV. Tranexamic acid update in trauma. Crit Care Clin. 2017;33(1):85–99.

Schulman S. Pharmacologic tools to reduce bleeding in surgery. Hematol Am Soc Hematol Educ Program. 2012;2012:517–21.

Transfusion Therapy and Massive Transfusions

14

Thomas G. DeLoughery

Many patients with bleeding disorders will require transfusion of blood products. This chapter will summarize the use of blood products for hemostasis. This chapter will also discuss the art of managing a massive transfusion.

Platelets

Description (Table 14.1) One *unit of random donor platelets* is derived from 1 unit of donor blood. *Single-donor plateletpheresis* can be used to harvest platelets. One unit of pheresis platelets is equivalent to 5–6 platelet concentrates. Pheresis platelets offer the advantage of exposure to only one blood donor. One random donor platelet unit can raise the platelet count by 5–7000/uL. Platelets are mildly "stunned" while in storage, and it takes 4 h for transfused platelets to be fully functional in the circulation. A pool of five platelet concentrates contains enough plasma to be the equivalent of a unit of FFP (all coagulation factors except the labile V and VIII). *HLA-matched platelets* are single-donor pheresis units

Table 14.1 Platelet products

Platelet concentrates
One donor
Dose: Adult 5–6 units, children 1 unit per 10 kg of body weight
Plateletpheresis platelet product
One donor
Dose: one per adult patient
HLA-matched platelets
One donor matched for one to four class I HLA antigens
Dose: one per adult patient

that are from an HLA-matched donor. This product should only be ordered if there is evidence of HLA antibodies in the recipient. If the response to platelet transfusion is poor, always check platelet counts 15 min after platelet infusion. A poor 15-min platelet count may be indicative of HLA antibodies. A good 15-min platelet count but poor 24-h count is more suggestive of increased consumption, as with fever, sepsis, drugs, etc. This scenario is not an indication for HLA-matched platelets.

Indications Risk of spontaneous severe bleeding rises only when the platelet count is below 5000/uL. Risk of intracranial hemorrhage is highest only when the count is below 1000/uL (risk 0.76%/day). The Gmur study demonstrated a rate of major bleeding of only 0.07%/day when platelet counts were 10–20,000/uL. This

T. G. DeLoughery (✉)
Division of Hematology/Medical Oncology, Department of Medicine, Pathology, and Pediatrics, Oregon Health & Sciences University, Portland, OR, USA
e-mail: delought@ohsu.edu

© Springer Nature Switzerland AG 2019
T. G. DeLoughery (ed.), *Hemostasis and Thrombosis*,
https://doi.org/10.1007/978-3-030-19330-0_14

risk of major bleeding rose to 1.9%/study day when platelet counts were less than 10,000/uL. Patients with chronic autoimmune thrombocytopenia can tolerate platelet counts in the 5–10,000/uL range for years. Considerable data from randomized trials now indicates that, for oncology patients, transfusing platelets when the morning platelet count is less than 10,000/uL is sufficient to prevent thrombocytopenic bleeding. Patient with chronic severe thrombocytopenia such as those with bone marrow disorders should only be transfused if bleeding or before a procedure.

One should order "single-donor plateletpheresis product" when giving patients platelets. Although not always available, use of this product will expose the patient to one donor instead of six to eight. It is best to give leukodepleted platelets to reduce the risk of alloimmunization. The dose of random donor units is 5–6 units in an adult patient or 1 unit per 10 kg in children.

In patients who are actively bleeding or who have DIC, one should consider a platelet transfusion trigger higher than 10,000/uL. A platelet count of 50,000/uL is recommended as there is some data that, at least for massive transfusions, this will stop microvascular bleeding.

Platelet transfusions are not indicated for stable thrombocytopenic patients with platelet counts over 10,000/uL. Also, transfusion of platelets may lead to complications in TTP patients.

Platelet Alloimmunization Patients exposed to blood cells with different HLA types will develop antibodies to HLA antigens. This is most common in patients who have received previous transfusions of blood that was not leukodepleted or in patients who have been pregnant. Since platelets carry class I HLA antigens, they will be rapidly destroyed by HLA antibodies. Historically, as many 90% of patients transfused for aplastic anemia or myelodysplasia became HLA-immunized. The incidence of HLA immunization is lower in patients receiving chemotherapy. In the older literature, this incidence was reported to be as high as 60–90% but is lower in

current studies. Patients who have developed HLA antibodies usually respond better to platelets matched for HLA antigens. Unfortunately, some patients will either have a rare HLA type or are so heavily immunized that they will not respond to any platelet transfusion.

The importance of alloimmunization centers on two concepts – recognition and avoidance. Patients with HLA antibodies will fail to have an immediate increment in platelet count with transfusions. One can test for anti-HLA antibodies if there is no rise in platelet count 15 min after transfusion. However, some patients have antibodies with specificity against specific platelet proteins and not HLA antigens. Patients with these types of antibodies will not respond to HLA-matched platelets. Patients who plan to undergo bone marrow transplant or aggressive chemotherapy, who have been pregnant, or who have been previously transfused should be evaluated for anti-HLA antibodies. This permits planning for transfusion needs. It is clear that transfused white cells are responsible for initiating the anti-HLA response. Trials have shown that giving leukodepleted blood products will reduce the incidence of alloimmunization; these products should be used for patients who are expected to have ongoing transfusion requirements. Given the other benefits of leukodepletion – reduced reactions, potentially less immunosuppression, and less CMV transmission – many blood centers offer only leukodepleted products.

Management of the Platelet-Refractory Patient

Patients who are refractory to platelet transfusion present a difficult clinical problem (Table 14.2). If patients are demonstrated to have HLA antibodies, one can transfuse HLA-matched platelets. Unfortunately, platelet transfusions do not work in 20–70% of these patients. HLA-matched platelets are matched for anywhere from one to four HLA loci. Some loci are difficult to match so good matches may be unavailable. As many as

Table 14.2 Evaluation and management of platelet alloimmunization

1. Check platelet count 15 min after platelet transfusion
2. If rise in platelet count is less than 5000/uL, check for HLA antibodies
3. Administer HLA-matched platelets and evaluate for response
4. If three HLA-matched platelet transfusions are ineffective, stop giving these.
5. In completely refractory patients:
   A. Evaluate for other causes of thrombocytopenia (HIT, drugs)
   B. Give 1 unit of platelets/day
   C. Consider antifibrinolytic therapy
     1. Epsilon aminocaproic acid 1 g/h iv or
     2. Tranexamic acid 10 mg/kg every 8 h

25% of patients have antiplatelet antibodies in which HLA-matched products will be ineffective. One can perform platelet cross-matching to find compatible units for these patients, but this may not always be successful. In the patient who is totally refractory to platelet transfusion, consider drugs as an etiology of antiplatelet antibodies (especially vancomycin). Use of antifibrinolytic agents such as epsilon aminocaproic acid or tranexamic acid may decrease the incidence of bleeding in these patients.

Fresh Frozen Plasma (FFP)

Description One unit of fresh frozen plasma is derived from 1 unit of donated whole blood. The average volume of FFP is 225 ml. One unit of FFP can raise coagulation factor levels by 5–7% and fibrinogen by 13 mg/dl in the average patient. FFP takes about 20 min to thaw.

Indications FFP should only be used when there is a documented coagulation defect that can be corrected by a reasonable amount of FFP. It is useful for the overdosed warfarin patient who is bleeding or needs immediate surgery. Otherwise, if reversal is necessary in a patient on warfarin, vitamin K should be used or, if the need is urgent, prothrombin complex concentrates. DIC with bleeding is another indication for FFP. FFP is used along with plasma exchange in thrombotic thrombocytopenic purpura. FFP may be useful in the bleeding patient with liver disease and documented coagulation defects, although most bleeding in this group of patients is due to "mechanical" reasons (i.e., hole in a varix). Since FFP contains the anticoagulant proteins C and S and antithrombin III, it is used to provide these anticoagulant factors for deficient patients undergoing surgery.

FFP is *not* indicated for most of the purposes for which it is commonly used. FFP seems often to be thought of as a "Super Glue" for any type of bleeding or any type of abnormality in coagulation testing (e.g., slightly prolonged PT). Use of FFP for any but the indications listed above is both a waste of product and a needless exposure of the patient to viral diseases. One example of inappropriate use is the stable patient with end-stage liver disease who has a coagulopathy. Assuming his factor VII is 25% of normal, it would take more than 6 units of FFP (1.2 l) to increase it to 75%. Since the half-life of factor VII is 7 h, keeping his factor VII above 50% would require 6 units of FFP every 6 h. This is almost 5 l of FFP per day. To keep the factor VII level above 100% would require 18 units of FFP every 6 h (15 l/day).

Cryoprecipitate

Description Cryoprecipitate is derived from 1 unit of fresh frozen plasma that is thawed at 4 degrees Celsius. The precipitate is resuspended with 10 ml of saline or FFP and refrozen for storage. One unit contains at least 150 mg of fibrinogen and 80 units of factor VIII, along with von Willebrand factor and factor XIII (Table 14.3). Cryoprecipitate takes about 20 min to thaw.

Indications Cryoprecipitate is useful to quickly increase the fibrinogen level in patients with DIC or in patients with massive transfusion and resulting hemodilution. It is third-line therapy in the treatment of Type 1 von Willebrand disease and is

Table 14.3 Components in cryoprecipitate

ADAMTS-13
Factor VIII
Factor XIII
Fibrinogen
Von Willebrand factor

second-line therapy in patients with other types of von Willebrand disease. Currently, Humate-P is the preferred replacement product for von Willebrand disease. Cryoprecipitate can be used as a source of factor VIII for hemophiliacs, but the preferred product for these patients is the super-pure factor VIII concentrates. Cryoprecipitate can also be used to shorten the bleeding time of uremic patients, but the results are variable for this indication.

Corrections of Defects Before Procedures in Patients with Liver Disease and Other Coagulopathies

Questions often arise with regard to the need to give FFP or platelets to a patient to correct coagulation abnormalities before procedures. This has been studied in several patient groups. In patients with liver disease, those undergoing paracentesis or thoracentesis with INRs of up to 3.8 and platelet counts as low as 50,000/uL had no increased incidence of bleeding. A retrospective study of liver transplant patients with coagulopathies revealed no bleeding complications with procedures or with transplant with no attempts at correcting coagulopathy. Data from our institution suggests a low incidence of bleeding with line placement in patients with coagulation defects **if** lines are placed by experienced operators who have placed more than 50 lines.

If a procedure is emergent, the person with the most experience should perform the procedure. If time permits, coagulation defects that are simple to correct such as thrombocytopenia should be corrected. However, coagulation factors will not compensate for poor procedural skills. If available, TEG can offer pre-procedure guidance for patients with liver disease.

Suggested Goals for Pre-procedure Correction of Coagulopathy

- Fibrinogen: >150 mg/dl
- INR: >1.8 before major procedures
- Platelets: >20,000/uL minor procedures (including line placement), 50,000/uL major procedures, 100,000/uL neurosurgery

Massive Transfusions

Massive transfusion is defined as giving more than one blood volume in 24 h or less, but it is more practically defined as giving one blood volume in 2 h or less. Patients requiring massive transfusion will require close attention to detail and careful monitoring for complications.

Managing Massive Transfusions

In the past decade, there has been a paradigm shift in management of massive bleeding with greater use of empiric therapy. This is based on analysis of resuscitation protocols used in military and civilian trauma centers showing that giving red cells and plasma units in a 1:1 ratio appears to be associated with improved outcomes in massive transfusion. Several studies have extended this concept to platelets, again suggesting improved survival with 1 unit of random donor platelets given one to one with red cells and plasma units. The PROPPR study compared a 1:1 to 1:2 ratio of what to what in trauma patients and found less exsanguination and faster achievement of hemostasis in the first 24 h with 1:1 ratios. Logistically this can be accomplished by the blood bank sending out boxes with 4–6 red cell units together with 4–6 units of FFP. Platelets should also be empirically transfused – either one random donor for every RBC unit or 1 platelet pheresis unit for every 6 red cell units.

There is still a key role for laboratory testing to ensure severe coagulation defects are corrected or do not develop. The laboratory approach to massive transfusions is to measure five laboratory tests which will reflect the basic parameters

Table 14.4 Five basic tests for management of massive transfusions

1. Hematocrit
2. Platelet count
3. Prothrombin time (INR)
4. Activated partial thromboplastin time
5. Fibrinogen level

essential for both blood volume and hemostasis (Table 14.4). The tests are:

1. Hematocrit
2. Platelet count
3. Prothrombin time (INR)
4. Activated partial thromboplastin time
5. Fibrinogen level

Replacement therapy is based on the results of these laboratories with these guidelines (Table 14.5):

- For platelet count less than 50–75,000/uL, a plateletpheresis concentrate or six packs of single-donor platelet concentrate are given to the patient. Since the platelets are suspended in plasma, this transfusion will also provide plasma to the patient.
- For a fibrinogen level less than 150 mg/dl, 10 units of cryoprecipitate should be given. This should raise fibrinogen by 100 mg/dl.
- For INR greater than/equal to 2.0 *with* an abnormal aPTT, give 2–4 units of FFP. Isolated elevation of the INR does not require replacement therapy.
- For an aPTT greater than 1.5 times normal, give 2–4 units of plasma.
- For a hematocrit below 21% – if the patient is bleeding or hemodynamically unstable – give red cells.

For centers that use thromboelastography:

- Elevated R time: give 2–4 units FFP
- Elevated K time: give 10 units cryoprecipitate
- Lowered alpha angle: give 10 units cryoprecipitate
- Low MA: give platelets
- Increased blood lysis: use tranexamic acid

Table 14.5 Management of massive transfusions

1. Start resuscitation with 1:1 ratio of red cells to plasma and to platelets
2. Rapidly obtain basic five tests
3. Assess need for products based on results of basic five tests:
   - A. Platelets <50,000/uL – give platelet concentrates or six to eight packs of single-donor platelets
   - B. Fibrinogen <150 mg/dl – give 10 units of cryoprecipitate
   - C. Hematocrit below 30% – give red cells

   Protime >INR 2.0 *and* aPTT abnormal – give 2–4 units of FFP

   Thromboelastography
   - Elevated R time: 2–4 units FFP
   - Elevated K time: 10 units cryoprecipitate
   - Lowered alpha angle: 10 units cryoprecipitate
   - Low MA: platelets
   - Increased blood lysis: tranexamic acid

Priority should be directed toward keeping the platelet count about 50–75,000/uL. Low platelet counts are the largest determinant of microvascular bleeding in massively transfused patients. The fibrinogen should be kept above 150 mg/dl. Low fibrinogen, along with preventing hemostasis, also results in prolongation of the INR and aPTT. Patients with marked abnormalities of the PT and INR (aPTT >2 times normal) should receive aggressive therapy with at least 4 units of plasma. Minor abnormalities of PT-INR and aPTT should be judiciously treated with plasma.

One should repeat the basic five laboratory tests frequently during resuscitation. This allows one to ensure that adequate replacement therapy was given for the abnormal laboratories. Frequent (every 4–6 h or more frequently if clinically indicated) checks of the coagulation laboratories also allow rapid identification and therapy of new coagulation defects before they become severe. A flow chart of the laboratories and the blood products administered should also be kept.

Two common abnormalities found after massive transfusions are isolated elevations of the PT and a massively prolonged aPTT. Factor VII is very labile, and often patients will have a mildly prolonged PT with normal INR for hours to days after massive transfusions. As mentioned before, this minor prolongation of the INR is irrelevant to bleeding risk and should not be treated. If both the PT and aPTT are very prolonged (aPTT>100 s), then the fibrinogen should be checked. Fibrinogen levels below 80 mg/dl interfere with the endpoints of the PT/aPTT determinations and will lead to spuriously high results. A very prolonged aPTT with only a minor elevation of the PT is suggestive of heparin contamination. This can be a common occurrence in the hectic management of massive transfusions.

Complications

The complications that can be seen with massive transfusions are hyperkalemia, hypothermia, and hypocalcemia. Hypothermia is the most common. Red cells are stored at 4 degrees Celsius and the infusion of red cells rapidly cools the patient. Rapid transfusers that also warm the blood should be used for these patients. Keeping the patient warm with thermal blankets is also useful. Core temperatures below 35 degrees have been associated with development of coagulopathies and a variety of metabolic disturbances.

Hyperkalemia is rarely seen. Massive amounts of citrate may lead to transient hypocalcemia. However, citrate is rapidly metabolized and clinical hypocalcemia is rarely a problem. One should not replace calcium empirically as this has been associated with worse outcomes. If calcium is of concern, measuring the ionized calcium can guide therapy.

Coagulation defects are common in massive transfusions. These may be due to dilution of the plasma by massive fluid resuscitation or by red cell transfusions. Packed red cells contain little plasma, and massive replacement of blood volume with only packed red blood cells can lead to a dilutional coagulopathy. Patients may also develop a coagulopathy due to underlying medical conditions or due to trauma.

Suggested Reading

Carson JL, Guyatt G, Heddle NM, Grossman BJ, Cohn CS, Fung MK, Gernsheimer T, Holcomb JB, Kaplan LJ, Katz LM, Peterson N, Ramsey G, Rao SV, Roback JD, Shander A, Tobian AA. Clinical practice guidelines from the AABB: red blood cell transfusion thresholds and storage. JAMA. 2016;316(19):2025–35. https://doi.org/10.1001/jama.2016.9185.

Holcomb JB, Tilley BC, Baraniuk S, Fox EE, Wade CE, Podbielski JM, del Junco DJ, Brasel KJ, Bulger EM, Callcut RA, Cohen MJ, Cotton BA, Fabian TC, Inaba K, Kerby JD, Muskat P, O'Keeffe T, Rizoli S, Robinson BR, Scalea TM, Schreiber MA, Stein DM, Weinberg JA, Callum JL, Hess JR, Matijevic N, Miller CN, Pittet JF, Hoyt DB, Pearson GD, Leroux B, van Belle G. PROPPR Study Group. Transfusion of plasma, platelets, and red blood cells in a 1:1:1 vs a 1:1:2 ratio and mortality in patients with severe trauma: the PROPPR randomized clinical trial. JAMA. 2015;313(5):471–82.

Schiffer CA, Bohlke K, Delaney M, Hume H, Magdalinski AJ, McCullough JJ, Omel JL, Rainey JM, Rebulla P, Rowley SD, Troner MB, Anderson KC. Platelet transfusion for patients with cancer: American Society of Clinical Oncology Clinical Practice Guideline Update. J Clin Oncol. 2018;36(3):283–99. https://doi.org/10.1200/JCO.2017.76.1734. Epub 2017 Nov 28

Stanworth SJ, Navarrete C, Estcourt L, Marsh J. Platelet refractoriness--practical approaches and ongoing dilemmas in patient management. Br J Haematol. 2015;171(3):297–305.

Stephens CT, Gumbert S, Holcomb JB. Trauma-associated bleeding: management of massive transfusion. Curr Opin Anaesthesiol. 2016;29(2):250–5.

Deep Venous Thrombosis and Pulmonary Embolism

15

Thomas G. DeLoughery

Natural History

At least 300–600,000 patients per year in the USA suffer a first deep venous thrombosis, with 5–10 per 10,000 population suffering a thrombotic event each year. More than 90% of pulmonary emboli occur as a complication of thrombosis in the deep venous system of the legs. Therefore, treatment and prevention of deep venous thrombosis will reduce the occurrence of pulmonary embolism. Another key point is that more than 90% of the deaths attributable to pulmonary embolism occur in the first hour. Thus, management is aimed toward prevention of a repeat embolism and not treatment of the initial embolus. It is estimated that the mortality rate of untreated pulmonary embolism is 30–40%, and the risk of pulmonary embolism from untreated proximal deep venous thrombosis is 50–80%.

Diagnostic Tests for Pulmonary Embolism and Deep Venous Thrombosis

Clinical Signs and Symptoms Patients first notice dyspnea and cough following a pulmonary embolism. Chest pain occurs hours to days after the event with development of lung infarction. One-third of patients will have hemoptysis, and 10–20% will have syncope. Most patients on exam will have tachypnea (70–92%), but less than half have tachycardia (30% of patients in the classic PIOPED study). Chest x-rays are normal in only 30%. A nonspecific infiltrate is seen in 50–70%, and an effusion is seen in 35%. In the PIOPED study, *15%* of patients had PO_2 greater than 90 mmHg, and *20%* had alveolar-arterial gradients less than 20 mmHg. These results demonstrate that patients with pulmonary embolism need not be hypoxic or have an abnormal a-A gradient.

Prediction Rules Recently there has been great interest in clinical prediction rules for deep venous thrombosis and pulmonary embolism. Using these rules, clinicians can better predict which patients are at higher risk of thrombosis, and this will guide testing. Several examples exist (Tables 15.1, 15.2a, and 15.2b). The best validated for DVT are the Wells criteria, and two prediction rules – Wells and Geneva – have also been validated for PE in multiple studies. Use of these prediction rules along with the D-dimer

T. G. DeLoughery (✉)
Division of Hematology/Medical Oncology,
Department of Medicine, Pathology, and Pediatrics,
Oregon Health & Sciences University,
Portland, OR, USA
e-mail: delought@ohsu.edu

© Springer Nature Switzerland AG 2019
T. G. DeLoughery (ed.), *Hemostasis and Thrombosis*,
https://doi.org/10.1007/978-3-030-19330-0_15

Table 15.1 Clinical probability score for deep venous thrombosis

Variable	Points
Active cancer	+1
Paralysis or recent plaster immobilization of the lower extremity	+1
Recently bedridden for >3 days or major surgery within 4 weeks	+1
Local tenderness	+1
Calf swelling greater than 3 cm than asymptomatic side (measured 10 cm below tibial tuberosity)	+1
Pitting edema in symptomatic leg	+1
Dilated superficial veins (non-varicose) in symptomatic leg only	+1
Alternative diagnoses as or more likely than DVT	−2

Low probability <0, moderate probability 1–2, and high probability >3
Used with permission *J Thromb Thrombolysis*. 2006 Feb;21(1):31–40

Table 15.2a Clinical probability score for pulmonary embolism (Wells) (1)

Variable	Points
Clinical signs and symptoms of DVT	+3
PE as likely or more likely than alternative diagnosis	+3
Immobilization or surgery in the past 4 weeks	1.5
Previous PE or DVT	1.5
Heart rate more than 100/min	1.5
Hemoptysis	1
Active cancer	1

Low probability <2, moderate probability 2–6, and high probability >6; PE unlikely ≤4; PE likely >4
Used with permission Streiff MB, Agnelli G, Connors JM, et al. *J Thromb Thrombolysis* (2016) 41: 32

determines whether patients should be evaluated for thrombosis. For the Wells PE criteria, results can be presented as "low," "intermediate," or "high" – alternatively as "PE likely" vs "PE unlikely." Taking a step back, the PERC rule (Table 15.3) evaluates whether the diagnosis of PE should even be considered. Patients who are felt to be at low risk already of PE and who answer negative on all eight questions have low (<1%) rates of being diagnosed with PE, and the evaluation can be halted without further testing. This test performs best in populations at low risk of PE such as young outpatients.

Table 15.2b Clinical probability score for pulmonary embolism (Geneva) (2)

Variable	Points
Previous DVT or PE	+2
Heart rate > 100	+1
Recent surgery	+3
Age	
60–79	+1
>80	+2
$PaCO_2$	
<36 mmHg	+2
36–40 mmHg	+1
PO_2	
<50 mmHg	+4
50–59 mmHg	+3
60–69 mmHg	+2
70–79 mmHg	+1
Atelectasis	+1
Elevated hemi-diaphragm	+1

Low probability 0–4, intermediate probability 5–8, high probability >9
Used with permission Streiff MB, Agnelli G, Connors JM, et al. *J Thromb Thrombolysis* (2016) 41: 32

Table 15.3 PERC rule

Eight questions
1. Age < 50 years
2. Heart rate less than 100 beats per minute
3. Room air oxygen saturations 95% or greater
4. No prior deep DVT or PE
5. No recent trauma or surgery in the past 4 weeks
6. No hemoptysis
7. No exogenous estrogen
8. No clinical signs suggestive of DVT such as unilateral leg swelling

In a population with low risk for PE, patients who answer "no" to all eight have a low (~1%) risk of PE
Used with permission Streiff MB, Agnelli G, Connors JM, et al. *J Thromb Thrombolysis* (2016) 41: 32

D-dimer A major advance in evaluation of patients with DVT/PE is the wide availability of rapid D-dimer assays. Thrombi contain areas which are growing and other areas which are undergoing fibrinolysis. It has been shown that all patients with clinically significant thrombosis will have levels of D-dimers above 500 ng/ml. Two most commonly used rapid assays are the point of care D-dimer and the high-sensitive D-dimer.

"Rapid" point of care D-dimer assays are slide assays (like pregnancy tests) devised to read positive if the D-dimer is above 500 ng/ml. These types of assays are less sensitive (80–90%) than the rapid ELISA but are simple to use and require no special equipment to run. The rapid D-dimer is most effective when used with a clinical prediction rule. Thus, a patient with a negative D-dimer and low probability of thromboembolic event has a remote chance of having thrombosis and need not be evaluated further. If a patient has either a not-low pretest probability or has a positive D-dimer, then they need further workup for DVT/PE.

The "rapid ELISA" or "high-sensitivity" assay for D-dimer offers nearly 100% sensitivity for DVT. Accordingly, a patient with a negative ELISA D-dimer requires no further evaluation unless they have a high pretest probability of thrombosis. The rapid ELISA often requires the test be performed in the central laboratory, increasing turnaround time.

The other drawback of the D-dimer test is its lack of specificity coupled with its high sensitivity. Therefore, patients with positive D-dimer assays require further testing to establish the presence of thrombosis. Patients with recent trauma, recent surgery, and pregnancy or those over age 70 have a higher baseline D-dimer level which greatly limits the use of D-dimers in these patients. There are recent data that an age-adjusted cutoff may improve the ability of D-dimers to exclude thrombosis in older patients. The formula for patients over age 50 is *D-dimer cutoff = age × 10* – so for a 65-year-old, this would be 650 ng/dl.

CT Angiography CT angiography (CTA) has become the diagnostic test of choice for pulmonary embolism. A CTA that is positive for thrombus in a segmental distribution and above pulmonary arteries is highly specific for PE, with it falling to 80% for subsegmental PEs. CTA is now the first-line test for PE, and there is much concern about its overuse since less than 10% of these tests are positive for PE in many institutions. This is why a diagnostic pathway utilizing assessment of clinical probability and D-dimers should be used before CTA to diagnose PE.

Ventilation/perfusion (V/Q) scans are sensitive but not specific for pulmonary embolism unless the result reads high probability. Interpretation is best viewed as "high probability," "negative," and "nondiagnostic." High-probability scans are specific if the patient has not had a previous pulmonary embolism, but specificity falls in patients with previous pulmonary emboli or pre-existing cardiac or pulmonary disease. Less than high-probability scans are not diagnostic unless the result is a normal scan or a low-probability scan in patients with a low pretest probability of thrombosis. V/Q scans are becoming less available as they have been mostly supplanted by CTA.

Leg studies are the definitive diagnostic test in patients with symptoms of deep venous thrombosis. Furthermore, leg studies aid in the patient with a nondiagnostic V/Q scan or in a patient for whom one wishes to defer CTA (pregnancy or renal disease). Deep venous thrombosis will be present in 50–70% of patients with proven pulmonary embolism. If deep venous thrombosis is present, this establishes the need for anticoagulant therapy and eliminates the need for CTA.

Venogram Used to be the gold standard. Venograms visualize both the calf and deep veins. Drawbacks of venography include dye load and a 5% risk of actually causing thrombosis. Given that very few venograms are currently performed, the accuracy and ability to perform technically adequate studies is greatly reduced.

Doppler ultrasound has very high sensitivity and specificity for diagnosing proximal deep venous thrombosis in symptomatic patients and is >90% for the calf veins, so a negative whole leg Doppler rules out DVT. Some institutions only perform Dopplers for proximal vein thrombosis, so if negative, one needs to perform follow-up duplex to rule out clot extension in high-probability patients.

Diagnostic Approach to DVT or PE

1. Assess pretest probability.
2. If high probability, then specific imaging (Doppler for DVT or CTA for PE).

3. If not high probability, then high-sensitivity D-dimer – if negative, no imaging.
4. If positive D-dimer, then specific imaging.

Immediate Therapy

Anticoagulation – See the following section.

Thrombolytic Therapy

PE Given the natural history of pulmonary embolism, the role of thrombolytic therapy is uncertain. The fact that thrombolytic therapy lyses clots faster than heparin was of no clinical significance in the large trials of the early 1980s or in more recent trials. Two trials showed that, in patients with right ventricular dysfunction, thrombolytic therapy failed to improve mortality or prevent long-term complications. Many patients with pulmonary embolism are poor candidates for lytic therapy due to recent surgery or other reasons. Finally of concern is the 1–2% risk of intracranial hemorrhage which accompanies thrombolytic therapy. The vast majority of patients with pulmonary embolism who survive long enough to be diagnosed will survive their thrombosis. Therefore only a small number of patients would benefit from thrombolytic therapy. However, for the patient in extremis due to a pulmonary embolism who is *not* a candidate for embolectomy, fibrinolytic therapy is an option.

If thrombolytic therapy is required, the agent of choice is tPA 100 mg IV over 2 h. There is no agreement on when to start heparin – some practitioners continue it during the tPA or restart after the bolus. In the USA it is more common to wait until the aPTT is less than twice control and then restart the heparin.

There is increasing interest in catheter-directed thrombolytic therapy for pulmonary embolism. Early studies have shown this is feasible, but to date there is little clinical trial data to suggest this is superior to heparin therapy.

DVT Systemic thrombolytic therapy for deep venous thrombosis has little effect on long-term outcomes such as post-thrombotic syndrome and has little role in management of these patients. However, there is increased interest in catheter-directed thrombolytic therapy in massive deep venous thrombosis involving the common femoral or iliac system. This approach uses catheter-guided lytic therapy to recanalize the vessel. Often there are anatomical issues such as May-Thurner syndrome (compression of the left iliac vein by the right iliac artery) that can be corrected with venoplasty and stenting. Unfortunately, data from a large clinic trial show no difference in development of post-thrombotic syndrome with this approach. However, patients with very severe DVT resulting in massive edema leading to arterial compromise (phlegmasia cerulea dolens) or with disabling symptoms despite adequate anticoagulation may benefit from directed thrombolytic therapy.

Embolectomy may be useful in the small subset of patients who are in unresponsive shock. Some series claim up to 70% survival. It has been suggested that if after an hour of medical management, a patient has persistent signs of massive PE such as a systolic blood pressure of less than 90 mmHg, urine output of less than 20 ml per hour, and/or PO$_2$ of less than 60 mmHg, that patient is a candidate for embolectomy. This approach obviously requires the presence of a qualified cardiac surgeon.

Vena Cava Filter The role of filters in treatment of thromboembolic disease is unclear due to lack of good trials. The clearest indication for filter placement would be PE/proximal DVT in a patient in whom anticoagulant therapy is contraindicated. In patients who can receive anticoagulation, clinical trials show no benefit in survival with filters. One common use of filters is as PE prevention in patients unable to receive prophylactic anticoagulation, but this is discouraged by guidelines and may increase complications. Another group of patients who should not receive filters are those who have recurrent thrombosis on warfarin. These patients need more aggressive anticoagulation and not another nidus for thrombosis.

Since filters do not protect against thrombosis, the patient needs to resume anticoagulation as soon as possible after filter placement. The risk of deep venous thrombosis is doubled with long-term filter placement, but this alone is not an indication for long-term anticoagulation if the patient had no other indications for long-term treatment.

Most filters placed now are removable filters which allow the filter to be taken out when the patient is back on stable anticoagulation. Unfortunately, many of these filters do not get removed; this can result in filter migration or breakage of the filter and strut embolization. All patients in whom a removable filter is placed need to have a plan for filter removal. Filters can be removed years after placement.

Compression stockings' role in DVT therapy is uncertain – studies have been inconsistent as to whether stockings prevent post-thrombotic syndrome. Some patients do derive relief from stockings so a trial of knee high stockings 30–40 mmHg at the ankle is always worthwhile.

Bed Rest Multiple studies have shown no benefit to bed rest and, in fact, demonstrate a trend for better outcomes the more active the patient with DVT is. Patients with DVT should ambulate as tolerated and be encouraged to exercise.

Home Therapy of PE There is now abundant data that patients at low risk of complications from a PE can be treated at home. There is a scoring system for PE that allows determination of risk of thrombosis (PESI – Table 15.4) with trial data showing patients in Classes I and II (score < 86) can be treated at home. Alternatively, patients who are not hypoxic, have normal blood pressure, and are not at risk of bleeding may be eligible for home treatment.

Table 15.4 PESI score

Add +1: Each year of age
Add +10: Male gender
Add +30: Cancer – active or past history
Add +10: Heart failure
Add +10: Chronic lung disease
Add +20: Heart rate > 110 bpm
Add +30: Systolic blood pressure < 100 mmHg
Add +20: Respiratory rate > 30 bpm
Add +20: Temperature < 36 C
Add +60: Altered mental status
Add +20: Oxygen saturation < 90%
Interpretation: Mortality at 30 days
Score < 65: Class I – Very low mortality risk (0–1.6%)
Score 66–85: Class II – Low mortality risk (1.7–3.5%)
Score 86–105: Class III – Moderate mortality risk (3.2–7.1%)
Score 106–125: Class IV – High mortality risk (4.0–11.4%)
Score > 125: Class V – Very high mortality risk (10.0–24.5%)

Used with permission Streiff MB, Agnelli G, Connors JM, et al. J Thromb Thrombolysis (2016) 41: 32

Anticoagulant Treatment of Venous Thromboembolism

There are now multiple options for treatment of DVT and PE with direct oral anticoagulants (DOACs) being recommended as first line in eligible patients.

Unfractionated Heparin

Standard heparin is fading from use – and is not recommended first-line therapy – due to its unfavorable pharmacokinetics and the demonstration of better outcomes with low molecular weight heparin (LMWH). If used, the absolute key in standard heparin use is to give enough. The standard bolus should be 5000 units (10,000 units for larger thrombi or pulmonary embolism). The initial drip should be 1400 units/h. The aPTT or heparin level should be checked 6 h after the bolus and the drip adjusted accordingly. A supratherapeutic aPTT/heparin level may just reflect the bolus. The drip should never be turned down until two consecutive aPTTs are supratherapeutic. If aPTTs are used to monitor heparin, the laboratory's aPTT must be standardized with heparin levels to determine the proper therapeutic range since the therapeutic range varies with different aPTT reagents. One must be very aggressive in rapidly achieving the proper aPTT when giving heparin. Patients should be on heparin for at least 5 days and have at least 24 h on both heparin and warfarin (in patients started on warfarin) once the INR is greater than 2.

Low Molecular Weight Heparin

The use of low molecular weight heparin (LMWH) for therapy in DVT/PE treatment is recommended because it is both safer and more effective than the use of standard heparin. As noted above, evidence is also clear that stable patients with DVT/PE can be treated at home with LMW heparin. For short courses of therapy, most patients do not need to have LMW heparin levels drawn. Patients who are very obese (greater than two times ideal body weight), pregnant, those with severe liver or heart failure, or those on long-term heparin therapy should have levels performed. Since LMWH is renally cleared, in patients with renal failure, dosing should be once per day. Levels are drawn 4 h after injection and the therapeutic range is 0.7–1.2 anti-Xa units. Like standard heparin, DVT/PE patients need at least 5 days of LMWH for acute thrombosis.

LMWH Options:

- Dalteparin 100 units/kg bid or 200 units/kg daily
- Enoxaparin 1 mg/kg bid or 1.5mg/kg daily (patients with low thrombotic burden)
- Tinzaparin 175 units/kg daily

Fondaparinux

Fondaparinux is a synthetic pentasaccharide that binds to antithrombin (like heparin). Due to the nature of fondaparinux binding to antithrombin, mainly factor Xa is inhibited. This agent is approved for therapy of DVT and PE. Dosing is 7.5 mg daily – rising to 10 mg in patients who weigh more than 100 kg. Fondaparinux has a half-life of 17–21 h and has high renal clearance so it should not be used in patients with renal disease.

Warfarin

Warfarin is started in the evening with a loading dose of 2.5–10 mg orally. Five milli gram is recommended in most patients. Young (under age 60) healthy patients will need a 10 mg loading dose, while the frail elderly (over age 85) should start with 2.5 mg. Warfarin is titrated to an INR of 2–3. Use of warfarin affects all the vitamin K-dependent proteins. Factor VII falls first, resulting in prolongation of the INR. However, the full antithrombotic effect of warfarin does not occur until factors X and II have fallen. This decrement will take an additional 24 t hours after factor VII levels fall. This explains why patients should overlap heparin and warfarin therapy for 24 h.

Direct Oral Anticoagulants

Four of the new direct oral anticoagulants have been studied as treatment for DVT/PE; all are equal to LMWH/warfarin in effectiveness, and the Xa inhibitors are safer.

In clinical trials, dabigatran and edoxaban were started after heparin therapy, but rivaroxaban and apixaban were started promptly at diagnosis without heparin – but both at initially higher doses. All of these agents are easier to use as they do not require INR monitoring and have no food and few drug interactions.

Direct Oral Anticoagulant Options (See Chapter for More Details).

- Apixaban 10 mg bid × 1 week, then 5 mg bid
- Dabigatran 150 mg bid – started 5 days after LMWH therapy
- Edoxaban 60 mg daily – started 5 days after LMWH therapy
- Rivaroxaban 15 mg bid × 3 weeks, then 20 mg daily.

Special Situations

In Patients with Cancer

Studies had shown that warfarin was inferior to LMWH in patients with cancer so LMWH has previously been recommended as first-line therapy. Clinical trials have shown DOACs to be just as effective to even more effective as LMWH in cancer patients. However, patients with upper GI cancers have a higher incidence of bleeding. One approach would be to offer DOAC to most patients, reserving LMWH for patients with upper GI cancers or other contraindications to DOAC such as mechanical cardiac valves. Patients who have recurrent thrombosis on DOAC should receive LMWH. Patients with recurrence on LMWH should have their dose increased by 20–25%.

In the Pregnant Patient

This is discussed in Chap. 28.

Calf and Muscular Vein Thrombosis

Patients with calf vein thrombosis are at risk for clot extension to proximal veins and subsequent pulmonary embolism. These patients – if safe to anticoagulate – should be anticoagulated for 12 weeks. Patients with calf vein thrombosis at high risk for bleeding on anticoagulation should be observed with serial ultrasounds. Patients with thrombosis in the muscular veins of the calf (soleus, gastrocnemius) can be treated with just 10 days of therapeutic LMWH or simply observed with serial ultrasounds if at high risk of bleeding with anticoagulant therapy.

Superficial Venous Thrombosis

Some superficial venous thrombosis can be treated with heat and anti-inflammatory agents. However, many patients – especially those with greater saphenous vein thrombosis – will go on to have thrombosis of the deep system. Many anticoagulation options exist to treat superficial venous thrombosis; common to all is the fact that prophylactic dosage of LMWH or fondaparinux is sufficient, and treatment duration can range from 12 to 42 days. One approach to treatment is for patients with superficial venous thrombosis over 5 cm or in the greater saphenous vein to be treated for at least 12–14 days with prophylactic-dose LMWH or fondaparinux. If still symptomatic, this treatment can be extended until resolution of symptoms.

"Incidental PE"

Pulmonary emboli may be found in patients receiving CT scans for other reasons. It is clear that in cancer patients, these PEs have the same negative prognostic implications as symptomatic PE and need to be treated aggressively. For other patients, the clinical situation needs to be assessed, but until data prove otherwise, all patients with incidental PE should receive antithrombotic therapy.

Subsegmental PE

The incidence of subsegmental PE has increased with high-resolution CT scans, and there is much controversy about therapy. Some retrospective data indicated a more benign outcome, but prospective studies showed the same natural history as more proximal PE. The diagnosis of subsegmental PE can be reduced by following diagnostic pathways (clinical predication rules, etc.) which allows for CTA only on a higher-risk population. There is a clinical trial underway, but until results of this are available, patients with subsegmental PE should receive the same therapy as any other patient with PE.

Duration of Therapy (Table 15.5)

The key questions to consider when determining duration of therapy are as follows: (1) what was

Table 15.5 Duration of treatment

Superficial venous thrombosis: 10–12-day course of prophylactic-dose LMWH or fondaparinux – repeat if still symptomatic

Muscular calf vein (soleus or gastrocnemius) thrombosis: 10 days of LMWH

Calf vein thrombosis: 12 weeks of therapy

Provoked first DVT or PE: 3 months

 Provoking factors: trauma, surgery, bed rest >72 h, pregnancy, estrogen, very long (>10 h) plane flights

Idiopathic first DVT or PE: 3 months of therapy and then strongly consider indefinite therapy for most patients due to high risk of recurrence

Two or more lower extremity proximal DVT or PE: Indefinite anticoagulation

DVT or PE during pregnancy: Duration – the entire course of pregnancy and at least 6 weeks after delivery – total should be at least 3 months. Can use LMWH or warfarin with breastfeeding

Cancer

 Use of DOAC or LMWH long-term should be considered especially with lung cancer or pancreatic cancer. Long-term LMWH is mandatory for warfarin/DOAC failures

the location of the thrombosis, (2) what were the circumstances of the thrombosis, and (3) are there any underlying hypercoagulable states?

Patients with thrombosis in unusual sites such as hepatic vein thrombosis or portal vein thrombosis should be indefinitely anticoagulated. An exception would be if there was a clear provoking factor such as an abdominal abscess leading to portal vein thrombosis. In these cases 3 months of therapy would be prudent. Also, as discussed in the next chapter, upper extremity thrombosis needs only limited therapy.

An important factor in determining risk of recurrence is assessing whether the thrombosis was idiopathic or provoked. Most studies indicate that, for a patient to be considered to have an idiopathic thrombosis, they should not have cancer, not have undergone surgery or had trauma in the previous 6 weeks, not be at bed rest, not be pregnant, or not have a major hypercoagulable state. Patients with idiopathic venous thrombosis are at substantial risk of recurrence with a risk that may be as high as 30% in the next 5 years. Many studies have indicated that long-term anticoagulation therapy is of benefit in these patients in preventing recurrent thrombosis. Patients with

idiopathic thrombosis, especially large thrombosis or pulmonary embolism, should be considered for indefinite anticoagulation. Trial data does show that warfarin at an INR of 2–3 is just as safe as and more effective than INR 1.5–2; therefore, INR of 2–3 should be the therapeutic range if warfarin is used. Studies have shown low-dose apixaban (2.5 mg bid) or rivaroxaban (10 mg) to be just as effective as standard doses when used for long-term anticoagulation 6–12 months after the initial thrombosis.

There are some data showing that checking a D-dimer 3 weeks after the patient has completed a course of therapy may help predict risk of recurrence. A patient who has a positive D-dimer 3 weeks off anticoagulation has an approximately 10% per year chance of recurrence. The problem is that a negative D-dimer still indicates a 3–5% per year risk of recurrence – which is higher than the risk of anticoagulation in most patients. The high recurrence rate even in low-risk patients plagues other prediction rules; currently the history of provoked vs idiopathic thrombosis remains most predictive of recurrence.

Patients with a provoked first proximal DVT or PE need only 3 months of treatment if the provocation has resolved. Patients who have two or more recurrences need to be treated indefinitely.

As discussed in Chap. 17, patients with inherited hypercoagulable states are at increased risk of first thrombosis but not recurrence. Therefore, the finding of factor V Leiden, etc. does not mandate indefinite therapy.

Prophylaxis of Venous Thromboembolic Disease

Overview

Etiology of Surgical Hypercoagulable States

The etiology of the surgically induced hypercoagulable state is complex. Certainly venous stasis during and after the operation is important. The surgery-induced inflammatory state will cause procoagulant changes in the blood and vessel endothelium. Direct venous trauma in orthopedic and pelvic surgery plays a role. Patients with a pre-existing hypercoagulable state (acquired or inherited), previous venous thrombosis, heart failure, malignancy, or estrogen use are at higher risk for thromboembolic disease in the operative period. Smokers have an increased risk as well.

The Need for Deep Venous Thrombosis Prophylaxis in Surgery

The first sign of thrombosis in 10–30% of patients is sudden death. The clinical signs of deep venous thrombosis tend to be unreliable. In most large screening studies, only 10–20% of patients with deep venous thrombosis are symptomatic. Prevention is crucial, not only to prevent DVT/PE but because up to 90% of patients with deep venous thrombosis will experience post-phlebitic syndrome. This included patients with asymptomatic thrombosis. Finally, it is better to prevent deep venous thrombosis since treatment in the postoperative period is associated with a higher risk of bleeding. Numerous studies have shown deep venous thrombosis prophylaxis to be medically sound as well as cost-effective. Failure of surgeons to use deep venous thrombosis prophylaxis is the largest cause of preventable operative death in the USA.

Who Is at Risk of Thrombosis?

Low-Risk Patients
- Patients under 40 with no other risk factors (including *negative* family history of deep venous thrombosis)
- Procedures lasting less than 30 min

Medium-Risk Patients
- Patients over 40 years of age with no other risk factors undergoing operations over 30 min long.

High-Risk Patients
- Previous history of venous thrombosis (or strong family history).
- Pelvic or abdominal surgery for malignancy. Lower limb orthopedic surgery.

Very High-Risk Patients

- Lower limb trauma and surgery.
- Surgery in patients with other risk factors – previous thromboembolic disease or cancer.

The Prophylactic Regimens

Intermittent Pneumatic Compression Mechanical means of preventing deep venous thrombosis by squeezing calves. Compression also stimulates fibrinolysis. Disadvantages of compression include patient discomfort, noncompliance, and risk of mechanical breakdown. Compression is effective for prevention of thrombosis in medium- and some high-risk patients.

Subcutaneous Heparin The standard (5000 units B-TID) prophylactic regimen. The dose is started 2–8 h before surgery and given until the patient is ambulatory. Low-dose heparin is effective in medium- but not high-risk patients. Bleeding increases from 3.8% in placebo patients to 5.9% in patients receiving heparin when all studies are considered, but this is far outweighed by prevention of both thrombosis and death.

Aspirin Studies using aspirin have not consistently shown that aspirin prevents deep venous thromboses, but it does lead to wound hematoma in 1 in 50 patients. Unlike heparin and warfarin, aspirin's antithrombotic effects are not reversible. Of additional concern is aspirin's gastrointestinal toxicity and prolonged inhibition of platelet function. Aspirin may be effective in thrombosis prevention when given after a 5-day course of LMWH or DOAC in hip and knee replacement patients.

Warfarin There are several regimens for warfarin in the literature. The "two-step" approach gives low doses of warfarin for 1–2 weeks before the operation to raise PT to 1.5–3 (INR 1.5) seconds above control. Post-op the warfarin dose is increased to raise the INR to 2–3. This approach is particularly effective in preventing deep venous thrombosis after elective hip or knee replacement. The other approach is to give

5 mg of warfarin daily starting immediately after surgery (or in some studies the night before) to achieve an INR of 2.0–3.0 as soon as possible after surgery. Anticoagulation is continued for 3–6 weeks. This was effective in reducing deep venous thrombosis after surgery for hip fractures. The prothrombin INR should be followed to monitor the patient's status and prevent overshooting of the INR. Rates of bleeding are as high as 30%, but most bleeding is seen in patients who are over-anticoagulated. In more recent studies, where therapy was closely monitored, significant post-op bleeding was not a problem.

Low molecular weight heparin is equal to or better than warfarin and subcutaneous heparin for high-risk patients. Low molecular weight heparin can also be given once a day in lower-risk patients and has a lower incidence of heparin-induced thrombocytopenia. Currently, for high-risk patients, LMWH is the standard to which the new anticoagulants are compared.

Fondaparinux is also effective in thrombosis prevention in high-risk patients. It is renally cleared and should not be used in patients with renal insufficiency. Also, given the fixed dose (2.5 mg), it should not be used in patients weighing less than 50 kilograms.

Direct Oral Anticoagulants All of the direct oral anticoagulants have been shown to be effective in thrombosis prevention in knee and hip replacement surgery. They have the benefit of being oral and less expensive than LMWH or fondaparinux.

The Situations

Low-Risk Patients

Patients under 40 and with no other risk factors (including a *negative* family history of deep venous thrombosis) or patients undergoing procedures less than 30 min long do not need prophylaxis.

Medium-Risk Patients

Patients over 40 years of age undergoing operations over 30 min long and with no other risk factors should receive low-dose heparin. Heparin, 5000 units TID, is started 2–8 h before surgery and given until the patient is ambulatory. Compression stockings, LMWH, and fondaparinux are also effective. LMWH or fondaparinux should be considered in patients undergoing surgery for abdominal cancers given their high risk of thrombosis.

High-Risk (Non-orthopedic) Patients

Previous history of venous thrombosis (or strong family history of thrombosis) or pelvic or abdominal surgery for malignancy puts a patient in a high-risk category. Low-dose heparin has been shown to be less effective in patients with previous thrombosis and malignancies (especially gynecological). In patients with a thrombotic history, use of LMWH or fondaparinux is effective. Pneumatic booties have been shown to be effective in patients with gynecological malignancies. Patients with very recent deep venous thrombosis who are ill and who absolutely need surgery require LMWH/fondaparinux along with consideration of an IVC filter.

Knee Surgery

High incidence of calf vein deep venous thrombosis (60%) but low incidence of pulmonary embolism accompanies knee surgery. LMW heparins, fondaparinux, and direct oral anticoagulants have been shown to be the most effective for deep venous thrombosis prevention. There is a high incidence of pulmonary embolism in bilateral knee surgery.

Elective Hip Surgery

In patients undergoing elective hip surgery, there is a high incidence of deep venous thrombosis

(50%), pulmonary embolism (11%), and fatal pulmonary embolism (2%). Low-dose heparin and aspirin are not effective in this situation. Although pneumatic booties are effective for prophylaxis, they have been recently shown to be inferior to two-step warfarin therapy. Effective in *all* patients are one of the warfarin regimens, LMW heparin, fondaparinux, or the direct oral anticoagulants. Prophylaxis should be started 24 h after surgery.

Hip Fractures

This is the highest-risk situation. Risk of deep venous thrombosis is 50–80%; risk of pulmonary embolism is 11–20%; and risk of fatal pulmonary embolism is 5–7%. Again, low-dose heparin and aspirin are *not* effective in this situation. Warfarin has been studied for over 30 years and had been found to be effective in reducing the risk of pulmonary embolism from 5–7% to 1%. Thus, for every two to six patients who have a wound hematoma, one patient's life will be saved. LMW heparin and fondaparinux are also very effective in these patients. There is currently no data at this time for the use of direct oral anticoagulants. The situation of the hip fracture patient is complicated by the fact that as many as 10% of patients have deep venous thrombosis before any hip surgery.

Trauma

These patients are at high risk not only for thromboembolic complications but also for bleeding. Once patients are stable (and if they do not have intracranial hemorrhage), enoxaparin 30 mg every 12 h should be used. Patients with spinal cord injury are at high risk for thrombosis and should receive low molecular weight heparin.

Neurosurgery

Patients are at risk for thrombosis, but until recently pharmacologic prophylaxis was not used due to fear of bleeding. However, studies indicate that enoxaparin 40 mg/day was more effective than pneumatic stockings with no associated higher incidence of bleeding. Patients undergoing neurosurgery for brain tumors are at particular risk of thrombosis and should receive LMW heparin.

Medical Patients

Medical patients are at risk for deep venous thrombosis. The range is from 20% in patients with heart failure or pneumonia to as high as 80% in stroke patients. The risk of deep venous thrombosis is increased in patients who smoke and have heart failure, cancer, and previous venous thrombosis. Studies involving thousands of medical patients have shown that low-dose heparin is effective for prophylaxis of venous thrombosis. It reduces deep venous thrombosis by 66%, pulmonary embolism by 50%, and fatal pulmonary embolism by 0.5%. Pneumatic booties may also be effective in these situations. Recent clinical trials have shown that LMW heparins are equal or superior to standard heparin for prophylaxis of the high-risk medical patient.

Patients over 40 and those with serious illnesses, especially heart failure and pneumonia, benefit from low-dose heparin. ICU patients should receive LMWH due to the high incidence of deep venous thrombosis in this population. Patients with strokes are at high risk for deep venous thrombosis, and consideration should be given to pneumatic booties plus low-dose heparin or LMW heparin.

Several studies have looked at DOACs for extended prophylaxis when patients leave the hospital, but reduction in thrombosis is offset by the increased risk of bleeding.

In Pregnancy

Most experience is with enoxaparin 40 mg every day or with dalteparin 5000 units every 12–24 h. See Chap. 28 for more details.

Suggested Reading

Anderson DR, Dunbar M, Murnaghan J, Kahn SR, Gross P, Forsythe M, Pelet S, Fisher W, Belzile E, Dolan S, Crowther M, Bohm E, MacDonald SJ, Gofton W, Kim P, Zukor D, Pleasance S, Andreou P, Doucette S, Theriault C, Abianui A, Carrier M, Kovacs MJ, Rodger MA, Coyle D, Wells PS, Vendittoli PA. Aspirin or rivaroxaban for VTE prophylaxis after hip or knee arthroplasty. N Engl J Med. 2018;378(8):699–707.

Chiu V, O'Connell C. Management of the incidental pulmonary embolism. AJR Am J Roentgenol. 2017;208(3):485–8.

Di Nisio M, van Es N, Büller HR. Deep vein thrombosis and pulmonary embolism. Lancet. 2016;388(10063):3060–73.

Kearon C, Akl EA, Ornelas J, Blaivas A, Jimenez D, Bounameaux H, Huisman M, King CS, Morris TA, Sood N, Stevens SM, Vintch JRE, Wells P, Woller SC, Moores L. Antithrombotic therapy for VTE disease: CHEST guideline and expert panel report. Chest. 2016;149(2):315–52.

Lim W, Le Gal G, Bates SM, Righini M, Haramati LB, Lang E, Kline JA, Chasteen S, Snyder M, Patel P, Bhatt M, Patel P, Braun C, Begum H, Wiercioch W, Schünemann HJ, Mustafa RA. American Society of Hematology 2018 guidelines for management of venous thromboembolism: diagnosis of venous thromboembolism. Blood Adv. 2018;2(22):3226–56.

Schünemann HJ, Cushman M, Burnett AE, Kahn SR, Beyer-Westendorf J, Spencer FA, Rezende SM, Zakai NA, Bauer KA, Dentali F, Lansing J, Balduzzi S, Darzi A, Morgano GP, Neumann I, Nieuwlaat R, Yepes-Nuñez JJ, Zhang Y, Wiercioch W. American Society of Hematology 2018 guidelines for management of venous thromboembolism: prophylaxis for hospitalized and nonhospitalized medical patients. Blood Adv. 2018;2(22):3198–225.

Tritschler T, Kraaijpoel N, Le Gal G, Wells PS. Venous thromboembolism: advances in diagnosis and treatment. JAMA. 2018;320(15):1583–94.

Vedantham S, Goldhaber SZ, Julian JA, Kahn SR, Jaff MR, Cohen DJ, Magnuson E, Razavi MK, Comerota AJ, Gornik HL, Murphy TP, Lewis L, Duncan JR, Nieters P, Derfler MC, Filion M, Gu CS, Kee S, Schneider J, Saad N, Blinder M, Moll S, Sacks D, Lin J, Rundback J, Garcia M, Razdan R, VanderWoude E, Marques V, Kearon C, Trial Investigators ATTRACT. Pharmacomechanical catheter-directed thrombolysis for deep-vein thrombosis. N Engl J Med. 2017;377(23):2240–52.

Wells PS, Ihaddadene R, Reilly A, Forgie MA. Diagnosis of venous thromboembolism: 20 years of progress. Ann Intern Med. 2018;168(2):131–40.

Thomas G. DeLoughery

Although the venous system is present throughout the body, the vast majority of thromboses occur in the deep veins of the legs. Thrombosis can occur in other locations and when it does, it is often a marker of underlying pathology.

Upper Extremity Thrombosis

Thrombosis of the upper extremity occurs commonly in two situations. The first is in the presence of a venous catheter. As discussed more thoroughly in Chap. 27, thrombosis is a common problem with long-term venous catheters for cancer care.

The second situation occurs with exertion. Vigorous use of the arm in such actions as throwing can compress the subclavian vein and result in thrombosis. Patients will note arm pain and swelling soon after the activity but ascribe it to muscle pain. These patients often have anatomic variants such as thoracic outlet syndrome which predispose them to thrombosis or venous scarring.

The incidence of classic hypercoagulable states in patients with upper extremity thrombosis is not higher than that of the normal population. This is consistent with the idea that most of these thromboses are due to mechanical factors. Also, the incidence of pulmonary embolism and clot recurrences are substantially less than those seen with lower extremity DVT.

Therapy of upper extremity thrombosis is with anticoagulation to prevent clot extension and pulmonary embolism. Data indicate that peripherally inserted central catheter (PICC) thrombosis is best treated with removal of the catheter, reserving anticoagulation for either very symptomatic thrombosis or for situations where the catheter remains in place. For tunnel catheters, anticoagulation for thrombosis is indicated for 3 months; rates of bleeding are increased in this setting.

Patients with non-catheter-related upper extremity thrombosis are treated with anticoagulation for 3 months. Given the high incidence of anatomical lesions, consideration should be given to early venography and thrombolytic therapy, especially in younger patients. Studies do suggest improved outcomes with lytic therapy – and imaging allows for identification of a vessel abnormality and its correction.

Cerebral Vein Thrombosis

Cerebral vein thrombosis commonly occurs in the cerebral sinuses, but some cases will occur in the deep cerebral veins. Risk factors for thrombosis in

T. G. DeLoughery (✉)
Division of Hematology/Medical Oncology,
Department of Medicine, Pathology, and Pediatrics,
Oregon Health & Sciences University,
Portland, OR, USA
e-mail: delought@ohsu.edu

© Springer Nature Switzerland AG 2019
T. G. DeLoughery (ed.), *Hemostasis and Thrombosis*,
https://doi.org/10.1007/978-3-030-19330-0_16

deep cerebral veins include the presence of venous hypercoagulable states, use of estrogen, and local factors such as trauma. Patients with acquired hypercoagulable states such as Behcet's disease also appear to be at increased risk. Another group of patients at risk are those suffering from severe dehydration with associated "sludging" of the cerebral blood flow. Finally, patients may have thrombosis due to local irritation of the venous sinuses. The classic presentation of infection-related thrombosis is cerebral vein thrombosis due to irritation of the transverse sinus by mastoiditis, so-called otic hydrocephalus.

Patients with cerebral vein thrombosis can present with one of two major patterns. The first is with focal neurologic defects due to venous thrombosis resulting in localized infarction. Infarctions are often hemorrhagic due to continued arterial blood flow, which pumps blood into the infarcted area. Patients with deep cerebral vein thrombosis may present with severe deficits and coma due to infarction of deep brain structures. Secondly and more commonly, patients with cerebral vein thrombosis will present first with signs of increased intracranial pressure due to obstruction of venous flow and cerebral spinal fluid reabsorption. Patients will have severe headaches, nausea, and vomiting which may progress to coma. Patients may also have reduced vision and blindness due to pressure on the optic nerve. Frequently, patients have a prolonged course lasting for days with gradual worsening of symptoms.

Especially early in the course of cerebral vein thrombosis, patients may present with nonspecific signs and symptoms. Patients may be misdiagnosed as having pseudotumor cerebri. This occurs if only scanning is done and found to be normal and the lumbar puncture shows high opening pressures. Diagnosis of cerebral vein thrombosis is best made by MRI and MR angiography which best show the venous obstruction.

Cerebral vein thrombosis requires anticoagulation. Despite the frequent presence of hemorrhagic transformation, immediate heparin therapy is associated with an improvement in outcome. In the Einhaupl trial, when patients received a small 3000 unit bolus and were anticoagulated with standard heparin, a dramatic improvement in outcome was seen compared to controls. Patients with severe neurological deficits may benefit from angiography and direct thrombolytic therapy of the venous obstruction. Patients with provoking factors such as ear infection or other local infections should be anticoagulated for 6 months. Recent data have shown that even patients with idiopathic cerebral vein thrombosis have low rates of recurrence and require only 6–12 months of therapy. The rates of recurrence are not influenced by whether the vessel recanalizes or not.

Adrenal Infarction

The adrenal gland contains a plexus of small veins and venules which receive the secreted hormones of the adrenal gland. This venous structure appears prone to thrombosis in several hypercoagulable states. Patients with purpura fulminans may present with adrenal crisis due to thrombosis and resultant hemorrhagic destruction of the gland. Patients with heparin-induced thrombocytopenia may rarely infarct the gland and have subsequent hemorrhage. Finally, patients with antiphospholipid antibody syndrome can have adrenal infarctions. The presentation in APLA patients is often one of adrenal insufficiency that initially may be overlooked due to nonspecific symptoms.

Budd-Chiari Syndrome

Patients with Budd-Chiari syndrome (hepatic vein thrombosis) present with the onset of a painful swollen liver and ascites which may progress to liver failure. Several hypercoagulable states are associated with Budd-Chiari syndrome (Table 16.1). These are myeloproliferative syndromes, antiphospholipid antibodies, paroxysmal

Table 16.1 Hypercoagulable states associated with Budd-Chiari syndrome

| Antiphospholipid antibodies |
| Behcet's disease |
| Myeloproliferative syndrome |
| Paroxysmal nocturnal hemoglobinuria |

nocturnal hemoglobinuria, and Behcet's disease. Budd-Chiari may be the presenting sign of a myeloproliferative syndrome and can occur with normal blood counts. This presentation is discussed further in Chap. 27.

Therapy is partially dictated by the severity of the liver disease. Since these patients have a hypercoagulable state and are at risk for further life-threatening thrombosis, anticoagulation should be initiated at the time of diagnosis of the thrombosis. Catheter-guided thrombolytic therapy can be considered for fresh clots in very ill patients. Patients who present with chronic obstruction may benefit from either surgical or catheter-placed shunts. Patients with myeloproliferative syndromes do poorly with surgery; therefore, catheter-based shunt approaches should be tried first. Despite the presence of hypercoagulable state, shunt thrombosis is uncommon in patients who are anticoagulated. Patients who undergo liver transplantation and have an identifiable hypercoagulable state should be aggressively anticoagulated to prevent thrombosis of the liver graft after transplant surgery.

Renal Vein Thrombosis

Renal vein thrombosis most often accompanies nephrotic syndrome. It is also associated with malignancy but is less often seen with the inherited hypercoagulable states. Patients can present with a clinical spectrum ranging from sudden onset of severe flank pain to a subtle deterioration of renal function. Patients with pre-existing renal disease may simply present with worsening renal function. Total venous occlusion will result in hemorrhagic infarction of the entire kidney. Acute thrombosis resulting in renal impairment can be treated with catheter-guided thrombolytic therapy. Patients with more chronic presentations require long-term anticoagulation.

Portal Vein Thrombosis

Portal vein thrombosis (PVT) can occur in several situations:

- Postsurgical – PVT is increasingly recognized following abdominal surgery. Often patients will have abdominal pain with nausea and vomiting. Short-term treatment for 3 months will often lead to recanalization of the portal vein.
- Idiopathic – most often due to severe hypercoagulable states such as myeloproliferative syndromes or paroxysmal nocturnal hemoglobinuria. These patients need indefinite anticoagulation.
- Cirrhosis – PVT is a common complication of cirrhosis. If the diagnosis is discovered incidentally during screening for hepatoma, patients can be observed without anticoagulation. Patients who appear to have hepatic decompensation due to acute PVT may benefit from anticoagulation.

Mesenteric Vein Thrombosis

The mesenteric veins are the third most common presenting site of thrombosis after deep venous thrombosis and cerebral vein thrombosis. Patients usually present with abdominal pain out of proportion to physical findings. Diagnosis can be established at the time of surgery or with CT scanning showing thrombus in the mesenteric vein. Patients may suffer extensive bowel infarction with mesenteric vein thrombosis. Patients with idiopathic mesenteric vein thrombosis should be treated indefinitely with anticoagulation, even in the absence of an identifiable hypercoagulable state, because this condition is strongly associated with recurrent thrombosis.

Retinal Vein Thrombosis

Retinal vein thrombosis is a not-uncommon cause of impaired vision. Despite the venous infarction, patients with retinal vein thrombosis do not appear to have a higher incidence of underlying hypercoagulable states. Instead, risk factors for arterial disease are often present, and these patients have a higher risk of developing arterial disease over the next 10 years. The retinal artery and vein share the same sheath in the eye, and a rigid atherosclerotic artery may predispose to compression of the vein. Patients with branch retinal vein thrombosis also tend to have the artery overlying the vein at the site of thrombosis. This gives further credence to the idea that local compression instigates thrombosis. Patients with retinal vein thrombosis should not be treated with anticoagulation as this may provoke retinal hemorrhage. Patients should not undergo a thrombophilia work-up; instead attention should be paid to arterial risk factors such as dyslipidemias and hypertension.

Priapism (Table 16.2)

Priapism is caused by one of two underlying mechanisms. The first is high-flow priapism due to increased arterial blood flow to the cavernosa. The penis is infused with well-oxygenated blood and permanent damage is not seen. This is most often seen with traumatic arterial-venous shunts.

Low-flow priapism results from blockage of the venous drainage of the cavernosa. This leads

Table 16.2 Priapism

High flow: Increased arterial blood flow to the penis
Low flow: Obstruction of venous drainage
Sickle cell disease
DIC with thrombosis
Venous trauma
Tumor infiltration
Medications
Diagnostic approach
Doppler ultrasound of vasculature
Aspiration of corporeal blood for blood gas analysis
pH less than 7.25 and oxygen less than 30 mmHg suggestive of low-flow state
Treatment of low-flow priapism
Corporeal aspiration of 60 ml of blood and injection of 200 ug of phenylephrine
Repeat for a total of three injections (if needed)
If this fails, patients should undergo corporo-spongiosum shunting
Patients with sickle cell disease should undergo exchange transfusion first to lower percentage of sickle cells to under 30%

to hypoxia and ischemia of the cavernosa and is an emergency. Patient may have low-flow priapism due to sickle cell disease, DIC with thrombosis, venous trauma, and tumor infiltrations or from medications such as trazodone or ecstasy.

Usually the history is helpful in differentiating low- vs high-flow priapism. If the cause is uncertain, Doppler ultrasound of the vasculature is indicated. High blood flows are suggestive of high-flow priapism. Another useful test is aspiration of corporeal blood with blood gas analysis. A pH of less than 7.25 and an oxygen level under 30 mmHg is diagnostic of a low-flow state.

Patients who present with low-flow priapism should undergo corporeal aspiration of 60 mL of blood and injection of 200 ug of phenylephrine. The phenylephrine can be repeated for a total of three injections. If this fails, patients should undergo corporo-spongiosum shunting.

Patients with priapism due to sickle cell disease should undergo exchange transfusion to reduce the percentage of sickle cells to under 30%. If this is unsuccessful, corporeal aspiration of 60 mL of blood and injection of 200 ug of phenylephrine can be tried, but this is rarely successful in sickle cell patients. Patients who fail therapy will require a corporo-spongiosum shunt.

Suggested Reading

Burnett AL, Bivalacqua TJ. Priapism: new concepts in medical and surgical management. Urol Clin North Am. 2011;38(2):185–94.

Dmytriw AA, Song JSA, Yu E, Poon CS. Cerebral venous thrombosis: state of the art diagnosis and management. Neuroradiology. 2018;60:669.

Intagliata NM, Caldwell SH, Tripodi A. Diagnosis, development, and treatment of portal vein thrombosis in patients with and without cirrhosis. Gastroenterology. 2019;. Epub ahead of print

Jonas JB, Monés J, Glacet-Bernard A, Coscas G. Retinal vein occlusions. Dev Ophthalmol. 2017;58:139–67.

Shatzel JJ, O'Donnell M, Olson SR, Kearney MR, Daughety MM, Hum J, Nguyen KP, DeLoughery TG. Venous thrombosis in unusual sites: a practical review for the hematologist. Eur J Haematol. 2019;102(1):53–62.

Inherited Thrombophilias

17

Thomas G. DeLoughery

Thrombophilia is defined as a condition in which, due to an inherited or acquired disorder, there is a propensity to form thrombosis. This hypercoagulability is manifested clinically by a greater number of thromboses, thrombosis at an early age, a familial tendency toward thrombosis, or thrombosis at unusual sites. The fundamental approach is to decide whether a thrombophilia is present by the logical ordering and interpretation of tests and then, if the patient has a thrombophilia, to decide on appropriate therapy.

When to Suspect a Thrombophilia (Table 17.1)

A thrombophilia is manifested clinically by:

- *Unprovoked thrombosis at an early age.* It is uncertain what age limit should be used for this criterion. Thrombosis in patients with inherited thrombophilias often starts in the teenage years. Despite the predilection for thrombosis early in life, the risk of thrombosis in patients with thrombophilias increases as the patient gets

Table 17.1 Markers of thrombophilias

Thrombosis at early age
Family history of thrombosis
Thrombosis at unusual site
Multiple thromboses

older. The Physician's Health Study showed a relative risk of thrombosis in carriers of factor V Leiden of 2 in patients less than 60 years of age and 7 in patients more than 60. An arbitrary age cutoff of 50 has been suggested, but older patients who have spontaneous thrombosis and a suggestive family history should also be evaluated for inherited thrombophilias.

- *Familial tendency toward thrombosis.* The penetrance of thrombophilias is variable so lack of a family history of thrombosis should not deter one from evaluating a patient.
- Thrombosis at *unusual sites* such as the hepatic or mesenteric veins. As noted in Chap. 16, upper extremity thrombosis is usually due to mechanical causes and should not provoke an evaluation for thrombophilias.
- *Recurrent thromboses* – especially if they are idiopathic.

Why Diagnose Thrombophilias?

The utility of diagnosing a specific thrombophilia has become controversial given that the therapy

T. G. DeLoughery (✉)
Division of Hematology/Medical Oncology,
Department of Medicine, Pathology, and Pediatrics,
Oregon Health & Sciences University,
Portland, OR, USA
e-mail: delought@ohsu.edu

© Springer Nature Switzerland AG 2019
T. G. DeLoughery (ed.), *Hemostasis and Thrombosis*,
https://doi.org/10.1007/978-3-030-19330-0_17

recommendations are often the same whether one is present or not. It is now agreed that thrombophilia workups should not be performed in patients with a first provoked thrombosis. Also, workup for classic genetic thrombophilias should not be performed for arterial disease. However, several arguments can be made for diagnosing the exact thrombophilia state(s). Thrombophilias do increase the risk of first thrombosis and may at least in part explain the thrombosis. Patients with antithrombin III deficiency will require concentrates during high-risk situations such as surgery. Also, patients found to be "triple positive" for antiphospholipid antibody disease should not receive DOACs as anticoagulation. It is still unsettled as to whether family screening is of value; the risk of first thrombosis is higher in affected relatives, and predictable additional stressors such as pregnancy, prophylactic measures can be taken.

Approach to the Patient Suspected of Having a Thrombophilia

Unfortunately – unlike with bleeding disorders – no screening tests for thrombophilias are available. The clinical setting should guide ordering a rational evaluation. When evaluating a patient one should ask the following questions:

Is the Thrombosis Arterial or Venous?

A critical piece in planning the evaluation is determining whether the thrombosis is arterial or venous. Most thrombophilias manifest themselves as predominantly venous thrombosis. Although anecdotal reports of arterial thrombosis associated with protein C, protein S, and antithrombin III deficiency exist, reviews of large patient cohorts have not proved an association. Arterial thrombosis is primarily either associated with atherosclerosis or embolism and not with the "classic" thrombophilias.

Where Is the Site of Thrombosis?

Although many thrombophilias present with deep venous thrombosis, certain thrombophilias have a predilection for visceral thrombosis. Myeloproliferative syndromes, paroxysmal nocturnal hemoglobinuria, and Behcet's disease are strongly associated with visceral thrombosis. Conversely, thrombosis of the upper extremity is rarely associated with a thrombophilia.

What Is the Age of the Patient?

Unlike presentations of inherited bleeding disorders, thrombophilias rarely present with thrombosis during the childhood years. Patients with inherited thrombophilias often have a first thrombosis in the late teens to thirties. A sudden onset of thrombosis in older patients raises the specter of neoplasm or of an acquired thrombophilia.

Were or Are There Any Associated Risk Factors for Thrombosis?

The suspicion of a thrombophilia needs to be tempered by the situation in which the thrombosis occurred. Thrombosis in older patients after surgery or during hospitalization is common and not necessarily a sign of a thrombophilia. In the younger patient, thrombosis with a stressor may be the first sign of an underlying thrombophilia, but since the presence of genetic thrombophilia will not influence the length of therapy, there is little utility in screening.

Is There a Family History of Thrombosis?

Since many thrombophilias are inherited, determining a family history of thrombosis is crucial. The thrombotic tendency has a variable penetrance and therefore the rate of thrombosis may be considerably lower than the 50% expected from an autosomal dominant trait. Thus, a detailed family history should be obtained.

Screening Family Members

Limited data now exist to suggest that asymptomatic carriers of inherited thrombophilias may have up to a 10% risk for thrombosis with stressors such as pregnancy or surgery. Thus, blood relatives of patients with inherited thrombophilias should be screened and offered prophylaxis before surgery and in other high-risk situations.

The Congenital Thrombophilias (Table 17.2)

- *Factor V Leiden (hereditary resistance to activated protein C)* is a defect in factor V which renders it unable to be degraded by activated protein C due to a mutation at amino acid 506, where substituting a glutamine for an alanine eliminate a protein C cleavage site. Factor V Leiden is only associated with venous thrombosis. This mutation is very common: it accounts for 40–60% of thrombophilias and 20% of first DVTs and is found in 2–8% of the normal population. It is estimated that the presence of factor V Leiden is associated with a threefold higher relative risk of thrombosis. Factor V Leiden is synergistic with estrogen, and this combination increases the risk of thrombosis over tenfold.
- *Prothrombin gene mutation* is a defect in the prothrombin gene (nt20210 G-->A). The pathophysiology of this thrombophilia is unknown but may be due to elevated levels of plasma prothrombin. The prothrombin gene

mutation is present in 1–2% of the normal population but is seen in perhaps 10–20% of patients with thrombophilias. Like factor V Leiden, it is associated with venous thrombosis and increases the relative risk of thrombosis threefold.
- *Protein C* is a protein which, when activated by thrombin, degrades factors V and VIII. Deficiency of protein C primarily causes venous thrombosis. The relative risk of thrombosis in those with protein C deficiency is estimated to be 10, while the risk in carriers ranges from 0.5% to 2.5% per year.
- *Protein S* is a cofactor for protein C. Protein S exists both in bound and unbound form. Deficiencies of total protein S and of unbound protein S (more common) can lead to a thrombophilia. Like protein C deficiency, the risk of thrombosis with protein S deficiency is increased tenfold, and the risk for carriers is 0.9–3.5% per year. Family studies indicated that only very low protein S levels (<42%) are associated with increased risk of thrombosis.
- *Antithrombin* inhibits activated clotting factors. Deficiency of antithrombin increases the risk of venous thrombosis up to 30-fold. Lack of antithrombin is usually not associated with heparin resistance.
- *Dysfibrinogenemia* is defined by a defective fibrinogen molecule that forms clots which are difficult to degrade by fibrinolytic agents. Dysfibrinogenemia can be associated with both venous and arterial thrombosis. Due to this difficulty with thrombus formation, some patients with dysfibrinogenemia may also have a bleeding diathesis.
- Elevated *factor VIII* – there is evidence implicating high levels of factor VIII (>150%) in venous thrombosis with a relative risk of 3 and

Table 17.2 Inherited thrombophilias

Defect	Incidence in population	Percent of thrombophilias	Relative risk of thrombosis
Factor V Leiden	2–8%	40–60%	3
Prothrombin gene mutation	1–2%	?10%	3
Protein C deficiency	1:200	5–10%	10
Protein S deficiency	?1:5000	5–10%	10
Antithrombin III deficiency	1:2–5000	1–3%	10
Dysfibrinogenemia	Rare	1	?

high risk of recurrence. The mechanism of the factor VIII elevation is unknown, but may be a combination of genetic factors and acquired risk factors such as inflammation.

- *Lipoprotein (a)* is a lipoprotein with uncertain function in thrombosis. High levels of lipoprotein (a) increase the risk of arteriosclerosis. The role of high levels of lipoprotein (a) in venous thrombosis remains controversial.
- *Fibrinolytic disorders* in theory should be classic causes of thrombophilias. However, the role of defects in fibrinolytic enzymes in congenital thrombophilias is controversial. No convincing relationship has been shown between defects in fibrinolysis and inherited thrombophilias.
- *Homocysteine* – high levels of homocysteine have in the past been reported to be associated with thrombophilia. This association is increasingly controversial as studies of lowering homocysteine have failed to show benefit in tendency for thrombosis, and animal models are not associated with an increased risk of thrombosis. It may be that high homocysteine levels are a marker of underlying inflammation or renal disease – both prothrombotic states.
- *MTHFR* – early studies suggested mutation in methyltetrahydrofolate reductase, an enzyme in the folate metabolic pathway, may be associated with thrombophilia. Large studies have convincingly shown that mutations of this enzyme do not play a role in either arterial or venous thrombosis.

Suggested Evaluation in Patients with Venous Thrombosis

The patient with venous thrombosis suspected of having a thrombophilia should be screened for diseases listed in Table 17.3.

The timing of the laboratory tests is a frequent concern. The decision is whether to test during the acute event or to wait until after the patient has completed a period of anticoagulation. Heparin only interferes with the first-generation coagulation assays for factor V Leiden and some assays

Table 17.3 Evaluation of patients with thrombophilias

Activated protein C resistance ratio (factor V Leiden)
Prothrombin gene mutation PCR assay
Protein C activity assay
Free protein S
Antithrombin activity assay
Antiphospholipid antibody assays
Anticardiolipin antibodies
Anti-beta2-glycoprotein
PTT-based assays such as hexagonal phospholipid assay and dilute Russell viper venom time
In selected patients
Dysfibrinogenemia evaluation
Fibrinogen activity level
Fibrinogen antigen level
Thrombin time
JAK2 mutation assay
Flow cytometry for paroxysm nocturnal hemoglobinuria
Limited evaluation for cancer

for antiphospholipid antibodies. Note that there is also a high incidence of false-positive lupus inhibitor with testing at the time of acute thrombosis. Also, certain coagulation factors, especially protein C, free protein S, and antithrombin, may be acutely lowered by the acute thrombosis. If the testing is performed early, one can decide at that time upon the duration of therapy if an abnormality is found. If the patient is to be tested later, one needs to ensure the patient has been off warfarin for at least two and preferably 3 weeks before testing, since proteins C and S are vitamin K-dependent proteins and their production will be reduced by warfarin therapy. The use of DOACs can also interfere with functional coagulation factor assays and testing for lupus inhibitors.

Although 3–20% of patients with thrombosis will have cancer diagnosed at the time of presentation, the patient and clinician are often concerned about the presence of an occult underlying malignancy. This situation is similar to the patient who presents with a metastatic lesion with an unknown primary where searching for the underlying primary malignancy is often futile. Although untested, one strategy in the absence of other clinical clues is to do a limited evaluation including chest x-rays (CT in smokers), mammography, colon cancer screening, and other age-appropriate screening.

Testing

Factor V Leiden The most cost-effective method is to perform a coagulation-based assay for resistance to activated protein C. The newer generation assays are not affected by anticoagulation. Given that the gene mutation is constant (ARG506GLN), one can perform a DNA assay via polymerase chain reaction. The DNA assay is useful in borderline cases or in patients who are suspected to have homozygosity for the mutation.

Prothrombin gene mutation is diagnosed by the polymerase chain reaction-based test which directly detects the mutation. Although plasma levels of prothrombin are higher in these patients, only measuring the prothrombin levels cannot detect carriers of the mutation.

Protein C and protein S deficiencies Since these are vitamin K-dependent proteins, their levels will be reduced by warfarin therapy. Blood for measuring these proteins should be drawn before starting warfarin or 2–3 weeks after stopping therapy. In patients who require lifelong therapy, one can perform family studies to pick up the deficiency or temporarily halt warfarin therapy for 2–3 weeks to determine the levels. Testing for "free protein S" levels should be requested since a deficiency in free protein S is more common than total protein S deficiency. Free protein S may be low (even under 30%) during a normal pregnancy. Both protein S and protein C may be low in acute thrombosis and with serious illness, so low levels obtained in these situations may be false positives.

Antithrombin deficiency Acute thromboembolism and rarely heparin therapy can lower levels. Thus, a normal antithrombin level drawn in these circumstances effectively rules this out as a cause of a thrombophilia. Low antithrombin levels performed in the acute setting should be repeated 6 weeks later (off heparin) before labeling the patient antithrombin deficient.

Therapy

The goal for warfarin anticoagulation is to keep the prothrombin time at an INR of 2.0–3.0. This ratio has been shown to provide the best risk-benefit ratio. The direct oral anticoagulants are also effective in inherited thrombophilia. As noted before, the presence of genetic hypercoagulable states increases the risk of first thrombosis but does not clearly increase the risk of recurrence. The duration of therapy should be decided by whether the thrombosis was provoked or if there have been multiple thromboses.

Suggested Reading

Carroll BJ, Piazza G. Hypercoagulable states in arterial and venous thrombosis: when, how, and who to test? Vasc Med. 2018;23(4):388–99.

Connors JM. Thrombophilia testing and venous thrombosis. N Engl J Med. 2017;377(12):1177–87.

Mannucci PM, Franchini M. Classic thrombophilic gene variants. Thromb Haemost. 2015;114(5):885–9.

Middeldorp S. Inherited thrombophilia: a double-edged sword. Hematology Am Soc Hematol Educ Program. 2016;2016(1):1–9.

Montagnana M, Lippi G, Danese E. An overview of thrombophilia and associated laboratory testing. Methods Mol Biol. 2017;1646:113–35.

Preston RJS, O'Sullivan JM, O'Donnell JS. Advances in understanding the molecular mechanisms of venous thrombosis. Br J Haematol. 2019.

Acquired Thrombophilias

Thomas G. DeLoughery

Acquired thrombophilias range from rare disorders such as Behçet's disease to the very common initial presentation of malignancy. Acquired hypercoagulable states may present at any age. Patients with acquired disorders often present with a "flurry" of thromboses. While patients with congenital disorders may have two thromboses separated by years, the patient with an acquired thrombophilia may present with repeated thrombosis even on anticoagulant therapy. In some patients, thrombosis may be the first manifestation of the underlying disease. In many patients, thrombosis is a well-recognized complication of the underlying disease.

Patients suspected of having an acquired thrombophilia should be carefully screened for the presence of classic underlying diseases such as cancer or inflammatory bowel disease.

The most common causes of acquired thrombophilias – cancer, antiphospholipid antibody disease, and pregnancy – are discussed in the appropriate chapters.

Inflammatory Bowel Disease

Patients with inflammatory bowel disease are at higher risk for thrombosis. Autopsy series show that 33% of patients had thrombi present at the time of death. It appears that the presence of inherited thrombophilias also raises the risk of thrombosis in these patients. Patients with inflammatory bowel disease complicated by thrombosis usually present with deep venous thrombosis of the lower extremity. An increased risk of visceral vein thrombosis has also been reported, perhaps due to local inflammation. Rarely, large arterial thrombi have also been reported.

Pathogenesis Patients with inflammatory bowel disease have been shown to have reduced levels of free protein S. This lower level of protein S is due to increased levels of its binding protein, C4B-binding protein, which is an acute phase reactant. Increased levels of the inflammatory cytokines such as IL-1 and TNF may also contribute to the thrombophilia by stimulating endothelial cells.

Diagnosis is by history. Rare patients may present with an unusual pattern of inflammatory bowel disease, but most thrombosis patients have the classic signs and symptoms of bowel disease.

Therapy is with anticoagulants. One obvious difficulty is that these patients are at risk for

T. G. DeLoughery (✉)
Division of Hematology/Medical Oncology,
Department of Medicine, Pathology, and Pediatrics,
Oregon Health & Sciences University,
Portland, OR, USA
e-mail: delought@ohsu.edu

© Springer Nature Switzerland AG 2019
T. G. DeLoughery (ed.), *Hemostasis and Thrombosis*,
https://doi.org/10.1007/978-3-030-19330-0_18

bleeding, and severe gastrointestinal hemorrhage can complicate therapy. Fear of bleeding should not discourage adequate anticoagulation to prevent fatal thrombosis or use of prophylaxis when patients are hospitalized. Therapy for the underlying bowel disease can also be helpful as thrombosis rates are lower when patients are in remission. Patients with ulcerative colitis experience resolution of their thrombophilia with total colectomy.

Surgery

The stress of undergoing surgery increases the risk of thrombosis in an otherwise normal patient by 10–30-fold. Recent surgery is the most common risk factor for deep venous thrombosis.

Pathogenesis of the surgical thrombophilia is complex. Venous stasis due to immobility during surgery and the recovery process certainly plays a role. The inflammatory response with the release of inflammatory cytokines is also important. The period of relative hypercoagulability can extend for weeks after surgery. The average time to presentation with postoperative deep venous thrombosis is over 2 weeks after the surgery. Smoking, oral contraceptives, previous history of thrombosis, genetic thrombophilia, and cancer all act synergistically to increase the risk of postoperative thrombosis.

Prevention is by two methods. The first is to try to reverse any risk factors before surgery (i.e., stop smoking or stop birth control pills). The other important step is to use appropriate prophylaxis for deep venous thrombosis which is discussed in detail in Chap. 15.

Nephrotic Syndrome and Other Renal Disease

Nephrotic syndrome has long been associated with a thrombophilia. Patients with nephrotic syndrome have an increased incidence of renal vein and other thrombosis. Less well-known is that patients with renal failure in general have a higher incidence of thrombosis. Thrombosis of

vascular grafts is one difficult problem. Occasional patients will suffer multiple graft thrombi which will impair their ability to undergo dialysis.

Pathogenesis of the thrombophilia in nephrotic syndrome is urinary loss of natural anticoagulants. Low levels of both antithrombin and protein S are commonly seen. The presence of concurrent autoimmune diseases such as lupus may add associated antiphospholipid antibodies to the mix. Pathogenesis of the thrombophilia seen in other renal disease is less well defined.

Therapy is with anticoagulation for established thrombosis. Duration is uncertain if the underlying renal disease is eliminated. Some authorities have argued that the risk of thrombosis is so high in nephrotic syndrome that these patients should be prophylactically anticoagulated; unfortunately, the associated risk of bleeding is higher in patients with renal disease due to the presence of the uremic bleeding diathesis.

Renal transplantation is also accompanied by a higher risk of thrombosis (Table 18.1). Patients with pre-existing thrombophilias, especially those with antiphospholipid antibodies, are at higher risk for graft thrombosis. Infusion of OKT3 has also been associated with thrombosis. Patients with a history of thrombosis should be evaluated for thrombophilias prior to undergoing transplantation. Patients with underlying autoimmune disease should also be evaluated for

Table 18.1 Renal transplants in hypercoagulable patients

Renal transplant patients at risk for graft thrombosis
Previous AV fistula thrombosis
Previous venous thrombosis
Presence of antiphospholipid antibodies or other thrombophilias
Previous large vein renal transplant thrombosis
Protocol for renal transplant patients at high risk of thrombosis
1. Two hours before surgery, enoxaparin 20 mg subcutaneously
2. Start daily enoxaparin 20 mg subcutaneously
3. Start warfarin evening after surgery with goal INR 2–3
4. Continue warfarin for at least 6 weeks after transplant

antiphospholipid antibodies. Patients should receive prophylaxis with low molecular weight heparin for the transplant, and consideration should be given to avoid routine use of OKT3 due to the associated risk of thrombosis.

No ideal solution exists for the problem of vascular graft thrombosis. One trial has suggested that antiplatelet agents may be of value in preventing occlusion, but this is associated with a high rate of bleeding.

Paroxysmal Nocturnal Hemoglobinuria (PNH)

PNH is a rare hematological disorder that most often presents with low blood counts, hypocellular bone marrow, and a high incidence of thrombosis which is the leading cause of death in untreated patients. The underlying problem is a mutation in a gene which encodes the enzyme phosphatidylinositol glycan A. This enzyme helps construct the glycosylphosphatidylinositol (GPI) that links cell membrane proteins with the phospholipid membrane. The loss of these membrane proteins causes a variety of clinical effects. The disease takes its name from the loss of red cell membrane proteins which inactivate complement, rendering erythrocytes more susceptible to lysis by the membrane attack complex.

Patients may present with thrombosis at any site. PNH is one of the few thrombophilias which classically presents with Budd-Chiari syndrome. The thrombosis associated with PNH may be refractory to oral anticoagulants, and rare patients may thrombose even on therapeutic doses of heparin. Another diagnostic clue is that many patients have elevated LDH which is reflective of red cell destruction.

Pathogenesis of the thrombosis is unknown. There is speculation that the platelets are also more likely to be activated by complement, leading to thrombosis.

The *diagnosis* of PNH should be suspected in patients with pancytopenia and thrombosis. The classic "nocturnal hemoglobinuria" is a rare finding. Most patients will have pancytopenia, although rare patients can present with elevated blood counts. Patients will usually have a high serum LDH. The older "Ham's test" and sucrose hemolysis tests have been replaced by flow cytometry. Flow cytometry will directly detect missing membrane proteins. Current technology uses fluorescein-labeled proaerolysin (FLAER) that directly binds GPI and is very sensitive to small cell populations that are missing this linker molecule.

Therapy The treatment of PNH has been revolutionized by eculizumab – a monoclonal protein that inhibits complement C5a. This prevents the formation of the membrane attack complex and blocks red cell lysis. This agent markedly decreases hemolysis and transfusion requirements. It also dramatically decreases the risk of thrombosis. Also available is ravulizumab which can be given every 2 months rather than eculizumabs every 2-week dosage interval. Patients with PNH clones over 10% and thrombosis should be started on anticomplement therapy. Patients who present with PNH and thrombosis should also be anticoagulated.

Behçet's Disease

Thrombosis is a frequent finding in patients with Behçet's. Patients may have both arterial and venous thrombosis. Patients with Behçet's have a predilection for both Budd-Chiari syndrome and cerebral vein thrombosis.

Pathogenesis is probably a combination of the underlying inflammatory disease and vasculitis. The arterial thrombosis is either at the site of vasculitis or due to aneurysm formation. Case reports have shown coexisting antiphospholipid antibodies in some patients with Behçet's.

The *diagnosis* of Behçet's disease should be considered in patients with thrombosis and any of the classic findings of Behçet's. The major criteria for diagnosis are presence of painful mouth ulcers, iritis or posterior uveitis, and genital ulcers. Patients may have skin manifestations, gastrointestinal bleeding, and central nervous system symptoms.

Therapy is with anticoagulation for the thrombotic complications. Patients with severe gastrointestinal bleeding will be challenging to treat. Immunosuppression is of benefit, especially in patients with arterial disease.

Hemolytic Disorders

Patients with a broad spectrum of acquired and congenital hemolytic diseases appear to be at a higher risk of thrombosis. Higher rates of thrombosis are also seen after splenectomy for hemolytic diseases.

Pathogenesis of the thrombosis associated with hemolysis is speculated to be due to damaged red cells. One constituent of the red cell membrane, phosphatidylserine, is very effective at promoting coagulation. Usually phosphatidylserine is on the inner red cell membrane but in some congenital hemolytic anemias, phosphatidylserine is exposed due to red cell damage. This exposed phospholipid may provide a surface for coagulation reactions.

Diagnosis is by diagnosing the underlying hemolytic anemia. Higher rates of thrombosis have been seen with all hemolytic anemias and with the thalassemic syndromes.

Therapy is with anticoagulation. Some have speculated that splenectomy will worsen the thrombophilia. However, this potential risk of splenectomy must be balanced by any relief this operation would provide for the anemia.

Air Travel

Much attention has been given to thrombosis due to airplane travel. Case-controlled studies suggest a relative risk of thrombosis of 3–4-fold with prolonged (over 4 hours) travel, with a higher risk for longer travel times – especially over 10 hours. It is uncertain what the absolute risk for thrombosis is. The overall risk of symptomatic pulmonary embolism is estimated to be 0.4 per million passengers, rising to 4 per million in the highest risk group. In contrast, a small prospective trial showed a calf vein thrombosis rate of up to 12%. The presence of risk factors such as a history of deep venous thrombosis is important. Up to 70–90% of those with travel-related thrombosis had other risk factors for thrombosis.

Pathogenesis is controversial. Venous stasis appears to be the primary risk factor. Relative hypoxia is uncertain given that most studies do not show activation of coagulation with mild hypoxic exposure. Pre-existing risk factors for thrombosis are also important. As noted above, most studies indicated that the people who develop travel-related thrombosis have other risk factors such as history of thrombosis, estrogen use, etc.

Prophylaxis Knee-high elastic compression stockings have the most data behind its use and are effective at reducing the risk of thrombosis by up to 90%. Another trial has shown benefit for LMWH heparin, but not for aspirin; LMWH is inconvenient for most people. A reasonable approach may be to recommend stockings and encourage foot movement for most people. It may be sensible to offer patients with a history of thrombosis or thrombophilias either LMWH or direct oral anticoagulant prophylaxis before very long (>10 hour) flights.

Suggested Reading

Alkim H, Koksal AR, Boga S, Sen I, Alkim C. Etiopathogenesis, prevention, and treatment of thromboembolism in inflammatory bowel disease. Clin Appl Thromb Hemost. 2017;23(6):501–10.

Audia S, Bach B, Samson M, Lakomy D, Bour JB, Burlet B, Guy J, Duvillard L, Branger M, Leguy-Seguin V, Berthier S, Michel M, Bonnotte B. Venous thromboembolic events during warm autoimmune hemolytic anemia. PLoS One. 2018;13(11):e020721.

Clarke MJ, Broderick C, Hopewell S, Juszczak E, Eisinga A. Compression stockings for preventing deep vein thrombosis in airline passengers. Cochrane Database Syst Rev. 2016;9:CD004002.

Gigante A, Barbano B, Sardo L, Martina P, Gasperini ML, Labbadia R, Liberatori M, Amoroso A, Cianci R. Hypercoagulability and nephrotic syndrome. Curr Vasc Pharmacol. 2014;12(3):512–7.

Hill A, DeZern AE, Kinoshita T, Brodsky RA. Paroxysmal nocturnal haemoglobinuria. Nat Rev Dis Primers. 2017;3:17028.

Lentz SR. Thrombosis in the setting of obesity or inflammatory bowel disease. Blood. 2016;128(20):2388–94.

Antiphospholipid Antibody Syndrome

Thomas G. DeLoughery

Antiphospholipid Antibodies (APLA)

APLA are antibodies directed against certain phospholipids. They are found in a variety of clinical situations. APLA are important to detect because in certain patients they are associated with a syndrome which includes a hypercoagulable state, thrombocytopenia, fetal loss, dementia, strokes, Addison's disease, and skin rashes.

The underlying mechanism leading to the clinical syndrome associated with APLA is still unknown. Perhaps the antibodies inhibit the function of proteins C or S, damage the endothelium, activate platelets, or inhibit prostacyclin. Despite several decades of research, the etiology of the thrombotic tendency associated with APLA remains unknown.

Definitions

- *APLA syndrome*: Patients with APLA and one "major clinical criterion" are said to have "APLA syndrome." The major clinical criteria

Table 19.1 Diagnosis of antiphospholipid antibody syndrome

Positive anticardiolipin, anti-beta2-glycoprotein, or lupus inhibitor test that is persistent when tested at least 12 weeks apart with at least one clinical feature:
• Arterial, venous, or small vessel thrombosis
• Frequent miscarriages
  • Three or more first trimester losses
  • One fetal death after 10 weeks
  • Premature birth due to early-onset eclampsia

include venous or arterial thrombosis (including neurological disease such as stroke), thrombocytopenia, and/or frequent miscarriages. (Table 19.1)

- *Secondary APLA syndrome* is APLA plus another autoimmune disease, most commonly lupus.
- *Primary APLA syndrome* is APLA syndrome occurring outside of the setting of lupus (SLE). In distinction to SLE-APLA patients, primary APLA patients are more often male and will have low-titer ANAs but no other criteria for SLE.
- *Anticardiolipin antibody* is an APLA in which the antibody is detected by an ELISA assay.
- *Anti-beta$_2$-glycoprotein (Anti-B$_2$GP)* is a subgroup of APLA also detected by ELISA assay. Anti-B$_2$GP are thought to be more specific for APLA that cause thrombosis.
- *Lupus anticoagulant and lupus inhibitor* are terms which are interchangeable. Lupus inhibitor is an APLA in which the antibody is detected by a coagulation test.

T. G. DeLoughery (✉)
Division of Hematology/Medical Oncology,
Department of Medicine, Pathology, and Pediatrics,
Oregon Health & Sciences University,
Portland, OR, USA
e-mail: delought@ohsu.edu

© Springer Nature Switzerland AG 2019
T. G. DeLoughery (ed.), *Hemostasis and Thrombosis*,
https://doi.org/10.1007/978-3-030-19330-0_19

Who Gets APLA?

Approximately 30–50% of patients with lupus will have APLA. The antibodies can also be found in patients with other autoimmune diseases. Patients without lupus or other autoimmune diseases can have symptomatic APLA ("primary APLA syndrome"). Children will often develop transient non-thrombotic APLA after viral infections. This laboratory finding often comes to attention during preoperative evaluation for tonsillectomy. Up to 30% of patients with HIV infection will also develop APLA. The infection-associated APLAs are not associated with thrombosis and are usually anti-B_2GP negative. Medication may also induce APLA. Chlorpromazine is the most commonly implicated drug, but APLA has also been associated with use of Dilantin and tumor necrosis factor inhibitors. In screening studies of blood donors and normal controls, up to 10–20% of asymptomatic people have APLA. However, the APLAs in these people are usually low titer and most often occur in young women.

APLA: Clinical Associations

APLAs are associated with a number of disease states (Table 19.2). The best described conditions are venous thrombosis, arterial thrombosis, neurological disease, frequent miscarriages, and thrombocytopenia.

Venous Thrombosis Venous thrombosis was the first described manifestation of APLA and is the most clinically predominant. Overall, retrospective studies show that 31% of patient with APLA have venous thrombosis. Patients with lupus and APLA have a thrombosis rate of 42%; patients with infectious or drug-induced APLA have a thrombosis rate of less than 5%. Patients with APLA are overrepresented in young patients with deep vein thrombosis. Prospective studies have demonstrated a relative risk for venous thrombosis of 5.3 for patients with IgG anticardiolipin antibodies. Patients with APLA-associated venous thrombosis may be difficult to

Table 19.2 Clinical syndromes

Venous thrombosis
Lower extremity
Cerebral vein thrombosis
Neurologic disease
Strokes
Dementia
Choreiform movements
Pregnancy complications
Second trimester miscarriages
HELLP syndrome
Thrombocytopenia
Adrenal insufficiency
Hypoprothrombinemia
Cardiac valve damage
Skin disease
Livedo reticularis
Livedo vasculitis
Superficial thrombophlebitis

treat. These patients have high rates of recurrent thrombosis (20–50% per year) if anticoagulation is stopped. Occasional patients may be refractory to warfarin and will need to be on long-term low molecular weight therapy.

Neurological Disease APLAs have been associated with stroke, especially in younger patients. A variety of other neurological disorders have been associated with APLA. The underlying cause of these disorders appears to be thrombosis. Some patients have large vessel disease while more often, patients have small vessel involvement. Patients with APLA often will have multiple MRI abnormalities consistent with small white matter infarcts. The neurological diseases include:

- *Stroke.* APLA is found in 10–46% of young patients with stroke and in 10% of stroke patients overall. Stroke patients with APLA tend to be younger (42 years vs 62 years). These patients also have a recurrence rate of 6–30% per year and a mortality rate of 10% per year. Certain groups of patients appear to be at even higher risk of recurrence. These would include SLE patients with APLA and patients with Sneddon's syndrome (described below).
- *Early-Onset Dementia.* This is becoming a well-recognized and feared feature of

APLA. The dementia is multi-infarct in nature and occurs often without a history of major stroke episodes. APLA-related dementia on the average occurs a decade earlier (average age 52 years) than non-APLA dementia. Sneddon's syndrome is a combination of livedo reticularis and cerebral ischemic events. Sneddon's syndrome is a form of APLA which often results in major morbidity and mortality. The skin involvement in Sneddon's may be severe enough to result in ulceration. Patients with Sneddon's syndrome seem also to have a high incidence of thrombocytopenia.

- *Ocular Events.* Amaurosis fugax, retinal artery thrombosis, and retinal vein thrombosis have been reported as part of APLA syndrome in multiple case reports.
- *Others.* APLA are found in as many as 50% of patients who get migraines. As will be discussed below, patients may have encephalopathy as part of severe APLA. Rare patients with choreiform movements with APLA have been reported; the movement disorder resolves with anticoagulation

Fetal Loss Fetal loss is seen in 38% of SLE patients with APLA. The incidence of fetal loss in non-SLE APLA is controversial. When women who have suffered recurrent fetal loss are screened, the incidence of APLA is 30%. The pathophysiology is thought to be placental microthrombosis. The incidence of HELLP syndrome is higher in these patients and tends to occur earlier in the pregnancy. Fetal growth retardation is also common due to placental infarctions.

Thrombocytopenia Certain APLA will react with activated platelets, leading to thrombocytopenia. Only activated platelets expose the proper phospholipid epitopes that react with the APLA. Therefore, it is the patients with the thrombotic manifestations of APLA who will also get the thrombocytopenia. The treatment of these patients is clinically challenging since the thrombocytopenia often occurs in patients who are anticoagulated for thrombosis. Danazol was used in the past and appeared to be uniquely effective for these patients;

recently, the use of rituximab to treat these patients is seen more frequently.

Hypoprothrombinemia Patients with APLA (almost always those with lupus inhibitors) may have an elevated prothrombin time (INR) for two reasons. The APLAs may be present in such high titers that they will also interfere with the PT/INR test. Alternatively, 10% of patients with lupus inhibitors will develop non-neutralizing antibodies to prothrombin. This leads to increased clearance of prothrombin from the plasma and hypoprothrombinemia. Since patients with hypoprothrombinemia can present with hemorrhagic complications, it is important to check for this when faced with an APLA patient with an elevated PT/INR. The workup includes a 50:50 mix on the PT and a measure of the plasma level of prothrombin. If the INR is due to the APLA, it will not correct on a 50:50 mix. If there is an antibody to prothrombin, the 50:50 mix corrects as the mechanism of action of the antibody is to speed degradation of prothrombin but not inhibit its activity. Plasma infusions and steroids are effective in raising the prothrombin level in patients with prothrombin antibodies.

Other Associated Diseases Patients with APLA may have an assortment of skin findings included livedo reticularis, Raynaud's phenomenon, ulcers, and superficial thrombophlebitis. Up to 26% of patients with SLE and APLA have cardiac valve vegetations and mitral regurgitation. Rarely, patients have valve destruction so extensive that it requires valve replacement. Myocardial dysfunction is seen in 5% of SLE-APLA patients. Primary pulmonary hypertension has been associated with APLA. Ten percent of patients with chronic thromboembolic pulmonary hypertension have APLA. Adrenal insufficiency from microvascular thrombosis has also been seen in APLA patients.

Catastrophic APLA (CAPS)

Rarely, patients with antiphospholipid antibody syndrome can present with fulminant multiorgan

Table 19.3 Catastrophic antiphospholipid antibody syndrome (CAPS)

Cardiac disease: cardiomyopathy
Pulmonary disease: pulmonary hemorrhage, ARDS
Neurologic disease: seizures, coma, encephalopathy
Renal disease: renal failure due to thrombosis
Skin disease: livedo reticularis, skin necrosis
Bone: necrosis
Severe thrombocytopenia

Table 19.4 APLA diagnosis

Anticardiolipin antibodies (>40 MPL or GPL)
Or
Anti-beta2-glycoprotein antibodies (>99th percentile)
Or
Demonstration of lupus inhibitor
Principles of demonstrating lupus inhibitor:
Prolongation of coagulation-based test
Failure of correction in 50:50 mix
Correction of abnormal test with addition of phospholipid
Coagulation-based tests for lupus inhibitor:
Dilute Russell viper venom time
Hexagonal phospholipid assay

system failure. CAPS is caused by widespread microthrombi in multiple vascular fields. These patients will develop renal failure, encephalopathy, adult respiratory distress syndrome (often with pulmonary hemorrhage), heart failure, dramatic livedo reticularis, and worsening thrombocytopenia (Table 19.3). Many of these patients have pre-existing autoimmune disorders and high titers of anticardiolipin antibodies.

It appears that the best therapy for these patients is aggressive immunosuppression with plasmapheresis and then (perhaps) IV cyclophosphamide monthly or rituximab. Early recognition of this syndrome can lead to rapid therapy and resolution of the multiorgan system failure.

Diagnostic Approach to APLA

As reviewed extensively in Chap. 2, there is unfortunately no one screening test for APLA. (Table 19.4) One must perform the entire diagnostic panel on patients suspected of having APLA. A good screen is to perform all of the following: (1) anticardiolipin antibodies, (2) anti-beta2-glycoprotein, and (3) lupus inhibitor screens – at least two different coagulation tests such as dilute Russell viper venom time and hexagonal phospholipid assay.

There are many confounding factors when testing for APLA. One is that there is a high rate of false positives with acute thrombosis – especially of lupus inhibitors. Most patients who have only an isolated positive lupus inhibitor at the time of diagnosis will on repeat testing have negative testing. Secondly, many patients will have low titers on these tests, especially anticardiolipin assays, so only titers >99th percentile or

anticardiolipin antibody titers >40 units are significant.

Currently, the *Sydney criteria* are used to diagnose APLA syndrome – this requires both clinical and laboratory findings:

- Clinical: one or more episodes of arterial, venous, or small vessel thrombosis (other than superficial thrombophlebitis) or pregnancy complications – either three or more miscarriages before 10 weeks, one or more fetal death after 10 weeks, or premature birth before 34 weeks due to preeclampsia
- Laboratory: one or more positive tests which are repeatedly positive when tested again in at least 12 weeks:
  - Lupus inhibitor
  - Anticardiolipin antibody – greater than either 99th percentile or greater than 40 MPL or GPL units
  - Anti-beta2-glycoprotein – greater than 99th percentile

Triple-positive patients are those with all three tests positive. These patients appear to be at high risk for thrombosis and are at higher risk of "breaking through" warfarin.

Occasional patients are seen who consistently have negative laboratory testing for APLA but have many of the clinical features of APLA such as thrombocytopenia, thrombosis, and miscarriages. It is probable that these patients do have "APLA-negative APLA syndrome," and they should be treated as such.

Table 19.5 APLA therapy

Venous or arterial thrombosis: warfarin with target INR 2.0–3.0

    Controversial: warfarin 3.0–4.0 for arterial disease or adding an aspirin

Warfarin-refractory cases: enoxaparin 1 mg/kg every 12 hours

DOACs contraindicated in "triple-positive" disease

Pregnancy

  History of thrombosis: enoxaparin 1 mg/kg every 12 hours

  No thrombosis: enoxaparin 40 mg/day + asa

Complications

  Thrombocytopenia:

    Short term: prednisone 60 mg/day ± immunoglobulin or anti-D

    Long term: danazol 200 mg po qid or rituximab

  Hypoprothrombinemia: prednisone 60 mg/day

  Catastrophic APLA syndrome:

    Plasma exchange

    Cyclophosphamide 1 gram/meter^2 IV every 28 days or rituximab

Therapy

Although there are few prospective trials of therapy in APLA, several lessons may be learned from retrospective studies (Table 19.5). While APLA does appear to be an autoimmune disease, immunosuppression does not prevent recurrent thrombosis, fetal loss, or neurological syndromes. Therefore, immunosuppression should not play a role in the therapy of thrombotic APLA. The only exception to this is "catastrophic APLA" where plasmapheresis and immunosuppression play a crucial role.

It used to be thought that anticoagulation with warfarin to an INR of 3.0–3.5 was effective in patients with APLA. However, randomized trials demonstrated that an INR range of 2.0–3.0 is just as effective as the higher INR range, especially for venous disease. Some still recommend INR 3–4 for arterial disease or adding an aspirin, but this remains controversial. Also controversial is stroke treatment as some studies indicate aspirin alone may be effective. For patients with major stroke or who are triple positive, warfarin is indicated. Patients with minor events and just one test positive may benefit from either warfarin or anti-

platelet therapy. For patients with thrombosis despite warfarin, the next choice is LMWH.

The role of direct oral anticoagulants (DOACs) is unclear. A clinical trial showed the use of DOAC was inferior to warfarin in "triple-positive" APLA. For patients with "single positive" testing, DOAC may be an option if there are issues with warfarin.

There are observational data that the use of hydroxychloroquine may prevent thrombosis and its use should be considered in patients with lupus or other autoimmune disease. Statins may also be protective and should be used in patients with APLA who otherwise meet criteria for statin use.

Thrombocytopenia Thrombocytopenia in patients with APLA occurs in those patients prone to thrombosis due to activated platelets expressing the epitopes for APLA. The low platelet counts make anticoagulation hazardous. In addition, patients with APLA are often high surgical risks. Thrombocytopenia may respond to steroids, immunoglobulin, and IV-anti-D. Danazol 200 mg po qid is effective in many patients with APLA-related thrombocytopenia as well as in treating with rituximab.

Pregnancy and APLA The approach is based on previous history. If there is a history of thrombosis, LMW heparin in therapeutic doses is used throughout the pregnancy. For frequent miscarriages, prophylactic doses of LMWH are used along with 81 mg of aspirin.

Difficulties in Monitoring Anticoagulation

Since APLA react with phospholipids, both the aPTT and the PT can be affected. If standard heparin is used to anticoagulate patients with APLA, treatment must be followed by monitoring heparin levels (target range 0.35–0.70 anti-Xa). The predictable dosing and anticoagulant effect is one advantage of using LMW heparin acutely for thrombosis in APLA patients. One should measure LMW heparin levels in patients with APLA on long-term therapy (goal is 0.5–1.1 anti-Xa units 4 hours after injection) or in those patients with renal failure.

Often patients with APLA will have minor elevations of PT/INR. Those few patients with elevated INR due to a lupus inhibitor can be very difficult to manage with warfarin. One option is to measure levels of factor X via a chromogenic assay (not affected by APLA). The therapeutic range of 15–30% has been shown to best correlate with therapeutic warfarin effect. Pairing factor X levels with INR, one can determine an INR range that is effective.

One difficult issue is that of the patient with APLA with no thrombotic manifestations. Although some of these patients are at risk, especially those with SLE, many will never develop thrombosis. The current recommendation would be to search thoroughly for thrombosis. The workup would include a brain MRI in patients with SLE or in patients with any neurological symptoms. If this workup is negative for prior thrombosis, then the patient is followed very closely. The only trial of aspirin for primary prophylaxis in APLA was negative.

Suggested Reading

Arachchillage DRJ, Laffan M. Pathogenesis and management of antiphospholipid syndrome. Br J Haematol. 2017;178(2):181–95.

Cervera R, Rodríguez-Pintó I, Espinosa G. The diagnosis and clinical management of the catastrophic antiphospholipid syndrome: a comprehensive review. J Autoimmun. 2018;92:1–11.

Garcia D, Erkan D. Diagnosis and management of the antiphospholipid syndrome. N Engl J Med. 2018;378(21):2010–21.

Pengo V, Denas G, Zoppellaro G, Jose SP, Hoxha A, Ruffatti A, Andreoli L, Tincani A, Cenci C, Prisco D, Fierro T, Gresele P, Cafolla A, De Micheli V, Ghirarduzzi A, Tosetto A, Falanga A, Martinelli I, Testa S, Barcellona D, Gerosa M, Banzato A. Rivaroxaban vs warfarin in high-risk patients with antiphospholipid syndrome. Blood. 2018;132(13):1365–71.

Schreiber K, Sciascia S, de Groot PG, Devreese K, Jacobsen S, Ruiz-Irastorza G, Salmon JE, Shoenfeld Y, Shovman O, Hunt BJ. Antiphospholipid syndrome. Nat Rev Dis Primers. 2018;4:17103.

Antithrombotic Therapy for Cardiac Disease

Joseph Shatzel

Cardiac Disease

Antithrombotic therapy is used for two major purposes in the treatment of cardiac disease. The first is the prevention of embolic disease in those with atrial fibrillation, mechanical heart valves, and ventricular assist devices; the other is for treatment or secondary prevention of ischemic heart disease (Table 20.1).

Ischemic Heart Disease

The underlying pathogenesis of ischemic heart disease is the gradual development of an atherosclerotic plaque. Patients develop clinical symptoms either through diminution of blood flow through a stenotic vessel or with acute ischemia due to thrombus formation on a ruptured plaque. The realization that acute thrombus formation underlies most acute presentations of ischemic heart disease is the driving idea behind the aggressive use of antithrombotic therapy for cardiac disease.

Primary Prevention

The long-held beliefs surrounding the benefit of aspirin for primary prevention have been challenged by recent trials examining healthy older individuals where benefits were not seen and in diabetic patients where increased bleeding mostly negated any benefit. Potential cancer prevention benefits have recently been challenged as well. The side effects of gastrointestinal bleeding and, more importantly, intracranial hemorrhage occur more frequently with aspirin use. More recent guidelines from the AHA reserve the use of aspirin for primary prevention to individuals with significant cardiovascular risk or known atherosclerotic disease.

Stable Angina

Patients with stable angina or with clinical evidence of coronary artery disease should receive aspirin 81 mg/day indefinitely. Clopidogrel 75 mg/day can be substituted in aspirin-intolerant patients.

Recently, the combination of low-dose rivaroxaban and aspirin has been approved for secondary prevention in patients with stable cardiovascular disease. Rivaroxaban (2.5 mg twice daily) plus aspirin resulted in better cardiovascular outcomes and more major bleeding events than aspirin alone in the trial leading to FDA approval for this indication.

J. Shatzel (✉)
Division of Hematology/Medical Oncology, Department of Medicine and Biomedical Engineering, Oregon Health & Sciences University, Portland, OR, USA
e-mail: shatzel@ohsu.edu

© Springer Nature Switzerland AG 2019
T. G. DeLoughery (ed.), *Hemostasis and Thrombosis*,
https://doi.org/10.1007/978-3-030-19330-0_20

Table 20.1 Therapy of ischemic heart syndromes

Primary prevention
  In high-risk patients: aspirin 75–100 mg/day
Stable angina
  Aspirin 75–100 mg/day or clopidogrel 75 mg/day
Unstable angina/NSTEMI
  Aspirin 160–325 mg initially and then 75–160 mg/day and
  P2Y12 antagonist
    Clopidogrel 600 mg and then 75 mg/day
    Prasugrel 60 mg and then 10 mg/day
    Ticagrelor 180 mg and then 90 mg
  Anticoagulation
    Enoxaparin, 30 mg loading dose followed by 1 mg/kg every 12 hours
    Unfractionated heparin, 60 IU/kg loading dose (max 4000 IU) followed by 12 IU/kg/h (max 1000 IU/h) with an aPTT target of 50–70 seconds (1.5–2 times control)
    Fondaparinux, 2.5 mg daily
    Bivalirudin, 0.10 mg/kg loading dose followed by 0.25 mg/kg/h (early invasive strategy only)
STEMI
Aspirin plus P2Y12 antagonist
PCI if available in <120 minutes
Thrombolytic therapy in patients with symptom onset <12 hours unable to receive timely PCI:
  Streptokinase – 1.5 million units IV over one hour
  tPA – 15 mg/kg bolus, 0.75 mg/kg over 30 minutes, then 0.5 mg/kg over next hour
  Reteplase – two 10-unit boluses 30 minutes apart
  Tenecteplase – is weight-based bolus over 5 seconds
    <60 kg = 30 mg
    60–69 kg = 35 mg
    70–79 kg = 40 mg
    80–89 kg = 45 mg
    >90 kg = 50 mg
Adjunctive therapy to thrombolytic therapy (to be continued for at least 48 hours or until PCI can be undertaken):
  tPA, reteplase, tenecteplase – heparin 75 units/kg bolus with start of tPA and 1000 units/h maintenance, adjusted to keep aPTT 1.5–2.0 times control *or* enoxaparin 30 mg IV and then 1 mg/kg every 12 hours
  SK – heparin 1000 units/h maintenance, adjusted to keep aPTT 1.5–2.0 times control starting 1–3 hours after SK

Non-ST Elevation MI (NSTEMI)

All patients with unstable angina or NSTEMI should receive aspirin 160–325 mg as soon as possible, and a dose of 75–100 mg daily should be continued indefinitely. Also, for true NSTEMI, a P2Y12 antagonist (clopidogrel, prasugrel, ticagrelor) should be considered as there are both short- and long-term (up to a year) benefits to dual antiplatelet therapy (DAPT) in acute coronary syndromes. If percutaneous coronary intervention (PCI) with placement of a bare metal stent (BMS) or drug-eluting stent (DES) is undertaken, DAPT is mandated for a period of time (as discussed in a later section of this chapter). In addition, in the acute setting all patients should receive anticoagulation therapy either with unfractionated heparin, LMWH, fondaparinux, or bivalirudin. For patients who are to undergo interventions, many cardiologists prefer unfractionated heparin as initial antithrombotic therapy; LMWH and bivalirudin are other choices. Fondaparinux is another choice, often reserved patients not destined for intervention, especially those at higher risk of bleeding. For patient receiving unfractionated heparin, most data are for using a recommended aPTT target of 50–70 seconds (1.5–2 times control) as bleeding and outcomes are worse with higher aPTTs.

With the advent of aggressive use of P2Y12 antagonists, GP IIb/IIIa inhibitors (abciximab, eptifibatide, and tirofiban) are being used less often. For high-risk patients (ST changes, positive troponins, previous infarct) scheduled for interventions, the use of GP IIb/IIIa inhibitors is rarely considered. During PCI, GP IIb/IIIa inhibitors may also be used as a bridge to oral P2Y12 antagonists.

Current recommendations for anticoagulation options from the American Heart Association/American College of Cardiology are listed below:

- *Enoxaparin*, 30 mg loading dose followed by 1 mg/kg every 12 hours
- *Unfractionated heparin*, 60 IU/kg loading dose (max 4000 IU) followed by 12 IU/kg/h (max 1000 IU/h) with an aPTT target of 50–70 seconds (1.5–2 times control)
- *Fondaparinux*, 2.5 mg daily
- *Bivalirudin*, 0.10 mg/kg loading dose followed by 0.25 mg/kg/h (early invasive strategy only)

Acute Myocardial Infarction: Acute Therapy

The patient who presents with suspicious chest pain needs to be rapidly evaluated for myocardial ischemia. Patients with evolving myocardial infarctions, particularly if ST elevations are present on electrocardiogram (STEMI), require rapid therapy to reopen the occluded coronary artery. Currently the treatment of choice is for percutaneous coronary intervention (PCI) as rapidly as possible to open the occluded vessel. Patients who cannot receive PCI in a timely manner – symptom onset within 12 hours and cannot receive PCI within 120 minutes – should be treated with thrombolytic therapy.

As with patients with NSTEMI/unstable angina, DAPT starting with a 162–325 mg of chewable aspirin should be started immediately. For patients going to PCI, a loading dose of P2Y12 antagonists – clopidogrel 600 mg, prasugrel 60 mg, or ticagrelor 180 mg – should be used to achieve maximal platelet inhibition before the procedure. Again, the use of GP IIb/IIIa inhibitor remains unsettled in the P2Y12 antagonists' age, and they may be considered during the PCI or in patients undergoing complex interventions.

Unfractionated heparin remains the preferred choice of antithrombotic therapy, with bivalirudin or LMWH as alternative agents.

Thrombolytic Therapy

Thrombolytic therapy reduces in-hospital mortality and increases 1-year survival in patients suffering from STEMI and is the therapy of choice if the patient cannot receive timely PCI.

Trials showing the benefits of thrombolytic therapy used these criteria to predict evolving STEMI: at least one-half hour of ischemic chest pain and either at least 1 mm ST elevation in two adjacent limb leads or 1–2 mm ST elevation in two adjacent precordial leads. Patients with pain and complete bundle branch block also showed benefit from thrombolytic therapy. Patients with pain and ST depression or a normal ECG do *not* benefit from thrombolysis. Thrombolytic therapy

should be started as soon as possible up to 12 hours from onset of STEMI. Thrombolytic therapy may be beneficial up to 24 hours after onset of STEMI in selected patients (i.e., ongoing pain without full evolution of Q waves). Patients with anterior MIs, those over 70 years of age and those with previous MI, have a higher mortality with STEMI and should be strongly considered for thrombolytic therapy (if immediate PCI is not available).

Choice of Drug and Dosing

The agents and recommended dosages:

- *Streptokinase* – 1.5 million units IV over one hour. Slightly less effective than tPA and potential for allergic reactions.
- *tPA* – 15 mg/kg bolus, 0.75 mg/kg over 30 minutes, then 0.5 mg/kg over next hour.
- *Reteplase* – two 10-unit boluses 30 minutes apart. Similar outcomes but easier to be given than tPA.
- *Tenecteplase* – weight-based (see table) and given as a bolus over 5 seconds. Most used thrombolytic therapy due to ease of use and slight decrease in bleeding complications.

Adjuvant Therapy to Thrombolytic Therapy

As noted above, all patients should receive DAPT. In addition, to preserve patency all patients who received thrombolytic therapy and who do not undergo PCI should receive antithrombotic therapy for a minimum of 48 hours or until reperfusion can be performed. Choices include:

- *Enoxaparin*, 30 mg loading dose followed by 1 mg/kg every 12 hours
- *Unfractionated heparin*, 60 IU/kg loading dose (max 4000 IU) followed by 12 IU/kg/h (max 1000 IU/h) to maintain an aPTT 1.5–2 times control
- *Fondaparinux*, 2.5 mg daily

Table 20.2 Acute myocardial infarction: indications for anticoagulation therapy

1. Mural thrombus on echocardiography
2. Atrial fibrillation (indefinite anticoagulation)
3. New-onset venous thrombosis
4. Anterior Q-wave infarction with high risk of mural thrombus (ejection fraction <40%, with significant wall motional abnormalities) (controversial)

STEMI: Long-Term Antithrombotic Therapy

Patients suffering from STEMI are at risk for a variety of thrombotic complications ranging from reinfarction to stroke. Therefore, some patients suffering from STEMI should be considered for anticoagulation (Table 20.2).

The following groups of patients specifically should be considered for therapeutic heparin or LMW heparin followed by warfarin (INR 2.0–3.0) or a DOAC for 1–3 months:

1. Mural thrombus on echocardiography
2. Atrial fibrillation (indefinite anticoagulation)
3. New-onset venous thrombosis
4. Anterior Q-wave infarction with high risk of mural thrombus (ejection fraction <40%, with significant wall motional abnormalities) (controversial)

Other patients should receive subcutaneous heparin 7500 units BID or prophylactic dose LMW heparin daily for either 7 days or until fully ambulatory.

In STEMI patients treated with medical therapy alone, a year of DAPT should be considered. Aspirin should be continued at 81 mg indefinitely. Clopidogrel may be considered in patients who cannot receive aspirin. Patients who undergo PCI with coronary stent placement should be treated as below based on the type of stent selected.

CABG

Aspirin 325 mg/day, started 6 hours after surgery, reduces the rate of graft closure and is recommended.

Coronary Stenting

Coronary stenting revolutionized PCI with outcomes showing improved long-term vessel patency. Currently there are two types of stents: "bare metal" (BMS) and "drug eluting" (DES). DES are impregnated with agents that inhibit cellular proliferation and vessel restenosis. The trade-off of DES is impaired healing of the antithrombotic endothelial cell layer and longer period of risk for stent thrombosis. The risk of stent thrombosis is highest for BMS in the first month after placement. DAPT has been shown to be effective at reducing the risk of stent thrombosis. This is important as stent thrombosis can be devastating, with risk of myocardial infarction of greater than 50% and death of 10–25%.

For BMS, dual antiplatelet therapy needs to continue for at least 1 month and for patients at low risk of bleeding for 1 year. For DES, the DAPT should ideally be continued for 1 year, although modern guidelines recommend tailoring the length of therapy to the patient's individual risks. For patients at very high risk of bleeding, consideration can be given to stopping DAPT after 6 months. DAPT for longer than 1 year can be considered for patients with history of stent thrombosis or at very high risk of stent complications – difficult coronary anatomy, multiple stents, or very proximal stent placement.

For the high-risk periods, DAPT should not be interrupted unless absolutely necessary. Elective procedures should be delayed, and for minor procedures (dental work, etc.) dual therapy should be continued. It is unclear whether GP IIb/IIIa inhibitors can "bridge" P2Y12 antagonists if they need to stop before major surgery. Cangrelor, which is an IV P2Y12 antagonist with short half-life of 3–5 minutes, may also be an option.

Stents and Anticoagulation

The management of patients with coronary stents who require anticoagulation is difficult as the use of "triple therapy" is associated with a 3–4-fold increase in the risk of serious bleeding. Recently, several trials (one with warfarin and three with DOACs) have compared triple therapy to "dual therapy" with P2Y12 antagonists + anticoagulation. Dual therapy universally leads to less bleeding without apparent compromise to protection from ischemic events. Although these trials were not powered for efficacy, the fact that numerical ischemic events appear similar, and at least one trial reports non-inferiority, has led to the more routine use of dual therapy. For atrial fibrillation patients who need a stent, a basic principle is to consider a bare metal stent if possible to limit the required time on DAPT.

Evaluation of the Young Patient with Acute Myocardial Infarction

Myocardial infarction in men under age 40 and women under age 50 is unusual. Myocardial infarction at these young ages can be due to reasons other than atherosclerosis. The most common other reasons are embolic occlusion, congenital defects in the coronary arteries, and vasculitis.

Unless the etiology is obvious, young patients with acute myocardial infarction should undergo coronary angiography to determine their coronary anatomy. Embolic occlusion of coronary arteries is common in patients with endocarditis and in under-anticoagulated patients with mechanical heart valves.

Patients with premature myocardial infarctions should be considered for a limited evaluation for hypercoagulable states. There is no evidence that deficiency of protein S, protein C, and antithrombin or the presence of the factor V Leiden mutation increases risk of MI or stroke. Patients should be evaluated for the presence of antiphospholipid antibodies and undergo a full lipid profile, and, given the association with premature atherosclerosis, levels of lipoprotein (a) may be considered. Workup for myeloproliferative neoplasms should be considered on an individualized basis.

Therapy is uncertain. Patients with an embolic source (unless due to endocarditis) should probably receive full anticoagulation with warfarin or a DOAC. Patients with premature atherosclerosis should undergo aggressive anti-lipid therapy and should be placed on antiplatelet therapy

Prevention of Embolism

Atrial Fibrillation

Atrial fibrillation is the most common cardiac condition leading to stroke or systemic embolism. The risk of stroke due to embolism in patients with atrial fibrillation varies with risk factors but can be up to 3–7%/year. As will be discussed below, several groups of patients have been identified as being at higher risk for embolism.

Past well-designed studies have clarified the role of anticoagulant therapy. These studies examined stroke prevention in patients with non-valvular atrial fibrillation. The warfarin trials have established the role of warfarin anticoagulation in reducing the risk of stroke from 5%/year down to 1%/year with low rates of hemorrhage; trials of the new direct oral anticoagulants have shown equivalence or superiority of stroke prevention over warfarin, with all showing reduction in major bleeding including intracranial hemorrhage. It is clear from reviewing these studies that anticoagulation is indicated for prevention of embolism in most patients with nonvalvular atrial fibrillation.

Prediction rules exist to risk-stratify patients and help the clinician choose whom to anticoagulate. (Tables 20.3 and 20.4) Data has been pooled from multiple clinical trials to make prediction rules including the initial CHADS2 score and the more current CHA2DS2–VASc score.

Table 20.3 Risk factors for stroke in patients with atrial fibrillation

Clinical risk factors
Hypertension
Recent congestive heart failure
History of embolism
Echocardiographic risk factors
Global LV dysfunction
Left atrial diameter ≥ 2.5 cm/m^2

Derived from data in The Stroke Prevention in Atrial Fibrillation Investigators. Predictors of thromboembolism in atrial fibrillation: echocardiographic features of patients at risk. *Ann Intern Med*. 1992;116:6–12

Table 20.4 CHADS2 and CHA2D2–VASc scoring system

CHADS2: One point each for recent heart failure, hypertension, age >75, and diabetes. Two points assigned for history of stroke

CHADS2 score	Yearly risk of stroke	Therapy
0	1.9	Aspirin
1	2.8	DOAC or warfarin
2	4.0	DOAC or warfarin
3	5.9	DOAC or warfarin
4	8.5	DOAC or warfarin
5	12.5	DOAC or warfarin
6	18.2	DOAC or warfarin

Used with permission: Freeman WD, Aguilar MI. Neurotherapeutics (2011) 8:488

CHA2D2–VASc: One point each for congestive heart failure, hypertension, diabetes, vascular disease, age 65–74, and female gender. Two points for stroke or age ≥75

Score	Yearly risk of stroke	Therapy
0	0	Aspirin
1	0.7	DOAC or warfarin
2	1.9	DOAC or warfarin
3	4.7	DOAC or warfarin
4	2.3	DOAC or warfarin
5	3.9	DOAC or warfarin
6	4.5	DOAC or warfarin
7	10.1	DOAC or warfarin
8	14.2	DOAC or warfarin
9	100	DOAC or warfarin

Used with permission: Nasser M, McCullough PA. (2014) Management of cardiovascular disease in chronic kidney disease. In: Arici M. (eds) *Management of chronic kidney disease.* Springer, Berlin/Heidelberg

CHA2DS2–VASc is better able to define a subgroup of patients at very low risk of stroke – <0.5%. Given the robust data of benefit from anticoagulants, patients with a CHA2D2–VASc score greater than or equal to 2 should be anticoagulated. No anticoagulation is recommended with scores of zero. Patients with a score of one should undergo a risk benefit discussion about the use of anticoagulation.

While aspirin is also a consideration in patients with a CHA2D2–VASc score of 1, it should be noted that trials comparing aspirin to DOACs note roughly similar safety profiles, but aspirin is significantly less effective at stroke prevention. Head to head studies of aspirin vs warfarin also strongly favor warfarin. Unfortunately, despite its docu-mented inferior stroke prevention, aspirin is often given to older patients because it is perceived as safer. The overall data suggest aspirin should not be preferentially used over anticoagulation.

Atrial Fibrillation: Special Situations

Patients with atrial fibrillation undergoing *cardioversion* are at risk for embolism with up to a 5% incidence. Consequently, patients with atrial fibrillation of greater than two days duration should receive warfarin to achieve an INR of 2.0–3.0 or a direct oral anticoagulant for a duration of 3–4 weeks prior to cardioversion. This should allow any thrombus present to organize. Since mechanical activity of the atria may not fully resume until sometime after resumption of normal sinus rhythm, patients should remain anticoagulated for 4 weeks after cardioversion. However patients at high risk of stroke as defined as CHA2D2–VASc score greater than or equal to 2 should consider indefinite anticoagulation. For patients who want faster cardioversion, trans-esophageal echocardiogram can be performed when the patient is on stable anticoagulation and, if no atrial thrombus is seen, can be cardioverted with at least a month of anticoagulation after. If thrombus is seen, then the patients require a month of anticoagulation before reimaging.

Atrial fibrillation in *thyrotoxic heart disease* is associated with a high rate of embolic phenomena. Therefore, these patients should receive warfarin to maintain an INR of 2.0–3.0 or a DOAC until 4 weeks after the resumption of normal sinus rhythm.

Rheumatic Valve Disease

Patients with rheumatic mitral valve disease are at a risk for stroke which may be as high as 20% per year. Thus, patients with rheumatic mitral valve disease should receive warfarin (INR 2.0–3.0) if they have one of the following:

1. History of embolism
2. Chronic or paroxysmal atrial fibrillation

3. Normal sinus rhythm and left atrial diameter >5.5 cm
4. Left atrial thrombus

Patients with recurrent emboli despite warfarin should receive 80–100 mg/day of aspirin in addition to their warfarin. Patients with significant mitral stenosis were generally excluded from major trials of DOACs, and as such warfarin is favored for this indication.

Mechanical Prosthetic Heart Valves

Patients with mechanical heart valves are at extremely high risk for embolization (12–30%/year without anticoagulation) and anticoagulation is strongly recommended (Table 20.5). It does appear that the newer generations of mechanical valves are less thrombogenic than the older ball-cage valves. Also, patients with mechanical aortic valves are at lesser risk of thrombosis than those with mitral valves, particularly in the absence of atrial fibrillation. However, the rates of embolism and valve thrombosis are still not trivial with newer valves and anticoagulation is still recommended.

Patients with mechanical prosthetic valves can be stratified by assessing the type of valve, valve position, and valve number. Using these clinical factors to risk-stratify patients, one can select an antithrombotic strategy:

- Bileaflet valve in aortic position: INR 2–3 with 80–100 mg/day aspirin
- Ball-cage valve: INR 2.5–3.5 with 80–100 mg/day aspirin
- All other valves: INR 2.5–3.5 with 80–100 mg/day aspirin

For all valve types and positions, the addition of antiplatelet therapy is useful for additional protection. The effect of antiplatelet therapy is most important for "high-risk" situations – older valves in the mitral position. The risk of bleeding is increased but is outweighed by the benefit of therapy. The addition of proton-pump inhibitor theory to aspirin will reduce the risk of gastrointestinal bleeding.

DOACs are considered contraindicated for this indication after a clinical trial of dabigatran for stroke prevention in mechanical valves was halted early for both increased stroke and increased bleeding compared to warfarin.

Bioprosthetic Heart Valves

Although the risk is lower, bioprosthetic heart valves still have a definite risk of associated embolization. This is highest immediately after surgery and in patients with bioprosthetic valves who have other risk factors such as atrial fibrillation. Warfarin should be considered for 3 months after implantation of a bioprosthetic valve, followed by aspirin indefinitely. Patients with atrial fibrillation and history of embolism or those with left atrial thrombi should be anticoagulated indefinitely. Newer forms of transcatheter aortic valve replacement (TAVR) require DAPT for 3–6 months followed by aspirin indefinitely.

Table 20.5 Risk stratification and therapy of mechanical valve patients

High risk: treat to INR 2.5–3.5 + ASA 80–100 mg/day
Valve implanted before 1980 (ball in cage or tilting disk valve)
Previous embolism
Vascular disease
Risk of stroke >2%/y on warfarin alone
Valves in the mitral position
Medium risk: INR 2.5–3.5
Low risk: INR 2–3
Bileaflet valve in aortic position without atrial fibrillation
Treatment and risk stratification of bioprosthetic valves
AVR or MVR: INR 2.5–3.5 for 3 months and then ASA
TAVR: DAPT for 3–6 months and then ASA
+ a fib: DOAC or warfarin with an INR 2–3
+ hx embolism or LA thrombus: INR 2.5–3.5 + ASA 80–100 mg/day

Chronic Heart Failure

Patients with left ventricular ejection fractions under 30% associated with global dysfunction appear to have a higher risk of stroke, but the use of warfarin or other antithrombotic agents to prevent stroke remains uncertain and should be guided by other clinical considerations. For example, if the patient has risk factors for coronary artery disease, aspirin would be appropriate. If the patient has atrial fibrillation or previous stroke, anticoagulation would be indicated.

Suggested Reading

January CT, Wann LS, Calkins H, et al. 2019 AHA/ACC/HRS focused update of the 2014 AHA/ACC/HRS guideline for the management of patients with atrial fibrillation: a report of the American College of Cardiology/American Heart Association task force on clinical practice guidelines and the Heart Rhythm Society. Heart Rhythm. 2019.

Larson EA, German DM, Shatzel J, DeLoughery TG. Anticoagulation in the cardiac patient: a concise review. Eur J Haematol. 2019;102(1):3–19.

Levine GN, Bates ER, Bittl JA, et al. 2016 ACC/AHA guideline focused update on duration of dual antiplatelet therapy in patients with coronary artery disease: a report of the American College of Cardiology/American Heart Association Task Force on clinical practice guidelines: an update of the 2011 ACCF/AHA/SCAI guideline for percutaneous coronary intervention, 2011 ACCF/AHA guideline for coronary artery bypass graft surgery, 2012 ACC/AHA/ACP/AATS/PCNA/SCAI/STS guideline for the diagnosis and management of patients with stable ischemic heart disease, 2013 ACCF/AHA guideline for the management of ST-elevation myocardial infarction, 2014 AHA/ACC guideline for the management of patients with non-ST-elevation acute coronary syndromes, and 2014 ACC/AHA guideline on perioperative cardiovascular evaluation and management of patients undergoing noncardiac surgery. Circulation. 2016;134(10):e123-155.

Lip GY. Stroke and bleeding risk assessment in atrial fibrillation: when, how, and why? Eur Heart J. 2013;34(14):1041–9. https://doi.org/10.1093/eurheartj/ehs435. Epub 2012 Dec 20.

Nishimura RA, Otto CM, Bonow RO, et al. 2017 AHA/ACC focused update of the 2014 AHA/ACC guideline for the management of patients with valvular heart disease: a report of the American College of Cardiology/American Heart Association Task Force on clinical practice guidelines. Circulation. 2017;135(25):e1159–95.

Vandvik PO, Lincoff AM, Gore JM, Gutterman DD, Sonnenberg FA, Alonso-Coello P, Akl EA, Lansberg MG, Guyatt GH, Spencer FA. American College of Chest PhysiciansPrimary and secondary prevention of cardiovascular disease: antithrombotic therapy and prevention of thrombosis, 9th ed: American College of Chest Physicians Evidence-Based Clinical Practice Guidelines. Chest. 2012;141(2 Suppl):e637S–68S.

Whitlock RP, Sun JC, Fremes SE, Rubens FD, Teoh KH. American College of Chest Physicians. Antithrombotic and thrombolytic therapy for valvular disease: antithrombotic therapy and prevention of thrombosis, 9th ed: American College of Chest Physicians Evidence-Based Clinical Practice Guidelines. Chest. 2012;141(2 Suppl):e576S–600S. https://doi.org/10.1378/chest.11-2305.

Stroke and Peripheral Vascular Disease

21

Thomas G. DeLoughery

Stroke

Cerebrovascular disease may be caused by atherosclerosis, embolism, or unusual causes such as vasculitis. Most strokes are due to either atherosclerosis or embolism, and discussion here will focus on these causes. However, the clinician must be alert to more unusual causes of stroke in selected cases.

Acute Stroke

The patient with acute neurological defects demands a swift decision as to whether the defect is ischemic in nature and, if so, what therapy should be instituted (Table 21.1). Most patients with symptoms less than 3 hours old are candidates for thrombolytic therapy, and for some this can be extended to 4.5 hours. The use of mechanical thrombectomy can be considered in patients presenting at 6 hours and in some causes out to 24 hours. Evaluation of these patients should be rapid. Patients should undergo imaging to rule out hemorrhage or mass lesion prior to treatment.

T. G. DeLoughery (✉)
Division of Hematology/Medical Oncology,
Department of Medicine, Pathology, and Pediatrics,
Oregon Health & Sciences University,
Portland, OR, USA
e-mail: delought@ohsu.edu

Table 21.1 Antithrombotic therapy of cerebrovascular disease

Acute stroke
Thrombolytic candidates: tPA 0.9 mg/kg (maximum 90 mg), with 10% of the dose given in 1 minute and the rest over 1 hour. Antiplatelet therapy started in 24 hours
No thrombolysis: antiplatelet therapy – for mild to moderate strokes or high risk TIAs, aspirin/ clopidogrel for 21–90 days
Embolic stroke: aspirin for 2 weeks then anticoagulation with warfarin or DOACs. Can consider earlier start in patients with very minor events
Long term: antiplatelet therapy with aspirin, clopidogrel, or extended release dipyridamole combined with aspirin

Evaluation for an underlying systemic process should also be undertaken.

Patients who meet the criteria should be considered for thrombolytic therapy (Table 21.2). Thrombolytic therapy is believed to be associated with an improvement in clinical outcome, but the rate of intracranial hemorrhage is high and patient selection is crucial. Absolute contraindications to thrombolytic therapy include evidence of intracranial hemorrhage, systolic blood pressure greater than 185 mmHg or diastolic greater than 110 mmHg, or active internal bleeding. Patients who undergo thrombolytic therapy should receive tPA 0.9 mg/kg (maximum 90 mg), with 10% of the dose given as a bolus over 1 minute and the rest given over 1 hour. Patients who receive

© Springer Nature Switzerland AG 2019
T. G. DeLoughery (ed.), *Hemostasis and Thrombosis*,
https://doi.org/10.1007/978-3-030-19330-0_21

Table 21.2 Criteria for tPA

Patients must have all the following:
 An ischemic stroke with a clearly defined time of onset
 Age over 18
Absolute contraindications
 Active internal bleeding
 Arterial puncture at a noncompressible site within the previous 7 days
 Brain tumor, vascular malformation, or aneurysm
 CT with large infarct (>1/3 of cerebral hemisphere)
 Current or past intracranial hemorrhage
 Direct oral anticoagulant use with measurable activity
 Glucose concentration below 50 mg/dl or above 400 mg/dl
 Patient on oral anticoagulants with INR >1.7
 Patients on heparin within the previous 48 hours and still with an elevated aPTT
 Platelet count below 100,000
 Prothrombin time higher than 15 seconds
 Rapidly improving or minor symptoms
 Recent brain or spine surgery
 Stroke or serious head trauma within the preceding 3 months
 Symptoms suggestive of subarachnoid hemorrhage
 Systolic blood pressure above 185 mm Hg or diastolic blood pressure above 110 mm Hg
Relative contraindications
 Gastrointestinal hemorrhage or urinary tract hemorrhage within the previous 21 days
 Major surgery in the past 14 days
 Myocardial infarction in past 3 months
 Pregnancy
 Rapidly improving or minor symptoms
Contraindications for thrombolytic therapy at 3–4.5 hours
 Age over 80
 Any oral anticoagulant use
 Diabetes and history of stroke
 NIHSS score over 25

thrombolytic therapy should not receive any other form of anticoagulation, including aspirin, for 24 hours. These patients should be carefully monitored for signs of bleeding.

For patients who present within 24 hours with stroke due to a large anterior artery thrombosis, mechanical thrombectomy should be considered; data show this results in a greater likelihood of less disability from the stroke. Patients presenting at 6 hours should be strongly considered for this procedure and receive thrombolytic therapy if

they are otherwise eligible for it. Those presenting at 6–24 hours who clinically appear to have more neurological deficits than their images suggest are also candidates. Patients who present early with stroke should be treated at or transferred to a center that can perform thrombectomy.

Patients who do *not undergo thrombolytic therapy or thrombectomy* and do not have an obvious embolic source for their stroke should be started on antiplatelet therapy. Two large trials have shown a small but real benefit of aspirin in preventing death or disability. Since patients with stroke also have risk factors for ischemic heart disease, the aspirin will be of benefit for this as well. Patients with mild to moderate disability from stroke should be started on dual antiplatelet therapy with aspirin/clopidogrel for 21–90 days and patients with major stroke should just be on aspirin.

Patients with a history of stroke or TIA should remain on antiplatelet therapy. Aspirin, aspirin combined with sustained release dipyridamole, or clopidogrel have all been shown effective at preventing stroke recurrence.

Patients who clearly have an *embolic source* for their stroke require lifelong anticoagulation, but initiation should be delayed due to increased risk of intracranial hemorrhage acutely. For small events, warfarin or direct oral anticoagulants can be started in a few days, but patients with large infarcts should wait for 2 weeks; covering with aspirin during this wait is prudent.

Dissection of the carotid or cervical artery is a more frequently recognized cause of stroke, especially in younger patients. Rates of new stroke are low (~ 2%) and antiplatelet therapy for at least 3 months is equivalent to anticoagulation in prevention of new strokes.

It is not clear how long the patient who suffers an *intracranial hemorrhage* on warfarin should remain off this drug. Recent data suggest that just 1 week off anticoagulation may be appropriate if the patient has a very strong indication for anticoagulation such as a mechanical valve. One should carefully investigate the circumstances around the time of the bleed to see if there are any reversible factors such as a very high INR. Given the lack of data, treatment should be tailored to the individual patient's circumstances. Several studies have shown that for most patients, restarting anticoagulation is associated with less thrombosis – and even death – after anticoagulation-induced intracranial hemorrhage outweighing the risk of rebleeding.

A frequent cause of morbidity and mortality in the stroke patient is deep venous thrombosis and pulmonary embolism. Stroke patients should receive prophylaxis with low molecular weight heparin, which has been shown to be safe and effective in these patients and does not increase the risk of bleeding.

Transient Ischemic Attacks

Patients with a transient neurological syndrome should be evaluated for the presence of arterial stenosis. Patients with ipsilateral carotid stenosis of over 70% should receive endarterectomy if they are surgical candidates, and patients with stenosis of 50–70% should be considered for surgery if they are at low risk of procedural strokes. For patients with several stenoses but at high risk of surgery or who have difficult surgical anatomy, carotid stenting can be used. All patients with TIA should be started on aspirin 75–100 mg/day. Risk of recurrence can be quantitated by the ABCD2 score (Table 21.3), and patients with a score of 4 or more should receive dual antiplatelet therapy for 21–90 days.

For patients who are intolerant of aspirin or who are aspirin failures, clopidogrel is of benefit. Patients with atherosclerosis should also receive aggressive treatment of risk factors such as smoking cessation, blood pressure control (aiming for less than 140/80), and a goal LDL less than 70.

Patients with Recurrent Strokes

Except for a small effect of aspirin, there is no good strategy for secondary prevention of non-embolic stroke. Patients who fail antiplatelet therapy and suffer a recurrent stroke are often placed on a different agent (i.e., patients who have a second stroke on aspirin are changed to clopidogrel) or to warfarin or direct oral anticoagulants, but there are scant data to guide therapy.

Patent Foramen Ovale and Stroke

Patent foramen ovale (PFO) exists in 20% of normal individuals, and the incidence of PFO in young stroke patients, especially those with idiopathic stroke, may be as high as 60%. Much controversy exists over the value of diagnosing PFO and the approach to management. In general, the PFO is more likely to be a source of embolism if:

- No evidence of atherosclerosis.
- Source of venous thrombosis.
- MRI shows areas of multiple infarcts.
- PFO shows significant shunting.
- Presence of atrial septal aneurysm.

Management options for PFO are to: (1) close the PFO surgically or with catheter devices,

Table 21.3 ABCD2 score

Points	0	1	2
Age	<60	>60	–
Blood pressure	normal	>140/90 mmHg	
Clinical features	No speech disturbances and no unilateral weakness	Speech disturbances	Unilateral weakness
Duration	<10 minutes	10–59 minutes	>60 minutes
Diabetes present	No	Yes	
ABCD2 score	2-day stroke risk (%)	7-day stroke risk	90-day stroke risk
Low (0–3)	1.0	1.2	3.1
Moderate (4–5)	4.1	5.9	9.8
High (6–7)	8.1	11.7	17.8

(2) use aspirin, or (3) use warfarin or other anti-coagulation. For patients younger than 60 with "cryptogenic stroke" (no atrial fibrillation, large vessel disease), closure of the PFO is currently recommended if there is evidence of right to left shunting. Patients are treated with dual antiplatelet therapy for 3 months, then aspirin therapy.

Stroke in Young Patients

Patients under age 50 with a stroke should receive aggressive evaluation (Table 21.4). In younger patients, premature atherosclerosis and embolism are still the two most common causes of stroke. Patients should undergo a transesophageal echocardiogram to look for cardiac abnormalities and vascular imaging to rule out abnormalities such as vasculitis, premature arthrosclerosis, dissection, or other vascular abnormalities. The use of long-term cardiac rhythm monitors has revealed a high incidence of silent atrial fibrillation in "cryptogenic stroke" patients.

Patients with premature strokes should receive a limited evaluation for hypercoagulable states. There is no convincing evidence that the classic thrombophilias such as deficiencies of protein S, protein C, antithrombin, etc., increase risk of stroke. Patients should be evaluated for the presence of antiphospholipid antibodies and have a full lipid profile and a homocysteine level determined. Given the association with premature atherosclerosis, levels of lipoprotein (a) should also be determined.

Children with sickle cell disease are at high risk of stroke and need to be screened with transcranial Doppler; patients with high velocities benefit from an aggressive transfusion program. Any patient with sickle cell disease who has a stroke will need indefinite therapy with transfu-

Table 21.4 Evaluation of the young patient with stroke

Angiogram
Antiphospholipid antibodies
Lipoprotein (a)
Long-term monitoring of heart rhythm
Plasma homocysteine
Transesophageal echocardiogram

sion to reduce and maintain the percentage of sickle hemoglobin to under 30%.

Peripheral Vascular Disease

Acute Ischemia

Patients who present with an acute occlusion of the arterial blood supply due to embolism or with sudden thrombosis of a preexistent atherosclerotic area in a limb require rapid intervention to save the limb. The time window for limb salvage is only 4–6 hours from onset of ischemia. Patients with embolic disease often just require removal of the thrombus, but those with thrombosis and atherosclerosis often require revascularization; therefore, differentiating between these two entities is important in order to formulate therapy. Patients who have embolic occlusion have sudden onset of symptoms and rarely have preexisting symptoms. Often there will be an obvious source of the embolism such as atrial fibrillation. Patients with underlying atherosclerosis will have previous symptoms of peripheral vascular disease.

The presentation of acute ischemia is the classic "five Ps": pain, pallor, paralysis paresthesia, and pulselessness. The affected limb should undergo evaluation to determine the degree of ischemia. Patients with mild weakness and sensory loss but without profound paralysis of the limb need emergent therapy to salvage the limb. The patient should undergo rapid evaluation for systemic disease. Although embolic occlusion can often be diagnosed on clinical grounds, angiography is indicated in many cases to determine the underlying cause by either demonstrating diffuse atherosclerotic disease or a discrete embolism.

Patients with acute ischemia require rapid anticoagulation with heparin. Catheter-based thrombolytic therapy is favored if the limb is viable and ischemia is less than 14 days from onset. tPA and its derivatives reteplase or tenecteplase are preferred, with infusion performed over 24–48 hours. A patient whose limb is reperfused after thrombolytic therapy often requires either angioplasty or surgical revascularization due to the severity of underlying vascular disease. A limb that is immediately threatened should undergo surgical revascularization. This is also the preferred approach to ischemia that has lasted more than 14 days.

Critical ischemia is signaled by rest pain. Pain is worsened by elevating the limb and may be relieved by putting the limb below the level of the heart. Patients most often require surgical revascularization to prevent tissue breakdown. Temporary control of symptoms may be achieved by a several day course of heparin therapy.

Chronic ischemia is by far the most common symptom of peripheral vascular disease, and with proper attention most patients will not progress to surgery. Patients with chronic ischemia due to peripheral vascular disease are at a higher risk of death from all vascular causes. These patients should receive full anti-atherosclerotic therapy, including help with smoking cessation and anti-lipid therapy. Smoking is the major risk factor for peripheral vascular disease and its progression. The other effective therapy is a supervised exercise program. Patients who follow such a program will have improvement of their exercise performance and a prolonged pain-free walking distance.

Blue toe syndrome is a distinct syndrome with the appearance of one or more blue toes. The differential of these lesions is vast (Table 21.5). The first step is to evaluate the patient for underlying diseases. Most causes of blue toe syndrome are associated with an underlying disease process and this can greatly aid in narrowing the differential. An atherosclerotic plaque that is "showering" fibrin-platelet emboli is the most common cause of blue toes in many series. These patients have underlying atherosclerosis and may have unilateral lesions. Patients with cholesterol embolization often (but not always) have an "instigating" event such as recent catheterization that sets off a shower of emboli. These patients also may have livedo reticularis and renal dysfunction. Patients rarely may develop blue toes during the first several weeks of warfarin therapy. This is thought to be due to disruption of plaque surfaces leading to cholesterol embolization.

Table 21.5 Blue toe syndrome (after O'Keefe)

Atheroembolism
Platelet aggregates
Cholesterol crystals
Warfarin-related cholesterol embolism
Cardiac embolism
Infective endocarditis
Non-thrombotic endocarditis
Cardiac myxoma
Atrial fibrillation
Prosthetic valve embolism
Hyperviscosity syndromes
Cryoglobulinemia
Cryofibrinogen
Cold agglutinins
Polycythemia rubra vera
Leukemias
Macroglobulinemia
Hypercoagulable states
Malignancy
Diabetes
Antiphospholipid antibodies
Essential thrombocytosis
Erythromelalgia
Disseminated intravascular coagulation
Deep venous thrombosis
Vasculitis
Microscopic polyarteritis
Classic polyarteritis nodosa
Lupus vasculitis

Therapy is dictated by the underlying disease. Patients with fibrin-platelet embolism often respond to antiplatelet therapy, although definitive therapy of the vascular lesion is often required. Patients with warfarin blue toe syndrome respond to heparin anticoagulation.

Antithrombotic Therapy for Peripheral Vascular Disease

Patients who have limb ischemia due to embolism require anticoagulation with warfarin or a direct oral anticoagulant.

The first line of therapy for all patients with atherosclerotic vascular disease is antiplatelet therapy with either aspirin or clopidogrel. Patients with peripheral vascular disease are at high risk for myocardial infarction and stroke in addition to their peripheral vascular disease, and they will benefit from antiplatelet therapy. Currently, single agent antiplatelet therapy is recommended with the exception of placement of a prosthetic below a knee graft – these patients may benefit from dual antiplatelet therapy for 1 year. When compared to aspirin, warfarin did not improve outcomes, nor did warfarin combined with aspirin. Rivaroxaban combined with aspirin did improve outcomes but at the cost of increased bleeding. This may be an option for high-risk patients or patients with recurrent thrombosis despite aspirin.

Suggested Reading

Farber A. Chronic limb-threatening ischemia. N Engl J Med. 2018;379(2):171–80.

Hankey GJ. Stroke. Lancet. 2017;389(10069):641–54.

Hasan TF, Rabinstein AA, Middlebrooks EH, Haranhalli N, Silliman SL, Meschia JF, Tawk RG. Diagnosis and management of acute ischemic stroke. Mayo Clin Proc. 2018;93(4):523–38.

Kuijpers T, Spencer FA, Siemieniuk RAC, Vandvik PO, Otto CM, Lytvyn L, Mir H, Jin AY, Manja V, Karthikeyan G, Hoendermis E, Martin J, Carballo S, O'Donnell M, Vartdal T, Baxter C, Patrick-Lake B, Scott J, Agoritsas T, Guyatt G. Patent foramen ovale closure, antiplatelet therapy or anticoagulation therapy alone for management of cryptogenic stroke? A clinical practice guideline. BMJ. 2018;362:k2515.

Markus HS, Levi C, King A, Madigan J, Norris J. Cervical Artery Dissection in Stroke Study (CADISS) Investigators. Antiplatelet therapy vs anticoagulation therapy in cervical artery dissection: the Cervical Artery Dissection in Stroke Study (CADISS) randomized clinical trial final results. JAMA Neurol. 2019; https://doi.org/10.1001/jamaneurol.2019.0072. [Epub ahead of print].

McNally MM, Univers J. Acute Limb Ischemia. Surg Clin North Am. 2018;98(5):1081–96.

Morley RL, Sharma A, Horsch AD, Hinchliffe RJ. Peripheral artery disease. BMJ. 2018;360:j5842.

O'Keeffe ST, Woods BO, Breslin DJ, Tsapatsaris NP. Blue toe syndrome. Causes and management. Arch Intern Med. 1992;152(11):2197 202.

Prasad K, Siemieniuk R, Hao Q, Guyatt G, O'Donnell M, Lytvyn L, Heen AF, Agoritsas T, Vandvik PO, Gorthi SP, Fisch L, Jusufovic M, Muller J, Booth B, Horton E, Fraiz A, Siemieniuk J, Fobuzi AC, Katragunta N, Rochwerg B. Dual antiplatelet therapy with aspirin and clopidogrel for acute high risk transient ischaemic attack and minor ischaemic stroke: a clinical practice guideline. BMJ. 2018;363:k5130.

Zerna C, Thomalla G, Campbell BCV, Rha JH, Hill MD. Current practice and future directions in the diagnosis and acute treatment of ischaemic stroke. Lancet. 2018;392(10154):1247–56.

Heparins and Heparin-Induced Thrombocytopenia

22

Thomas G. DeLoughery

Heparin functions as an antithrombotic agent by binding antithrombin (AT) and promoting inactivation of the active serine proteases involved in blood coagulation (factors IIa, VIIa-TF, IXa, Xa, and XIa). Heparin is a blend of saccharide polymers ranging in molecular weight from 3 to 30,000 daltons. A specific pentasaccharide sequence is required for promoting AT activity. This sequence is found in only one-third of the heparin molecules in the heparin currently used. Other polymers found in heparin may have platelet-inhibitory effects or fibrinolytic effects.

The low-molecular-weight heparin (LMW heparin or LMWH) compounds are derived by breaking up either enzymatically or chemically the long heparin chains into smaller fragments. These small chains have greater specific antithrombotic activity and less antiplatelet activity. They also have the virtues of being easier to dose and safer to use. LMW heparin is the treatment of choice over standard heparin for most thrombotic disease.

Given that only a specific five monomer sequence is essential for promotion of antithrombotic activity, synthetic molecules called pentasaccharides which bind to antithrombin and promote its ability to inactivate factor Xa have been developed. Currently, only one – fondaparinux – is in clinical use.

Antithrombotic Use of Standard Heparin

The key to the use of standard heparin is to give enough. The strongest predictor of repeat thrombosis is failure to achieve adequate anticoagulation *at 24 hours*. The bolus should be 5000 units (10,000 for larger thrombi or pulmonary embolism). The initial drip should be *1400* units/h. The traditional regimen of starting with 1000 units/h resulted in woefully inadequate anticoagulation and higher risk of repeat thrombosis in the vast majority of patients. Either anti-Xa levels ("heparin levels") or aPTT can be used to monitor heparin.

If the aPTT is used, it is checked 6 hours after the bolus, and the drip is adjusted accordingly if the aPTT is subtherapeutic. Since a supratherapeutic aPTT may just reflect the bolus, one should never turn down the drip until two consecutive aPTTs are supratherapeutic 6 hours apart. When using standard heparin, one must be very aggressive in rapidly achieving a therapeutic aPTT. Unlike the relationship of subtherapeutic heparin levels to recurrent thrombosis, there is no association between supratherapeutic aPTTs and bleeding. Thus, one should not overreact to high

T. G. DeLoughery (✉)
Division of Hematology/Medical Oncology,
Department of Medicine, Pathology, and Pediatrics,
Oregon Health & Sciences University,
Portland, OR, USA
e-mail: delought@ohsu.edu

© Springer Nature Switzerland AG 2019
T. G. DeLoughery (ed.), *Hemostasis and Thrombosis*,
https://doi.org/10.1007/978-3-030-19330-0_22

aPTT values. Recently, several nomograms have been published for adjusting heparin to achieve therapeutic anticoagulation. If a nomogram is used, it must be calibrated for the particular aPTT reagent used in your lab and not simply copied from a book or article. Therapeutic range varies with different aPTT reagents and must be standardized at each laboratory with heparin levels.

Measuring anti-Xa levels as a reflection of plasma heparin activity is being performed more frequently because these levels are less likely to be influenced by inflammation and allow for more precise titration of heparin infusion.

Duration of therapy with any heparin can be as short as 5 days for patients with deep venous thrombosis, assuming that the patient has been adequately anticoagulated with warfarin at that time for at least 24 hours. Subcutaneous heparin is usually not used for treatment of venous thrombosis; however, there are data that, if dosed as 333 U/kg bolus followed by a fixed dose of 250 U/kg every 12 hours, this is as effective as LMWH for therapy of venous thrombosis.

Standard heparin is also used for prevention of venous thrombosis and given as 5000 units BID or TID. Standard heparin is also used for a variety of other uses, such as in dialysis or cardiac bypass machines, due to its short half-life and provider familiarity.

Antithrombotic Use of Low-Molecular-Weight Heparin

Low-molecular-weight heparins are derivatives of heparin with improved anti-Xa effect and less antiplatelet effect (Tables 22.1 and 22.2). Several trials have shown that the LMW heparins have an improved risk-benefit ratio over regular heparin. Since LMW heparins do not bind to acute phase proteins or endothelial cells, their pharmacokinetics are more predictable than that of standard heparin. For prophylactic use, LMW heparins can be administered once or twice daily without the need for laboratory monitoring. There is now abundant evidence that using LMW heparin for therapy in DVT/PE treatment is both safer and more effective than standard heparin. Evidence is

Table 22.1 Standard heparin vs low-molecular-weight heparin

Standard heparin	Low-molecular-weight heparin
Binds nonspecifically to plasma proteins	Lacks nonspecific binding
Increased plasma half-life with increased dose of drug	Stable plasma half-life
Binds platelet factor 4	Does not bind platelet factor 4
In therapeutic use must follow aPTT	Most patients can be treated without levels
aPTT used to monitor	Need specific plasma levels if levels are deemed necessary
Neutralized by protamine	Only 50% neutralized by protamine
Short half-life	Longer half-life

Table 22.2 Agents and dosing

Heparin
Route of administration: Subcutaneous or intravenous
Prophylactic: 5000 units BID-TID
Therapeutic: Bolus 5–10,000 units followed by 1–2000 units/h to achieve heparin levels of 0.35–0.7 anti-Xa units

Low-molecular-weight heparins
Dalteparin
Prophylactic: 2500 units q day (low risk); 5000 units q day (high-risk abdominal surgery)
Therapy: 100 units/kg every 12 hours or 200 units/kg daily
Enoxaparin
Prophylactic: 40 mg/day or 30 mg every 12 hours (orthopedic indications)
Therapy: 1 mg/kg every 12 hours or 1.5 mg/kg in low-risk patients
Nadroparin
Prophylactic: 2850 units every 24 hours (38 units/kg in high-risk patients)
Therapy: 86 units/kg every 12 hours or 171 units/kg every 24 hours
Tinzaparin
Prophylactic: 3500 units every 24 hours (4500 units in high-risk patients)
Therapy: 175 units every 24 hours

Pentasaccharide
Fondaparinux
Prophylaxis: 2.5 mg every 24 hours
Therapy: 7.5 mg every 24 hours (5.0 mg in patients under 50 kg and 10 mg in patients over 100 kg)

also clear that stable patients with DVT/PE can be treated at home with LMW heparin.

For acute venous thrombosis, LMWH agents are dalteparin, enoxaparin, or tinzaparin. For short courses of therapy, most patients do not need to have LMW heparin levels drawn. Patients who are very obese (>two times ideal body weight), who have severe liver or heart failure, who are pregnant, or who are on long-term LMWH therapy should have levels performed.

LMWH are renally cleared, and the dose needs to be adjusted for renal function. For patients with creatinine clearance between 10 and 30 ml/min, the dose of enoxaparin is 0.65 mg/kg q12 hours, and levels should be followed. In these patients, the dose of enoxaparin should be 1 mg/kg/day. The pharmacokinetics of LMWH are not affected by weight, and there should be no capping or adjusting of doses for overweight patients. Levels are drawn 4 hours after injection, and the therapeutic range for enoxaparin is 0.7–1.2 anti-Xa units.

For treatment of venous thrombosis, the first dose of LMW heparin is given as soon as possible after diagnosis, and warfarin is started the first evening after diagnosis. The second dose of LMWH should be a "transition" to get the patient on an 8 AM and 8 PM dosing schedule. This is derived by multiplying the patient's usual dose of 1 mg/kg by the time of the first dose until the second subtracted from 12. For example, if a 60 kg patient received his first dose at midnight, at 8 AM the patient would get 40 mg and from then on 60 mg every 12 hours. Patients should be followed every day with a visit or phone check. One still needs to overlap LMW heparin and warfarin by 24 hours once the INR is therapeutic. Five days of LMW heparin is also recommended before starting dabigatran or edoxaban if these are to be used for long-term therapy of venous thrombosis.

Antithrombotic Use of Pentasaccharides

Currently only one pentasaccharide – fondaparinux – is on the market. It has been shown to be effective in surgical venous thrombosis prevention and in treatment of venous thrombosis as well as acute coronary syndrome. Prophylactic dosing is 2.5 mg daily. For therapy of venous thrombosis, the dose is 7.5 mg daily (5.0 mg in patients under 50 kg and 10 mg in patients over 100 kg). Dosing for acute coronary syndromes is 2.5 mg daily. Fondaparinux is

highly renally cleared – a prophylactic dose of 1.5 mg daily has been shown to be safe in patients with creatine clearance 50–20 ml/min and is contraindicated in severe renal disease. Also, since the drug is given as a fixed dose, it should not be used in patients weighing under 50 kg for thrombosis treatment or prevention. A final consideration is that the half-life of fondaparinux is 17–21 hours; this drug is not an option if quick dissipation of anticoagulant effect is needed as in bridging therapy before surgery.

Special Problems

Patients with lupus inhibitors who require heparin are difficult to monitor since their aPTTs are already prolonged. One option is to use LMW heparin due to its predictable dosing. The other choice is to directly assay for heparin by measuring its ability to inhibit factor Xa; this assay is insensitive to lupus inhibitors. Therapeutic range for standard heparin is 0.35–0.7 anti-Xa units. Heparin assays are also valuable in patients where an acute-phase inflammatory process may lead to nonspecific heparin binding to inflammatory proteins, resulting in the aPTT not reflecting heparin levels. This can be seen in patients on cyclosporin. In pregnant women, the acute rise in factor VIII may also lead to a misleading aPTT; thus, one should use heparin levels to guide therapy in those patients – even with prophylactic doses of standard heparin.

Pregnant women with prothrombotic states pose a special problem. Pregnancy adds to the thrombotic risk but is an absolute contraindication to warfarin therapy. The use of heparin was once also feared, but now it is clear that heparin can be safely used in pregnancy. There is abundant experience with LMW heparin; it is safe and effective in pregnant women for both prophylaxis and therapy. LMW heparin does not cross the placenta and is associated with less osteoporosis than standard heparin. For therapy, one should follow LMW heparin levels every 4 weeks. Experience shows that levels are more stable than with standard heparin as the pregnancy progresses. For patients who are allergic to any heparin, fondaparinux may be substituted, but less data are available in pregnant women.

Table 22.3 4 T's score for heparin-induced thrombocytopenia

Points	2	1	0
Thrombocytopenia	>50% fall or nadir 20–100,000/ul	30–50% fall or nadir 10–19,000/ul	Fall <30% or nadir do you mean nadir >10,000 instead of <10,000/ul
Timing of platelet fall	Onset day 5–10 of heparin or <1 day if patient recently exposed to heparin	Consistent but not clear records or count falls after day 10	Platelets fall <5 days and no recent (100 days) heparin
Thrombosis	New thrombosis or skin necrosis or systemic reaction with heparin	Progressive or recurrent thrombosis or suspected but not proven thrombosis	None
oTher cause for thrombocytopenia	No	Possible	Definite
Pretest score 6–8 high, 4–5 intermediate, 0–3 low			

Warkentin, Heddle Current Hematology Reports 2:148, 2003
If HIT score is ≥6 *or*
patient has documented new thrombosis on heparin *or*
platelets fall by over 50% for no other reason than heparin exposure,
then stop heparin and substitute argatroban
If HIT score is 4–5, then obtain HIT test. If test positive, stop heparin, and substitute argatroban
If HIT score is 0–3, no need to obtain HIT test

Heparin resistance is where there is an unusually high dose of heparin needed to raise the aPTT or other measures of heparin affect. It often can be seen in patients with intense inflammatory states. High levels of factor VIII can blunt the aPTT response to heparin, while other proteins such as fibrinogen may absorb heparin. In a patient suspected of heparin resistance the first step is to use an anti-Xa level to monitor heparin. If the patient is still resistant then checking an antithrombin level and supplement if very low (< 50%) may help. Finally use of an alternative anticoagulant such as bivalirudin or argatroban may be necessary.

Complications of Heparin

Bleeding Approximately 5% of patients placed on therapeutic heparin will bleed. Some patients appear to be more at risk than others. Patients without risk factors for bleeding have a complication rate of 1%, whereas those with risk factors have rates of bleeding of 10–23%. Risk factors include use of aspirin, age greater than 60, liver disease, and other severe illness (cancer, heart disease). The risk of bleeding is small in patients receiving prophylactic heparin. Multiple double-blind trials have shown no increase in major or fatal bleeding with the use of prophylactic heparin.

Protamine is used to reverse heparin and low-molecular-weight heparin. The dose for heparin reversal is dependent on timing of the last heparin dose. For immediate reversal (30 minutes or less since the last heparin dose), 1 mg of protamine should be given for every 100 units of heparin. A suggested nomogram is given in Table 22.3. One should avoid giving over 50 mg of protamine at one time and ensure that the infusion does not exceed 5 mg/min.

Protamine does not fully reverse low-molecular-weight heparin but does appear to be effective at reducing bleeding. Due to the longer half-life of low-molecular-weight heparin, sometimes a second dose of protamine is required. The dose is 1 mg per 100 units of dalteparin or tinzaparin or 1 mg of protamine per 1 mg of enoxaparin. If the aPTT is prolonged 4 hours later, one-half of the initial dose of protamine should be given. Protamine is not effective for fondaparinux – only rVIIa 90 ug/kg may be effective.

Heparin-Induced Thrombocytopenia (HIT)

HIT occurs due to the formation of antibodies directed against the complex of heparin bonded to platelet factor 4 (PF4) which, in a minority, binds to the FcγRIIA receptor and activates platelets and macrophages. The incidence of HIT is 1–5% with unfractionated heparin use but is less than 1% with low-molecular-weight heparin.

HIT should be suspected when there is a sudden onset of thrombocytopenia – either at least a 50% drop in the platelet count from baseline or the platelet count falling to less than 100,000/uL in a patient receiving heparin in any form. HIT usually occurs 4 days after starting heparin but may occur suddenly in patients with recent (less than 3 months) exposure. A scoring system – the Four Ts – that combines several clinical factors into a scoring system has been validated. One advantage is that patients who score very low (0–3) on this scale are very unlikely to have HIT and can forgo testing and empiric therapy. Another historical clue is a biphasic platelet pattern after cardiac surgery – recovery from the postsurgical thrombocytopenia followed by recurrent thrombocytopenia; this pattern is strongly predictive for HIT.

The diagnosis of HIT can be challenging in the patient who has multiple reasons for being thrombocytopenic. In this situation, the laboratory assay for HIT is essential. Two types of HIT tests exist. One is a platelet aggregation assay where patient plasma, donor platelets, and heparin are added. If added heparin induces platelet aggregation, the test is considered positive. The test is technically demanding but, if performed carefully, can be sensitive and specific. Increasingly, an ELISA assay for the presumed pathogenic anti-PF4 antibodies is being used. This test is very sensitive but in some populations – cardiac surgery and dialysis patients – not specific. While treatment for HIT is mandatory, cardiovascular, dialysis, and vascular surgery patients should have positive anti-PF4 antibody assays confirmed by a serotonin release assay before being permanently labeled as having HIT.

The first step in therapy of HIT consists of stopping all heparin. Low-molecular-weight heparins cross-react with the HIT antibodies, and therefore these agents are also contraindicated. Institution of warfarin therapy alone has been associated with an increased risk of thrombosis and is also contraindicated. For immediate therapy of HIT, several antithrombotic agents are available (Table 22.4).

Argatroban is a synthetic thrombin inhibitor with a short half-life of 40–50 minutes. Dosing is 2 ug/kg/min with the infusion adjusted to keep the aPTT 1.5–3 times normal. One advantage of argatroban is that it is not renally excreted and no dose adjustment is necessary in renal disease. However, argatroban must be used with caution in patients with severe liver disease by giving an initial dose of 0.5 ug/kg/min. Also, metabolism appears to be decreased in patients with multi-organ system failure, and these patients should receive a dose of 1.0 ug/kg.

Table 22.4 Treatment of heparin-induced thrombocytopenia

Argatroban

Therapy: Initial dose of 2 ug/kg/min adjusted to an aPTT of 1.5–3.0 times normal

Reversal: No antidote but half-life is approximately 40 minutes

In severe liver disease (jaundice), dose at 0.5 ug/kg/min adjusted to an aPTT 1.5–3.0 times normal

Multi-organ system failure: 1 ug/kg/min adjusted to aPTT 1.5–3.0 times normal

Post-CABG – 0.5–1 ug/kg/min adjusted to aPTT 1.5–3.0 times normal

Fondaparinux

Prophylaxis: 2.5 mg every 24 hours

Therapy: 7.5 mg every 24 hours (consider 5.0 mg in patients under 50 kg and 10 mg in patients over 100 kg)

Reversal: Protamine ineffective; rVIIa (90ug/kg) may be of use

Bivalirudin

Bolus: 1 mg/kg

Infusion: 0.15 mg/kg/h

Renal adjustment:

    For creatinine clearance of 30–59 ml/min, decrease dose by 20%

    For creatinine clearance of 10–29 ml/min, decrease dose by 60%

    For creatinine clearances less than 10 mg/min, decrease dose by 90%

Direct oral anticoagulant

Apixaban

    10 mg bid × 7 days then 5 mg bid

Rivaroxaban

    15 mg bid × 21 days then 20 mg daily.

Immune globulin

1 gram/kg IV × 2 days

Argatroban prolongs INR, making the initiating of warfarin therapy difficult. Options are:

1. Chromogenic X assay will measure the warfarin-sensitive factor X, and this can be used to adjust warfarin; therapeutic levels are ~15–35%.
2. If the patient is on a drip of 2 ug/kg/min or less, one can simply aim for a PT/INR of more than 4.0 as therapeutic.
3. When the platelets have recovered, change the patient to fondaparinux or a direct oral anticoagulant.

Fondaparinux does not cross-react with HIT antibodies and may be useful for prophylaxis in HIT and, as clinical experience accumulates, for therapy as well. The long half-life of the drug and its renal clearance make it unsuitable for acute therapy in most patients.

Increasingly, the direct oral anticoagulants are being used for HIT. They are clearly suitable for long-term management of HIT patients, and there are more data showing that they can be used in acute management in selected patients. However, patients who may need procedures or have renal impairment should receive argatroban.

Platelet transfusions in the past were felt to be contraindicated, but recent reports have challenged this notion. A prudent approach would be to reserve transfusion for the rare patient with severe thrombocytopenia and life-threatening bleeding.

Some patients, even with alternative anticoagulation, may have persistent thrombocytopenia. Intravenous immune globulin – 1 gram/kg for 1–2 days – has been shown to result in an acute rise in platelet count.

As mentioned above, initiation of warfarin alone has been associated with limb gangrene and should not be started as the sole antithrombotic agent in HIT. In patients receiving specific antithrombin therapy, warfarin can be started with small doses (2–5 mg) once the platelets have recovered. These often-malnourished patients tend to have a dramatic response to warfarin therapy, and excessive anticoagulation can easily occur. One should overlap warfarin and parenteral therapy by 2–3 days as there is evidence patients may do worse with shorter specific antithrombin therapy.

Patients with HIT but without evidence of thrombosis are at a high risk of thrombosis and should be considered for antithrombotic therapy aiming for therapeutic levels. Patients with HIT should also be carefully screened for any thrombosis; this should include obtaining lower extremity dopplers. Patients with HIT who are negative for thrombosis should be anticoagulated for 3 months (unless they are at high risk of bleeding) to prevent thrombosis.

Patients with a history of HIT ideally should never again be exposed to heparin. The only exception is situations such as cardiac bypass where heparin is the anticoagulant of choice. If feasible, one can wait until antibody testing is negative and then use heparin for the surgery. If surgery cannot wait, then alternative anticoagulation can be used as discussed in Chap. 10.

Suggested Reading

Cuker A, Arepally GM, Chong BH, Cines DB, Greinacher A, Gruel Y, Linkins LA, Rodner SB, Selleng S, Warkentin TE, Wex A, Mustafa RA, Morgan RL, Santesso N. American Society of Hematology 2018 guidelines for management of venous thromboembolism: heparin-induced thrombocytopenia. Blood Adv. 2018;2(22):3360–92.

Garcia DA, Baglin TP, Weitz JI, Samama MM, American College of Chest Physicians. Parenteral anticoagulants: Antithrombotic Therapy and Prevention of Thrombosis, 9th ed: American College of Chest Physicians Evidence-Based Clinical Practice Guidelines. Chest. 2012;141(2 Suppl):e24S–43S.

Kearon C, Akl EA, Ornelas J, Blaivas A, Jimenez D, Bounameaux H, Huisman M, King CS, Morris TA, Sood N, Stevens SM, Vintch JRE, Wells P, Woller SC, Moores L. Antithrombotic therapy for VTE disease: CHEST guideline and expert panel report. Chest. 2016;149(2):315–52.

Laposata M, Green D, Van Cott EM, Barrowcliffe TW, Goodnight SH, Sosolik RC. College of American Pathologists Conference XXXI on laboratory monitoring of anticoagulant therapy: the clinical use and laboratory monitoring of low-molecular-weight heparin, danaparoid, hirudin and related compounds, and argatroban. Arch Pathol Lab Med. 1998;122(9):799–807.

Warkentin TE, Pai M, Linkins LA. Direct oral anticoagulants for treatment of HIT: update of Hamilton experience and literature review. Blood. 2017;130(9):1104–13.

Other Parenteral Anticoagulants

23

Thomas G. DeLoughery

Introduction

Although heparin and its derivatives are the most commonly used parenteral anticoagulants, other agents are also used for this purpose. Since clinical trials showed most of these had no major advantages over heparin, use of most of these agents is restricted to patients with heparin-induced thrombocytopenia. The exception is bivalirudin which is also used in some patients with acute coronary syndromes undergoing interventions.

Danaparoid

Danaparoid is a mixture of various glycosaminoglycans that can also promote the anticoagulant activity of antithrombin. Unfortunately, its half-life is 25 hours, there is no antidote, and monitoring must be done by specific danaparoid levels. It is no longer available in the United States but is used in other countries as another option for treatment of heparin-induced thrombocytopenia.

Direct Thrombin Inhibitors

Given thrombin's central part in coagulation, direct inhibition of thrombin is a potent mechanism for achieving anticoagulation. The first thrombin inhibitor, hirudin, was derived from leech saliva, and it is marketed clinically as the agents lepirudin and desirudin. Also currently available are bivalirudin which is a large molecular inhibitor (MW 2180) and argatroban which is a small molecular inhibitor (MW 526).

Thrombin inhibitors share certain properties. They raise both the INR and aPTT since thrombin is part of the common pathway of blood coagulation. Clinically they are monitored by the aPTT, usually aiming for a goal of 2–2.5 times normal control. More precise monitoring can be achieved by using the ecarin time. No effective antidote exists for these agents.

Since all the parenteral thrombin inhibitors prolong the prothrombin time/INR, initiation of warfarin therapy is difficult if patients are receiving these drugs. The chromogenic factor X assay can be used to adjust warfarin therapy. This assay is not affected by the thrombin inhibitor. Warfarin is started at a low dose of 2.5–5 mg/day, and a daily factor X assay is performed. When the factor X assay level is down to 15–30%, the thrombin inhibitor is stopped. If argatroban is used, there is a nomogram in the package insert to guide warfarin therapy doses of 2 ug/kg/min and under are used.

T. G. DeLoughery (✉)
Division of Hematology/Medical Oncology,
Department of Medicine, Pathology, and Pediatrics,
Oregon Health & Sciences University,
Portland, OR, USA
e-mail: delought@ohsu.edu

© Springer Nature Switzerland AG 2019
T. G. DeLoughery (ed.), *Hemostasis and Thrombosis*,
https://doi.org/10.1007/978-3-030-19330-0_23

Argatroban

Argatroban is a synthetic thrombin inhibitor derived from L-arginine that binds only to the thrombin active site. It has a short half-life of 40–50 minutes. The dosing for anticoagulation is 2 ug/kg/min with the infusion adjusted to keep the aPTT 1.5–2.5 times normal. Argatroban can also be used for percutaneous coronary intervention with a bolus of 350 ug/kg being given followed by a continuous infusion of 25 ug/kg/min.

One advantage of argatroban is that it is not renally excreted, and therefore no dosage adjustment is necessary in renal insufficiency or failure. These characteristics make it the most useful agent for patients who require thrombin inhibitors. However, argatroban must be used with caution in patients with severe liver disease. An initial dose of 0.5 ug/kg/min is used and titrated upward guided by the aPTT. For critically ill patients or following major cardiac surgery, starting at a lower dose of 1.0 ug/kg/min is recommended.

Bivalirudin

Bivalirudin is a synthetic thrombin inhibitor that binds to the thrombin active site and also to the substrate binding site. It also has a short half-life of 30 minutes. Its use is best studied for cardiac indication, and it is currently approved for percutaneous cardiac intervention. Bivalirudin is renally excreted, and dosage adjustments should be made for patients with renal insufficiency. Bivalirudin is also used in patients with heparin-induced thrombocytopenia who need cardiac procedures or surgery or who are placed on ECMO (see Chap. 10).

Hirudin

Hirudin is derived from leech saliva. It binds both the active site of thrombin and the substrate binding site. Currently hirudin is made using recombinant technology, and two forms have been developed for clinical use – desirudin and lepirudin.

Although off the market currently, lepirudin was once used for heparin-induced thrombocytopenia. It can be monitored by using the commonly available aPTT. The half-life of lepirudin is short, ~90 minutes, but the drug accumulates in renal insufficiency with the half-life increasing to up to more than 50 hours. Patients with even mild renal insufficiency (creatinine greater than 1.5) must have lepirudin doses adjusted to avoid over-anticoagulation. Up to 80% of patients receiving long-term lepirudin therapy will develop antibodies. These antibodies reduce the metabolism of hirudin *and increase* the therapeutic effect of lepirudin. Patients on long-term (greater than 6 days) lepirudin therapy should still continue to be monitored to avoid over-anticoagulation.

Desirudin is available and approved for use as deep venous thrombosis prophylaxis with a dose of 15 mg sub-q bid. Like lepirudin, the dosing of desirudin is renal-dependent, and adjustment is needed if the creatinine clearance is less than 60 ml/min. Desirudin has also been studied in heparin-induced thrombocytopenia with dosing of 15 mg bid in patients without thrombosis and 30 mg bid for those with clot.

Argatroban

Therapy 2 ug/kg/min infusion with dose adjustments to keep aPTT 1.5–3 times normal.

For patients with severe liver disease, start with 0.5 ug/kg/min infusion, and follow aPTT to same goal of aPTT 1.5–3 times normal.

For PCI

Bolus with 350 ug/kg over 3–5 minutes, and then infuse with a maintenance drip of 25 ug/kg/min adjusting to an ACT of 350–400 minutes.

Bivalirudin

Bolus: 1 mg/kg

Infusion: 2.5 mg/kg/hour for 4 hours and then 0.2 mg/kg/hour for 14–20 hours.

Renal adjustment:

- For creatinine clearance of 30–59 ml/min, decrease dose by 20%
- For creatinine clearance of 10–29 ml/min, decrease dose by 60%
- For creatinine clearances less than 10 mg/min, decrease dose by 90%

Danaparoid

Therapeutic: Bolus of 2250 units (1500 units <60 kg, 3000 units 75–90 kg, 3750 units >90 kg), then a 4-hour infusion of 400 units/hour, then 4 hours of 200 units/hour, then a drip at 150–200 u/h to maintain an anti-Xa level of 0.5–0.8 anti-Xa units.

Desirudin

Prophylaxis: 15 mg BID

- If CrCl 30–60: 5 mg BID – check am aPTT and hold if >2× control
- If CrCl <30: 1.7 mg BID – check am aPTT and hold if >2× control

Hirudin

Therapy Bolus of 0.4 mg/kg followed by 0.15 mg/kg/hour to maintain an aPTT of 1.5–3.0 times normal. Can be omitted if not life- or limb-threatening thrombosis

Adjustments for renal dysfunction:

- For creatinine of 1.6–2.0 mg/dl: Bolus of 0.2 mg/kg followed by a 50% reduction in infusion rate
- For creatinine of 2.0–2.5: Bolus of 0.2 mg/kg followed by a 75% reduction in infusion rate
- For creatinine of 2.6–6.0: Bolus of 0.2 mg/kg followed by a 90% reduction in infusion rate
- For creatinine of greater than 6.0 mg/ml: Bolus of 0.1 mg/kg on alternate days only when the aPTT is less than 1.5 times normal; no continuous infusion

Suggested Reading

Garcia DA, Baglin TP, Weitz JI, Samama MM, American College of Chest Physicians. Parenteral anticoagulants: Antithrombotic Therapy and Prevention of Thrombosis, 9th ed.: American College of Chest Physicians Evidence-Based Clinical Practice Guidelines. Chest. 2012;141(2 Suppl):e24S–43S.

Kelton JG, Arnold DM, Bates SM. Nonheparin anticoagulants for heparin-induced thrombocytopenia. N Engl J Med. 2013;368(8):737–44.

Shah R, Rogers KC, Matin K, Askari R, Rao SV. An updated comprehensive meta-analysis of bivalirudin vs heparin use in primary percutaneous coronary intervention. Am Heart J. 2016;171(1):14–24.

Van Cott EM, Roberts AJ, Dager WE. Laboratory monitoring of parenteral direct thrombin inhibitors. Semin Thromb Hemost. 2017;43(3):270–6.

Direct Oral Anticoagulants

24

Thomas G. DeLoughery

Introduction

The direct oral anticoagulants are drugs that represent a new class of anticoagulants working by directly blocking active coagulation enzymes either thrombin or factor Xa (Table 24.1). All have been shown to have a lesser rate of intracranial hemorrhage in atrial fibrillation patients and all the Xa inhibitors have less bleeding when used as therapy for venous thrombosis.

Table 24.1 Direct oral anticoagulants

Direct thrombin inhibitor
Dabigatran
Pharmacology
Time to maximum concentration: 1–2 hours
Half-life: 12–17 hours
Renal elimination: 80%
Dosing:
Prophylaxis 220 mg or 110 mg dDay
Venous thrombosis treatment: 150 mg bid (acute thrombosis after 5 days parenteral heparin)
Stroke prevention atrial fibrillation: 150 mg bid
Renal clearance: dose reduced to 75 mg bid if CrCl <30 and contraindicated CrCl <15
Affects aPTT – can use to see if patient still has drug effect – 1.5–2 × 0.5–2 hours after dose

T. G. DeLoughery (✉)
Division of Hematology/Medical Oncology,
Department of Medicine, Pathology, and Pediatrics,
Oregon Health & Sciences University,
Portland, OR, USA
e-mail: delought@ohsu.edu

Table 24.1 (continued)

Drug-drug interaction – P-gp inhibitors: Dronedarone, ketoconazole – dose reduced to 75 mg bid or contraindicated if renal impairment. P-gp inducers: rifampin. St. John's wort – contraindicated
Reversal agent: Idarucizumab 5 g IV
Factor Xa inhibitors
Apixaban
Pharmacology
Time to maximum concentration: 3–4 hours
Half-life: 12 hours
Renal elimination: 25%
Dosing
Prophylaxis 2.5 mg bid
Venous thrombosis treatment: Initial treatment for acute thrombosis of 10 mg bid × 7 days and then 5 mg bid, contraindicated if CrCl <25
Stroke prevention atrial fibrillation: 5 mg bid 2.5 mg bid if 2 out of the 3: age over 80, creatine >1.5, weight less than 60 kg – contraindicated with CrCl <15
Drug-drug interaction: CYP 3A4 agents (azole antifungals (except fluconazole) or HIV-protease inhibitors) – reduced dose to 2.5 mg bid
Does not effect INR – use anti-Xa or specific levels to monitor
Reversal agents: PCC 50 units/kg or andexanet 400 mg IV bolus and then 4 mg/min for 120 minutes (if 10 mg apixaban dose within 8 hours, then 800 mg IV bolus followed by 8 mg/min for 120 minutes)
Betrixaban
Pharmacology
Time to maximum concentration: 3–4 hours
Half-life: 19–27 hours
Renal elimination: 20%

(continued)

© Springer Nature Switzerland AG 2019
T. G. DeLoughery (ed.), *Hemostasis and Thrombosis*,
https://doi.org/10.1007/978-3-030-19330-0_24

Table 24.1 (continued)

Dosing
    Prophylaxis: First day 180 mg, then 80 mg daily for
    35–42 days

Drug-drug interaction: P-gp inhibitors – cut dose by
50%

Does not affect INR/aPTT – use anti-Xa or specific
levels to monitor

Reversal: PCC 50 units/kg

Edoxaban

Dosing
    Prevention: 15 mg/day
    Thrombosis therapy: 60 mg/day or 30 mg/day if
    weight <60 kg, CrCl 30–60, or on strong P-gp
    inhibitors
    Stroke prevention in atrial fibrillation: 60 mg/day or
    30 mg/day if weight <60 kg, CrCl 30–60, or on
    strong P-gp inhibitors

Drug-drug interactions: dose reduced 50% – verapamil,
quinidine, erythromycin, azithromycin, clarithromycin,
ketoconazole, or itraconazole. Contraindicated –
protease inhibitors and cyclosporine

Affects INR – use anti-Xa or specific levels to monitor

No specific antidote: PCC 50 units/kg

Rivaroxaban

Pharmacology
    Time to maximum concentration: 2–4 hours
    Half-life: 5–9 hours
    Renal elimination: 66%

Dosing
    Prophylaxis 10 mg qD
    Therapy venous thrombosis: DVT 15 mg BID × 3
    wks and then 20 mg/day, contraindicated CrCl <30
    Stroke prevention in atrial fibrillation 20 mg/
    day – dose reduced to 15 mg/day CrCl 50–15

Drug-drug interaction: CYP 3A4 agents (azole
antifungals (except fluconazole) or HIV-protease
inhibitors)

Affects INR – use anti-Xa or specific levels to monitor

Reversal Agents – PCC 50 units/kg or andexanet
800 mg IV bolus and then 8 mg/min for 120 minutes
(if >8 hours since dose, then 400 mg IV bolus followed
by 4 mg/min for 120 minutes)

General Considerations

The advantage of the DOACs are no food interactions, fewer drug interactions, and no need for monitoring in most patients. However, there are certain caveats to use. One is they are absolutely contraindicated in patients with mechanical cardiac valves. The other is being fixed-dose drugs, they need to be used with caution with extremes of weight (see Chap. 28). Finally, these drugs are more expensive than warfarin, and this can be an issue for many patients.

Thrombin Inhibitor: Dabigatran

Generation of thrombin is a pivotal step in hemostasis. Thrombin not only cleaves fibrinogen into fibrin to form a thrombosis; it also activates platelets and many procoagulant factors including V, VIII, XI, and XIII. Thus, it represents a potent target for antithrombotic agents. Clinical studies of the direct thrombin inhibitor ximelagatran provided proof that novel oral anticoagulants could replace warfarin in therapy of thrombosis, but a high incidence of liver toxicity kept this drug off the market. Dabigatran is a direct thrombin inhibitor that has been tested in phase III trials to be effective for stroke prevention in atrial fibrillation and for venous disease prophylaxis and therapy.

Dabigatran reaches a peak activity after 2–3 hours after ingestion with a half-life of 12–14 hours. Dabigatran is 80% renally excreted, so for patients with creatinine clearances less than 30 ml/min, a lower dose should be used. It does not require activation by cytochromes, but its metabolism is affected by P-glycoprotein (P-gp) interactions.

For stroke prevention, the dosing is 150 mg bid. In countries where the 110 mg dose is available, this dose bid is often used for patients felt to be at higher risk of bleeding such as the frail elderly. In the United States, a 75 mg dose is approved for patients with creatine clearances between 30 and 15 ml/min. For prevention of venous thrombosis after orthopedic surgery, the dose is 220 mg daily to 150 mg in patients with creatine clearances of 15–30 ml/min. Therapy of acute venous thrombosis is 150 mg bid after patients have received an initial 5 days of low-molecular-weight heparin.

Drug interactions are with agents that are strong inhibitors of P-gp such as dronedarone or ketoconazole, especially in the setting of renal disease.

Studies have shown the bleeding risks of dabigatran are the same as warfarin with two exceptions. In atrial fibrillation patients with risk of gastrointestinal bleeding is higher, but the risk of intracranial hemorrhage is lower. It does appear that dabigatran – like other thrombin inhibitors – has a slight risk of myocardial infarctions (relative risk 1.3 – an absolute risk increase 0.2–0.3%). The other notable side effect is that 15% of patients will complain of dyspepsia.

The aPTT is sensitive to dabigatran – usually peak levels are twice normal controls and trough 1.2–1.5 times control. Animal studies suggest reversal of anticoagulant effect can be achieved with use of prothrombin complex concentrates 50 units/kg. A specific neutralizing antibody – idarucizumab – is approved for reversal. The dose is 5 g IV for life-threatening bleeding. In patients with renal disease, a thrombin time should be checked after the idarucizumab dose to ensure complete reversal. Dabigatran can also be dialyzed off, but this seems impractical for most acute bleeding issues.

For surgeries dabigatran is held for 48 hours before procedures and 3–4 days if there is renal impairment.

Factor Xa Inhibitors

Factor Xa is responsible for generating thrombin. Inhibition of coagulation at this step prevents thrombin generation and its powerful positive feedback for coagulation. Animal studies suggested that Xa inhibitors also can be inhibited by prothrombin complex concentrates dosed at 50 units/kg. A specific antidote – andexanet – for Xa inhibitors has been approved for use. Andexanet is a modified factor Xa that cannot support coagulation but has a higher affinity for Xa inhibitors and neutralizes the anticoagulant effect of these drugs. The dose is dependent on both the anticoagulant used and time from last dose (Table 24.1). There may be a prothrombotic effect, so feasible patients should resume anticoagulation once they are stable.

Apixaban

Apixaban is a factor Xa inhibitor that is 66% bio-available and has a peak onset of action in 1–3 hours after ingestion with a half-life of 8–15 hours. It is only ~25% renally excreted but is metabolized by CYP 3A4 and P-gp. Apixaban has been shown to be effective for prevention and treatment of venous thromboembolic diseases as well as stroke prophylaxis in atrial fibrillation. Studies have shown that rates of bleeding – including intracranial hemorrhage – are decreased with apixaban with no other apparent side effects.

Dosing for venous thromboembolic prevention is 2.5 mg bid. For treatment of acute venous thrombosis, a higher initial dose is used – 10 mg bid times for 1 week and then 5 mg bid. Six to 12 months after the thrombosis, the dose can be cut to 2.5 mg bid. For stroke prevention in atrial fibrillation, the dose is 5 mg bid – 2.5 mg bid if the patient has two or more of these risk factors: age over 80, creatinine over 1.5 mg/mL, or weight less than 60 kg.

Only drugs that are strong inhibitors of both CYP 3A4 and P-gp interfere with apixaban metabolism. These would be azole antibiotics and HIV antiviral agents. For patients taking 5 mg bid, one would need to cut the dose in half to 2.5 mg bid.

Apixaban does not affect classic tests of hemostasis (INR and aPTT) but can be measured using anti-Xa assay. Given the wide availably of this test once standards are made, there should be widespread availability of specific assays.

For surgery apixaban is held for 48 hours and for patients with renal impairment 72 hours.

Betrixaban

This Factor Xa inhibitor is 47% bioavailable with a peak onset in 2–3 hours. Its two unique features are a long half-life of 19 hours and minimal renal excretion. Another potential advantage is the lack of metabolism by CYP3A4. Betrixaban has been the subject of few clinical studies and is currently approved for prevention of thrombosis in medical patients. Dosing is a 160 mg dose on the first day followed by 80 mg daily for 35–42 days. If patients are on P-gp inhibitors, the dose should be halved. The dose should be also halved if the creatinine clearance is less than 30 ml/min.

Edoxaban

Edoxaban is 45% bioavailable and has a peak onset of action in 1–1.5 hours with a half-life of 9–11 hours. It is 33% renally excreted. Clinical trials show effectiveness in the treatment and prevention of venous thromboembolism plus stroke prevention in atrial fibrillation.

30 mg daily of edoxaban is the dose for prevention of venous thrombosis. For therapy the dose is 60 mg daily with a dose reduction to 30 mg for patients with creatinine clearance between 30 and 60 min/ml, weight less than 60 kg, or on P-gp agents. Like dabigatran, in clinical trials edoxaban was started after 5 days of parenteral heparin in patients with acute venous thrombosis.

As noted above, drug interactions with edoxaban are with the P-gp inhibitors, and the dose should be reduced by 50% when taking verapamil, quinidine, erythromycin, azithromycin, clarithromycin, ketoconazole, or itraconazole. The use of the P-gp inhibitors protease inhibitors and cyclosporine is contraindicated.

Edoxaban dose affects the INR, and this can be used to determine if there is a significant drug effect. For surgery drug should be held for 24–48 hours depending on the bleeding risk of surgery.

Rivaroxaban

Rivaroxaban is readily absorbed, being 80–100% bioavailable, and has a half-life of 5–9 hours. It is metabolized by cytochrome CYP 3A4 and P-gp. It has been shown to be effective for prevention and treatment of venous thromboembolic diseases as well as stroke prophylaxis in atrial fibrillation and acute coronary syndromes. Besides bleeding there appears to be no unique side effects of rivaroxaban.

The dose for prevention of venous thrombosis is 10 mg daily. For treatment of venous disease, a higher initial dose is used for acute events 15 mg bid for 3 weeks and then 20 mg daily. Six to 12 months after the thrombosis, the dose can be cut to 10 mg daily. For stroke prevention in atrial fibrillation, the dose is 20 mg daily – 15 mg for patients with creatine clearances between 50 and 15 ml/min.

Like apixaban, drugs that are strong inhibitors of both CYP 3A4 and P-gp – azole antibiotic and HIV antiviral agents – interfere with rivaroxaban metabolism.

Rivaroxaban does affect the protime and INR so these can be used to detect drug effect. Like apixaban, soon specific monitoring should be available via anti-Xa levels.

For surgery rivaroxaban is held for 24–48 hours for patients with renal impairment.

Diseases Where the Direct Oral Anticoagulants Have Been Studied

Atrial Fibrillation

For stroke prevention in atrial fibrillation, apixaban and dabigatran have shown superiority over warfarin in stroke prevention, while edoxaban and rivaroxaban are non-inferior. All showed decreased rates of intracranial hemorrhage. Apixaban has also been shown to be superior to aspirin with no worsening of bleeding. The direct agents also have the advantage of no monitoring and much reduced drug interactions.

Prevention of Venous Thrombosis

For orthopedic thrombosis prevention in hip and knee replacement, apixaban and rivaroxaban have been shown to be superior to enoxaparin with dabigatran being non-inferior. Edoxaban has been tested in a Japanese orthopedic population and also shown effective. The direct agents have been widely accepted for this indication due to ease of use (oral and not injection) and cost.

Treatment of Venous Thrombosis

All agents have been shown to be effective in treatment of venous thrombosis with the three Xa inhibitors shown to have less bleeding. In clinical trials apixaban and rivaroxaban were used as initial therapy of acute thrombosis – using higher doses at the initiation of therapy – while dabigatran and edoxaban used an initial course of heparin. Three agents – apixaban, dabigatran, and rivaroxaban – have also been studied for long-term therapy of venous thromboembolism with all being safe and effective.

Cancer Patients

Previous clinical trials have shown that warfarin was inferior to LMWH in cancer patients. Despite recommendations for LMWH, only a minority of cancer patients received this agent long term for treatment of venous thrombosis. There is increasing data that DOACs as just as – if not more – effective as LMWH in treatment of cancer related thrombosis and appear to be as safe. The only exception is that patients with upper gastrointestinal cancers appear to have an increased rate of bleeding with DOACs compared to LMWH.

Acute Coronary Syndrome and Coronary Arterty Disease

Three direct oral anticoagulants – apixaban, dabigatran, and rivaroxaban – have been tested in patients with acute coronary syndromes. All had shown increased rates of bleeding, but the low-dose rivaroxaban 2.5 mg bid did show improved cardiac outcomes but at the cost of increased bleeding including intracranial hemorrhage.

There are studies with apixaban, dabigatran, and rivaroxaban showing that when combined with a P2Y12 inhibitor such as clopidogrel in patients with both recent coronary stents and atrial fibrillation, the rates of bleeding were decreased with minimal loss of antithrombotic effectiveness compared to "triple therapy" with warfarin/aspirin/P2Y12 inhibitors. This may be a useful option for most patients except those at high risk of stent thrombosis such as those with recent myocardial infraction and complex coronary anatomy.

Monitoring

Although designed to be used without monitoring, there are occasions when it will be useful to know if patients have a measurable drug effect. One indication is with the patients with recurrent thrombo-embolic event to see if they have been compliant. Another is a bleeding patient or a patient needing to go to surgery to see if there is a persistent drug effect. Currently for dabigatran, the PTT is the best test. Some reference laboratories have used a modified thrombin time to quantitate levels. For rivaroxaban, the pro-time/INR is used, but for apixaban neither the PTT nor INR appears to be sensitive. As noted above, soon specific levels should be obtainable by using anti-Xa levels.

Suggested Reading

Barnes GD, Kurtz B. Direct oral anticoagulants: unique properties and practical approaches to management. Heart. 2016;102(20):1620–6.

Barr D, Epps QJ. Direct oral anticoagulants: a review of common medication errors. J Thromb Thrombolysis. 2019;47(1):146–54.

López-López JA, Sterne JAC, Thom HHZ, Higgins JPT, Hingorani AD, Okoli GN, Davies PA, Bodalia PN, Bryden PA, Welton NJ, Hollingworth W, Caldwell DM, Savović J, Dias S, Salisbury C, Eaton D, Stephens-Boal A, Sofat R. Oral anticoagulants for prevention of stroke in atrial fibrillation: systematic review, network meta-analysis, and cost effectiveness analysis. BMJ. 2017;359:j5058.

Samuelson BT, Cuker A, Siegal DM, Crowther M, Garcia DA. Laboratory assessment of the anticoagulant activity of direct oral anticoagulants: a systematic review. Chest. 2017;151(1):127–38.

van Es N, Coppens M, Schulman S, Middeldorp S, Büller HR. Direct oral anticoagulants compared with vitamin K antagonists for acute venous thromboembolism: evidence from phase 3 trials. Blood. 2014;124(12):1968–75.

Weber J, Olyaei A, Shatzel J. The efficacy and safety of direct oral anticoagulants in patients with chronic renal insufficiency: a review of the literature. Eur J Haematol. 2019;102(4):312–8.

Warfarin

Thomas G. DeLoughery

Warfarin works by blocking vitamin K-dependent gamma-carboxylation of coagulation proteins II, VII, IX, and X. As a result of warfarin therapy, these coagulation factors cannot bind calcium. This causes impairment of these factors' binding to membranes and its folding into the proper configuration leading to decreased activity and synthesis.

Therapy with warfarin is initiated by giving the patient 5–10 mg in the evening for the first 2 nights (2.5 mg in those over 75 years) and adjusting the dose to achieve an adequate prothrombin time. Although the use of a 10 mg loading dose has been traditional in the past, for many patients – especially older ones or ones with comorbidities – this may lead to overshooting the INR and delay in achieving a stable therapeutic INR. A practical approach is to use 5 mg in loading patients over the age of 50 or in patients with albumin under 3 and 10 mg in young healthy patients. The elderly patient (over age 75) only needs a 2.5 mg loading dose. Nomograms for 5 and 10 mg warfarin loading doses are given in Table 25.1. The effect of warfarin on the INR takes 36 hours to occur, so the morning INR reflects the effect of the warfarin dose taken 36 hours before.

Table 25.1 Nomograms for warfarin loading

5 Mg warfarin nomogram		
Day	INR	Dosage (Mg)
1		5.0
2	<1.5	5.0
	1.5–1.9	2.5
	2.0–2.5	1.0–2.5
	>2.5	0.0
3	<1.5	5.0–10.0
	1.5–1.9	2.5–5.0
	2.0–2.5	0.0–2.5
	2.5–3.0	0.0–2.5
	>3.0	0.0
4	<1.5	10.0
	1.5–1.9	5.0–7.5
	2.0–3.0	0.0–0.5
	>3.0	0.0
5	<1.5	10.0
	1.5–1.9	7.5–10.0
	2.0–3.0	0.0–5.0
	>3.0	0.0
6	<1.5	7.5–12.5
	1.5–1.9	5.0–10.0
	2.0–3.0	0.0–7.5
	>3.0	0.0

Used with Permission: Hadlock GC, Burnett AE, Nutescu EA. Warfarin. In: Lau J, Barnes G, Streiff M, editors. Anticoagulation therapy. Cham: Springer; 2018

T. G. DeLoughery (✉)
Division of Hematology/Medical Oncology,
Department of Medicine, Pathology, and Pediatrics,
Oregon Health & Sciences University,
Portland, OR, USA
e-mail: delought@ohsu.edu

© Springer Nature Switzerland AG 2019
T. G. DeLoughery (ed.), *Hemostasis and Thrombosis*,
https://doi.org/10.1007/978-3-030-19330-0_25

10 mg warfarin nomogram		
Day	INR	Dosage (Mg)
1		10.0
2	<1.5	7.5–10.0
	1.5–1.9	2.5
	2.0–2.5	1.0–2.5
	>2.5	0.0
3	<1.5	5.0–10.0
	1.5–1.9	2.5–5.0
	– 2.0–2.5	0.0–2.5
	2.5–3.0	0.0–2.5
	>3.0	0.0
4	<1.5	10.0
	1.5–1.9	5.0–7.5
	2.0–3.0	0.0–0.5
	>3.0	0.0
5	<1.5	10.0
	1.5–1.9	7.5–10.0
	2.0–3.0	0.0–5.0
	>3.0	0.0
6	<1.5	7.5–12.5
	1.5–1.9	5.0–10.0
	2.0–3.0	0.0–7.5
	>3.0	0.0

Table 25.2 Maintenance warfarin adjustment nomogram

INR	Dose change
1.1v1.4	Day 1: Add 10–20% total weekly dose (TWD)[a]
	Weekly: Increase TWD by 10–20%
	Return: 1 week
1.5–1.9	Day 1: Add 5–10% of TWD
	Weekly: Increase Twd by 5–10%
	Return: 2 weeks
2.0–3.0	No change
	Return: 4 weeks
3.1–3.9	Day 1: Subtract 5v10% TWD
	Weekly: Reduce TWD by 10–20%
	Return: 2 weeks
4.0–5.0	Day 1: No warfarin
	Weekly: Reduce TWD by 10–20%
	Return: 1 week
> 5.0	Stop warfarin until INR <3.0
	Decrease TWD by 20–50%
	Return daily

Modified from: Wilson SE, Costantini L, Crowther MA. *J Thromb Thrombolysis*. 2007;23:195
[a]*TWD* total weekly dose

Factor VII has the shortest half-life, and so it is the first factor reduced as a result of warfarin therapy. However, the full anticoagulant effect does not occur until there is a reduction in prothrombin (factor II) and factor X, which may take several days. Thus, in acute thrombosis, heparin needs to be continued for at least 24 hours after the prothrombin time is therapeutic to allow for factors II and X to fall. For chronic indications such as atrial fibrillation, warfarin can be started at lower daily doses (2.5–5.0 mg). This allows for the initiation of warfarin therapy without the use of heparin. Table 25.2 gives guidelines for adjusting warfarin doses in patients once therapeutic prothrombin times have been reached.

Unfortunately the dose of warfarin required for achieving therapeutic anticoagulation varies tremendously among patients. This is due to a combination of the patient's genetic ability to metabolize warfarin, concurrent medications, illnesses, and diet. Patients who are older require less warfarin with patients over age 65 requiring one-half to one-third of the warfarin doses of younger patients. Some of the variation in warfarin dosing is due to genetic factors. Polymorphisms in CYP2C9 can affect warfarin metabolism with a variant found in 6–10% of the population (2C9*3) leading to reduced warfarin dosing. There are also polymorphisms in vitamin K epoxide reductase complex subunit 1 (VKORC1) that can influence warfarin dosing. Although clinical testing is available for these polymorphisms, clinical trials have shown little if any advantage to use of genetically guided dosing protocols to other monograms for warfarin dosing.

Since warfarin is metabolized in the liver by the cytochrome P450 system, the INR may change with starting or stopping other medications that affect CYP2C9. Multiple agents can augment or decrease warfarin effect and are listed in Table 25.3. Unfortunately, many drugs may have an unpredictable effect on the INR. The most prudent strategy is to check the INR several days after starting a new drug and then weekly to ensure the INR is stable. If the patient is started on a drug which results in predictable changes in the INR, then the warfarin dose may be adjusted, usually by 50%, when starting that drug.

Vitamin K is found in many foods (Table 25.4), especially green vegetables. Patients will often

Table 25.3 Medication effects on warfarin effect

Increased warfarin effect

Acetaminophen

Allopurinol

Amiodarone (may last for months after drug is stopped)

Anabolic steroids

Aspirin

Azithromycin

Cephalosporins (NMTT group)

Cimetidine

Ciprofloxacin

Clarithromycin

Clofibrate

Cyclophosphamide

Diltiazem

Disulfiram

Erythromycin

Fluconazole

Furosemide

Gemcitabine

Gemfibrozil

Isoniazid

Itraconazole

Ketoconazole

Metronidazole

Micronase

Omeprazole

Propafenone

Propranolol

Quinidine

Quinine

Quinolones

Ropinirole

Serotonin re-uptake inhibitors

Simvastatin

Sulfinpyrazone

Sulfonylureas

Tamoxifen

Tetracycline

Thyroid hormones

Tramadol

Tricyclic antidepressants

Vitamin E

Voriconazole

Decreased warfarin effect

Alcohol

Barbiturates

Carbamazepine

Corticosteroids

Phenytoin (may potentiate warfarin at initiation of drug)

Cholestyramine

Estrogens

Griseofulvin

Rifampin

Table 25.3 (continued)

Sucralfate

Vitamin K

Mercaptopurine

Bosentan

Azathioprine

Ribavirin

Table 25.4 Vitamin content of foods

Item	Vitamin K content (ug/100 ug)
Green tea	712
Avocado	634
Turnip greens	408
Brussels sprouts	317
Chickpeas	220
Broccoli	200
Cauliflower	192
Lettuce	129
Cabbage	125
Kale	125
Beef liver	92
Spinach	89
Watercress	57
Asparagus	57
Lettuce (iceberg)	26
Green beans	14

avoid any vegetables due to fear of reversing their anticoagulation. This will result in those patients having lower vitamin K stores and will make them prone to unstable INRs. Patients should be instructed that *consistency* of diet is more important than avoiding vitamin K. A diet rich in vegetables and fruits is beneficial, especially for patients being anticoagulated, and should be encouraged. Patients should be advised of the vitamin K content of common foods and should be encouraged to be consistent with their diet. For patients with unstable INR, adding a known amount of vitamin K (75–150 ug) daily may improve stability.

Therapeutic Range of the INR

Warfarin therapy is guided by the prothrombin time reported as the INR. Separate laboratories use thromboplastin from different manufacturers which results in variability of the prothrombin time. The international normalized ratio (INR) is the prothrombin time ratio that would be obtained if the "WHO reference thromboplastin reagent" was used to test the plasma. Laboratories convert their local prothrombin time ratios to INRs by using the ISI (international sensitivity index) by the formula INR = PT RATIO^{ISI}. The advantage of the INR is that it reflects a constant level of anticoagulation despite the different thromboplastins used to perform the prothrombin time. The ISI of thromboplastin used in the United States ranges from 1.4 to 2.8. Given this, an INR of 3.0 can be equivalent to a prothrombin time of anywhere from 18.1 to 26.8 seconds. Thus it is meaningless to use the prothrombin time, and INR should always be used for guiding warfarin therapy, especially when dealing with different laboratories.

The therapeutic INR range for most indications for warfarin is an INR of 2.0–3.0. Some patients with mechanical heart valves will require higher doses of warfarin. To avoid subtherapeutic doses of warfarin, it is better to aim for a "target" INR of 2.5 and use the range of 2–3 as indicating acceptable values. Use of the mid-range target as a therapeutic goal results in a lower incidence of subtherapeutic INRs. Increasingly, home monitors are being used – this allows the patient greater freedom to check their INR and offers improved control.

Complications of Warfarin Therapy

Bleeding Studies have shown that physicians consistently overestimate the risk of bleeding with warfarin. Past studies of the bleeding risk are marred by an inconsistent approach to anticoagulation, use of nonstandardized measures prior to INRs, and retrospective analysis. Newer studies have shown that the risk of bleeding with warfarin is highly dependent on several factors. The most significant risk factor is over-anticoagulation especially with INRs of 4.5. In addition, these are additional risk factors that increase the risk of bleeding:

- Variability of the INR resulting in frequent dose changes
- Excess alcohol use
- Anticoagulated for arterial reasons
- First 3 months of anticoagulation therapy
- Three or more comorbid conditions

In general the risk of major bleeding with warfarin in an average patient is 1%/year; the risk of fatal bleeding is 0.2–0.25%/year. For younger patients being anticoagulated for venous disease, this is lower, and for older patients being anticoagulated for arterial disease, this is higher.

Although age may not be a risk in and of itself, certain conditions associated with aging increase the risk of bleeding. Older patients require less warfarin to achieve the desired anticoagulation effect. Secondly, many older patients are on a variety of medicines that can interfere with warfarin. Finally, the very old (>80) may be at increased risk of intracranial hemorrhage.

There is increasing evidence that assessing a limited set of pretreatment variables can help predict the risk of bleeding. The best studied is the HAS-BLED prediction rule (Table 25.5). With this rule, patients with HAS-BLED scores of 3 or more had bleeding rates of over 3.74 bleeds per 100 patient years reported. This prediction rule appears to be most prognostic for bleeding with warfarin therapy for atrial fibrillation but not as predictive for bleeding with treatment of venous thrombosis. Another benefit of this scores is that some factors (concurrent antiplatelet agents) are modifiable.

Table 25.5 HAS-BLED score

Assign point for:
H – Hypertension – 1
A – Abnormal renal and liver function (1 point each) 1 or 2
S – Stroke – 1
B – Bleeding – 1
L – Labile INRs – 1
E – Elderly (>65) – 1
D – Drugs (antiplatelet agents or NSAIA) or alcohol (1 point each) 1 or 2

Score	Risk group	Yearly risk of major bleeding
0	Low	0.59–1.13
1	Low	1.02–1.51
2	Intermediate	1.88–3.2
≥3	High	3.74–21.43

Used with permission: Nantsupawat T, Nugent K, Phrommintikul A. *Drugs Aging.* 2013;30:59

Warfarin Skin Necrosis This is an extremely rare but devastating complication of warfarin therapy. Classically it starts 4 days after initiation of therapy with pain and skin discoloration. Then frank necrosis occurs in the affected area. The most common sites are the breast and buttocks in women and the penis in men. Most reported cases have occurred in post-surgical or post-partum patients with venous thrombosis. Many (but not) all patients had protein C or protein S deficiencies when tested. The etiology of the skin necrosis is still debated, but it appears that protein C or S deficiency and an inflammatory state are prerequisites for occurrence. The entity has not been described in patients anticoagulated for arterial events. A prudent approach is to overlap warfarin therapy with heparin for 24 hours whenever anticoagulating patients with venous thrombotic events. When starting warfarin for arterial events or for prophylaxis in atrial fibrillation, heparin coverage is probably not required if the patient does not have a personal or family history of venous thrombosis or evidence of antiphospholipid antibodies. Warfarin should be started gradually at 2.5–5.0 mg/day in these patients.

Addition to Antiplatelet Agents to Warfarin

Many patients on warfarin – up to 20–30% in some studies – for atrial fibrillation are also taking aspirin. Most of the time, this is because of a perceived need to treat concurrent coronary artery disease. However the evidence is clear that the addition of aspirin does not provide any further antithrombic effect but does definitely increase the risk of bleeding. Warfarin is an excellent agent in both the primary and secondary prevention of myocardial infarction. Patients do not obtain any more antithrombotic risk reduction with combined therapy, but this will increase their risk of serious bleeding. Combined therapy needs to be avoided unless there are clear indications – recent acute coronary syndrome, stroke despite warfarin therapy, recent stent placement, or mechanical valves (discussed more in Chap. 10).

Warfarin Resistance and Unstable INRS

Two common problems complicate warfarin therapy. One is the patient who requires large doses of warfarin, and the other is the patient with erratic INRs.

Rarely, the clinician is faced with a patient in whom massive doses of warfarin are required for anticoagulation or, more disturbingly, the patient who seems to be resistant to even large doses of warfarin. A careful evaluation of such a patient is needed to determine the cause of the warfarin resistance.

True genetic warfarin resistance is extremely rare, with only a few affected kindred reported. These patients are always difficult to anticoagulate and may only respond to very large doses (i.e., 150 mg) of warfarin. More common is acquired resistance to warfarin. The three major causes of acquired resistance are medications, ingestion of vitamin K, and non-compliance.

It is less common for medicines to inhibit the action of warfarin than to potentiate it. Common drugs which inhibit warfarin action are barbiturates, rifampin, and nafcillin. Patients on these medications may require 20 mg of warfarin per day to maintain a therapeutic INR. Since most drug-warfarin interactions are mediated through induction of liver enzymes, it may take several days for the warfarin resistance to be noticed after starting the drug and several days for the effect to wear off after stopping the drug. Cholestyramine uniquely interferes with warfarin absorption.

Vitamin K is found in several nutritional supplements and often in generic multivitamins, and use of these products can result in warfarin resistance. For example, Ensure contains 80 ug of vitamin K per 1000 kcal and Sustacal 230 ug/1000 kcal. In patients who depend solely on these products for nutrition, large doses of warfarin or anticoagulation with heparin may be required. If a patient changes supplements or starts ingesting regular food, the warfarin requirement will change dramatically. Patients may also be ingesting large amounts of vitamin K-containing food that can induce warfarin resistance. Even 1 or 2 days of high intake of vitamin K-rich food can dramatically lower INRs.

Some patients who present with warfarin resistance are simply not taking the medicine as prescribed. These patients initially require the usual doses of warfarin therapy but then present with normal INRs despite massive warfarin doses. Measuring serum warfarin levels is useful in patients suspected of non-compliance. Patients with undetectable warfarin levels despite allegedly taking large doses of warfarin are most likely not taking the drug. In the patient who has a non-detectable warfarin level, a level should be repeated after the patient is witnessed taking the drug to ensure that the patient is not suffering from rare malabsorption of warfarin. One case has been described of a patient who could not absorb warfarin but could absorb phenindione, a non-coumarin vitamin K inhibitor. Curiously, this malabsorption occurred after 2 years of stable warfarin therapy.

Patients with erratic INRs are at greater risk for both bleeding and thrombosis. Patients need to be questioned about the use of all other medications including "natural" remedies and over-the-counter medicines. A good dietary history as well as a frank discussion about compliance should be performed. As noted above, adding vegetables and other sources of vitamin K to the diet will stabilize the INR in some patients. Unless there is a compelling reason to stay on warfarin (i.e., mechanical heart valve), patients with erratic INRs should be switch to direct oral anticoagulants.

Management of High INRs and Bleeding

The risk of bleeding with an elevated INR depends on the degree of elevation of the INR and on the reason for anticoagulation therapy. An older patient being anticoagulated for an arterial reason (stroke, valve, etc.) is at higher risk for bleeding than a younger patient being anticoagulated for a venous indication. The rate of INR correction depends upon whether the patient is bleeding.

For nonbleeding patients with high INRs less than 5, one can simply omit or lower the dose of warfarin with the goal of getting the INR back

into range. There is a delay of 12–36 hours after stopping warfarin before the INR begins to fall, so for INRs in the 5–10 range, one can hold the next 1–2 doses and give 1.0–2.5 mg of vitamin K orally to achieve faster reversal. For INRs of more than 10, one should give 2.5–5.0 mg of vitamin K with the expectation that the INR will be lowered in 24–48 hours.

If the patient requires rapid full reversal because of bleeding or the need for surgery, one can give vitamin K by the intravenous route in addition to fresh frozen plasma. Since one unit of plasma on average raises coagulation factors by only 5%, one must give large doses (15 mg/kg or 4–5 units) to attempt to completely correct the INR. Risks in transfusing this amount of plasma are volume overload and transfusion reactions.

In the patient with intracranial or other life-threatening hemorrhage, correction of the INR with vitamin K and plasma is too slow. The use of prothrombin concentrates (which contain all the vitamin K-dependent clotting factors) results in a more rapid correction of coagulation than plasma and in some studies better outcomes. The ideal products are the "4-factor" concentrates which contain all the vitamin K procoagulants – factors II, VII, IX, and X. Use of these agents have been shown to rapidly decrease the INR to normal (Table 25.6).

Table 25.6 Mangagment of high INRs

Warfarin	
Not bleeding: goal is INR in 2–3 range	
INR	**Action**
3–4.5	Hold dose until INR decreased
4.5–10	1.25 mg vitamin K PO
> 10	2.5–5 mg vitamin K PO
Should see INR back in therapeutic range in 24–48 hours	
Bleeding: goal is INR under 2	
INR	**Action**
2–4.5	2.5 mg vitamin K ± FFP (15 ml/kg)
4.5–10	5 mg vitamin K ± FFP (15 ml/kg)
>10	5–10 mg vitamin K ± FFP (15 ml/kg)
FFP fresh frozen plasma	
Warfarin life or brain-threatening bleeding:	
4-factor PCC	
If INR 2–4: 25 units/kg (not to exceed 2500 units)	
If INR 4–6: 35 units/kg (not to exceed 3500 units)	
if INR > 6: 50 units/kg (not to exceed 5000 units)	

In the past there was much enthusiasm for rVIIa in reversing warfarin. However, studies suggest despite normalization of the INR that bleeding is not affected and there is a higher incidence of both arterial and venous thrombosis, particularly in patients over the age of 75. rVIIa should only be used if PCCs are not available for the patient with warfarin-induced intracranial hemorrhage.

When to Restart Anticoagulation After Serious Bleeding?

The key decision point in restarting anticoagulation is to review the patients' indications for therapy. Patients with atrial fibrillation and high CHADS2 definitely require therapy, while a patient with a remotely provoked venous thrombosis can just stop therapy. Although people are more fearful about resuming anticoagulation after a cerebral bleeding event, data show that gastrointestinal bleeding has the higher rate of recurrence. Rebleeding after intracranial hemorrhage is low – perhaps 1–2% over the next few years. For most patients this risk is outweighed by the benefits of anticoagulation as studies show patients who are reanticoagulated after cerebral or gastrointestinal bleeding have better outcomes including less thrombosis and mortality. The exception to this is the patient with evidence of cerebral amyloid angiopathy who should never be re-anticoagulated given their very high (>30%) risk of rebleeding. The patients often present with deep lobar bleeds and have MRI evidence of the angiopathy.

The timing of the resumption of anticoagulation is also not settled. Studies do indicate that with intracranial hemorrhage, only a short period off anticoagulation is needed. There is enough data to suggest that once the INR is normal only 4–7 days off, anticoagulation is necessary before restarting some form of anticoagulation. There is also increasing data for gastrointestinal hemorrhage; 7 days also suffices to stay off anticoagulation. For other bleedings holding 1–2 weeks may be appropriate. Patients with genitourinary or gastrointestinal bleeding while on warfarin should be worked up aggressively since pathological lesions will be found in over 50% of anticoagulated patients who have this type of bleeding.

Temporary Cessation of Warfarin for Procedures

Many patients on warfarin will require procedures. The approach for surgery needs to take into account the reason the patient is being anticoagulated and the risk of bleeding with the procedure.

In theory, the risk of thrombosis with holding anticoagulation should be low. For example, if the 1-year risk of thrombosis/embolism with a mitral ball-cage valve is 30%, then simple math yields a daily risk of 0.08% and a 2-week risk of 1.15%. For less thrombogenic valves presumably the risk would be lower. However, this calculation does not take into account the clotting stimulus of surgery which appears to significantly increase the risk of thrombosis. Retrospective data suggests an overall risk as high as 1–2% of thrombotic arterial events in patients if their anticoagulation is held before surgery.

One can approach perioperative anticoagulation in several ways. The simplest is to *continue the warfarin* and perform the procedure with the patient anticoagulated. This is the standard approach for dental procedures, cataracts, and endoscopy and is a safe and effective approach even for complex surgeries including hip replacements. This approach is associated with the lowest risk of strokes (0.4%) but does carry the risk of increased bleeding. For patients requiring pacemaker and implantable defibrillators, this approach has been shown to be associated with less bleeding than bridging with low-molecular-weight heparin with an equal risk of thrombosis.

The next simplest approach would be to *stop the warfarin* 4–5 days before surgery, allow the INR to drift back to normal, and then restart oral anticoagulation after surgery. This would expose the patient to a thrombotic risk for up to 4–6 days but would have the lowest risk of bleeding.

In recent years, the concept of *bridging therapy* has been proposed with the idea of using low-molecular-weight heparin to "bridge" the patient when the warfarin effect is gone. This presumably would have the lowest risk of thrombosis but may expose the patient to bleeding, especially postoperatively. For these patients the risk of thrombosis or embolism needs to be balanced by the risk of surgical bleeding. However, this approach is associated with the most bleeding especially in the perioperative periods. Two factors promote excess bleeding are to late stopping and early restarting of LMWH. LMWH be stopped at least 24 hours before surgery (longer in patients with renal disease). For complex procedures one should not give therapeutic LMWH for at least 48 hours or more to prevent bleeding. Recent data suggests that the low rate of thromboembolism in patients not bridged was outweighed by the three- to fivefold increased risk of significant bleeding in patients who were bridged calling into question this approach for most patients. Currently bridging should be limited to only the highest-risk patient group.

Given the above a suggested approach is, for low bleeding risk procedures (and modest risk ones if the surgeon agrees), warfarin is continued with an INR goal in the 2–2.5 range. For patients with low risk of thrombosis – i.e., primary stroke prevention in atrial fibrillation – the warfarin can be held before surgery and restarted afterward. For patients at higher risk of bleeding, bridging therapy such as suggested in Table 25.7 can be used. These patients would be:

- Recent (<3 months) proximal venous thrombosis or pulmonary embolism
- Mechanical cardiac valves (except low risk bileaflet)
- Atrial fibrillation with recent (12 weeks) history of stroke or CHADS2 score >4

Table 25.7 Management of patient anticoagulated with warfarin who needs a procedure

Consider bridging for patients with mechanical cardiac valves (except low-risk tilting disk valve in the aortic position), bioprosthetic valve with history of thrombosis, patients with atrial fibrillation who have suffered a stroke/TIA in the last 12 months or CHADS2 >4, and patients with recent (<3 months) venous thrombosis

Method

Day 5: Stop warfarin 5 days before procedure

Day 3: Start therapeutic LMWH every 12–24 hours

Day 1: Give last LMWH dose this am. If patient has renal insufficiency, stop last dose 48 hours before surgery

Day 0: Check PT-INR/aPTT morning of surgery. For most procedures can start warfarin the night of surgery. If very minor procedure, restart therapeutic LMW heparin that night. Otherwise start LMWH at prophylactic doses, and change to therapeutic when safe from a surgical standpoint but no sooner than 48 hours

Suggested Reading

Ageno W, Gallus AS, Wittkowsky A, Crowther M, Hylek EM, Palareti G, American College of Chest Physicians. Oral anticoagulant therapy: Antithrombotic Therapy and Prevention of Thrombosis, 9th ed: American College of Chest Physicians Evidence-Based Clinical Practice Guidelines. Chest. 2012;141(2 Suppl):e44S–88S.

Douketis JD, Spyropoulos AC, Kaatz S, Becker RC, Caprini JA, Dunn AS, Garcia DA, Jacobson A, Jaffer AK, Kong DF, Schulman S, Turpie AG, Hasselblad V, Ortel TL, BRIDGE Investigators. Perioperative bridging anticoagulation in patients with atrial fibrillation. N Engl J Med. 2015;373(9):823–33.

Hunt BJ, Levi M. Urgent reversal of vitamin K antagonists. BMJ. 2018;360:j5424.

Vazquez SR. Drug-drug interactions in an era of multiple anticoagulants: a focus on clinically relevant drug interactions. Blood. 2018;132(21):2230–9.

Witt DM, Nieuwlaat R, Clark NP, Ansell J, Holbrook A, Skov J, Shehab N, Mock J, Myers T, Dentali F, Crowther MA, Agarwal A, Bhatt M, Khatib R, Riva JJ, Zhang Y, Guyatt G. American Society of Hematology 2018 guidelines for management of venous thromboembolism: optimal management of anticoagulation therapy. Blood Adv. 2018;2(22):3257–91.

Antiplatelet Agents

Thomas G. DeLoughery

Aspirin

Aspirin is the oldest and still the most widely used antiplatelet agent. Aspirin exerts its anti-thrombotic effect by irreversibly inhibiting platelet cyclooxygenase (COX) through acetylation of serine at position 529 leading to steric hindrance of the enzyme. This prevents the formation of the platelet agonist thromboxane A_2 leading to inhibition of platelet function.

In most patients, platelet cyclooxygenase can be inhibited by aspirin doses as small as 30 mg per day. In clinical trials, aspirin doses ranging from 1200 to 30 mg daily have been shown to be effective for prevention of thrombosis. Gastrointestinal side effects are diminished by the lower doses. Currently, the recommended dosage of aspirin is 81–325 mg/day with less side effects seen with doses less than 100 mg. Aspirin is rapidly metabolized by the liver, and when the drug is taken in low doses, most platelet inhibition occurs in the portal vein. Since the platelet inhibition lasts the life of the platelet, the biological half-life of aspirin of 5–7 days is considerably longer than the plasma half-life of 20 minutes. The only drug interactions are with COX-1 inhibitor such as ibuprofen and naproxen which block aspirin from acetylating COX-1. This interaction is not seen with more COX-2 selective drugs such as celecoxib and diclofenac. This negative interaction can be lessened with taking aspirin before other COX-1 inhibitors or if chronic use is required using more COX-2 selective agents.

Aspirin is the initial therapy for any arterial ischemic disorder. Clinical trials have shown aspirin to be effective in ischemic heart disease, angioplasty, coronary artery bypass surgery, and cerebrovascular disease.

Aspirin is effective in secondary prevention of myocardial infarctions. In a meta-analysis by the Antiplatelet Trialists' Collaboration, aspirin use after myocardial infarction reduces the risk of non-fatal strokes by 42%, non-fatal MI by 31%, and vascular death by 13%. Aspirin use in acute myocardial infarction reduces strokes by 45%, re-infarction by 49%, and vascular death by 22%.

Recent clinical trials looking at aspirin for primary prevention of vascular events have found little to no benefit and a consistent risk of bleeding. While older trials suggested a use of aspirin in primary prevention, in the current era of good blood pressure control and statin use, aspirin is no longer recommended for primary prevention except for patients who have evidence of vascular disease – angina, claudication, etc.

Aspirin effect is achieved very rapidly with oral ingestion of more than 160 mg; this dose or higher should be used when a rapid antiplatelet

T. G. DeLoughery (✉)
Division of Hematology/Medical Oncology,
Department of Medicine, Pathology, and Pediatrics,
Oregon Health & Sciences University,
Portland, OR, USA
e-mail: delought@ohsu.edu

© Springer Nature Switzerland AG 2019
T. G. DeLoughery (ed.), *Hemostasis and Thrombosis*,
https://doi.org/10.1007/978-3-030-19330-0_26

effect is desired such as in acute myocardial infarction. Since platelet cyclooxygenase is permanently inhibited, the antiplatelet effect of aspirin will last until the majority of circulating platelets have been replaced; this may take up to 5 days. Coated aspirin – especially enteric coated – may not be as well-absorbed especially in obese patients. Consideration should be given to either using higher (>81 mg) doses or chewable aspirin.

The major side effect of aspirin is bleeding. Minor bleeding complications are increased by 5%. Randomized trials suggest that the incidence of severe or fatal bleeding with aspirin use is increased by 0.5%/year of use with chronic use.

There has been interest in identifying patients who in testing appear to be "aspirin-resistant." Several difficulties with this concept are that the incidence of aspirin resistance varies with the techniques used to study this and true biochemical resistance appears to be rare. Far more common is the "resistance" of the patient to taking aspirin.

Uncertainty now exists for management of a bleeding emergency in the patient taking aspirin. In a study of patients with non-traumatic intracranial hemorrhage on aspirin, the transfusion of platelets significantly worsened outcomes. Also, studies have suggested transfused platelets do not reverse the impaired platelet function in patients taking aspirin. It has been reported that DDAVP will reverse aspirin inhibition and may be effective for emergency surgery or for patients with minor bleeding.

Platelet P2Y12 Receptor Antagonists

Clopidogrel

Clopidogrel is the most widely use thienopyridine and is dosed at 75 mg once per day. Clopidogrel takes 4–7 days to achieve full platelet inhibition, so for acute situations, a loading dose of 300–600 mg is used. The antiplatelet effect can last for 7 days after cessation of therapy. In early trials, single-agent clopidogrel was found to be slightly better than aspirin in prevention of myocardial infarctions and strokes than aspirin, so it can substitute for aspirin in patients who are aspirin-intolerant or aspirin failures.

Most studies have looked at clopidogrel in combination with aspirin. For patients with acute coronary syndromes, this combination leads to improved outcomes and should be continued for a year. Patients with stents also benefit from combined therapy – bare metal for 4 weeks and drug eluting up to a year as described in Chap. 20. Combined therapy for acute coronary syndromes after 1 year, chronic ischemic heart disease, or primary prevention appears not to be effective. For patients with strokes, combined therapy has been shown to be harmful. The only exception is immediately after a stroke or TIA, combined therapy does reduce the risk of new events.

Two factors in theory may decrease effectiveness of clopidogrel. One is that many proton pump inhibitors (especially omeprazole) in theory block conversion of clopidogrel to the active metabolite, but this appears to be clinically irrelevant as most clinical data from large trials do not support lowered effectiveness. Second is that up to 30% of people carry a CYP2C19 loss-of-function polymorphism that also decreased the conversion of drug to the active form. While this appears to translate into these patients having less platelet inhibitor by clopidogrel, again overall clinical significance of this appears not to be relevant.

The amount of platelet inhibition by clopidogrel is more variable than that seen with aspirin. While the notion of using platelet testing such as the VerifyNow P2Y12 to identify low-responding patients and then altering therapy is appealing, clinical trials to date have shown no benefit to this approach.

Although it first appeared that, like ticlopidine, clopidogrel was also associated with the development of TTP, the incidence now appears to be much lower than that seen with ticlopidine at 0.0001%.

Management of patients on clopidogrel who are bleeding is uncertain for the same reasons as discussed for aspirin and use of DDAVP may be helpful.

Prasugrel

Prasugrel is a thienopyridine that binds and blocks the ADP receptor. Unlike clopidogrel it requires one, not two, step for activation resulting in quicker platelet inhibition within 30 minutes of ingestion. It is dosed as a 60 mg loading dose and then 10 mg daily in combination with aspirin. The Triton-TIMI 38 trial showed that prasugrel is more effective than clopidogrel in therapy of acute coronary syndromes undergoing PCI but is associated with an increased risk of bleeding – including fatal bleeding, especially in patients over the age of 75, with history of stroke, or who weigh less than 60 kg. In a trial of patients with acute coronary syndrome not undergoing an intervention, the outcomes with prasugrel and clopidogrel were similar.

Prasugrel has also been reported to rarely cause TTP – perhaps an incidence similar to clopidogrel.

Ticagrelor

Ticagrelor is a non-thienopyridine that reversibly binds and blocks the ADP receptor. A loading dose of 180 mg of ticagrelor is used, and the maintenance dose is 90 mg twice a day. The PLATO trial showed that this drug combined with aspirin is more effective in acute coronary syndrome than aspirin plus clopidogrel and even reduced mortality. A peculiarity of this trial was that this benefit was only seen if the aspirin dose was less than 100 mg. The major non-bleeding side effect of ticagrelor is dyspnea which can be seen in 10% or more of patients. Despite its reversibility, the platelet inhibition caused by ticagrelor does persist for up to 5 days. Since ticagrelor is metabolized by CYP3A4 inducers or inhibitors, it should not be used with these types of drugs. It is also contraindicated in patients with a history of intracranial hemorrhage as the rate of recurrence of bleeding is high. Its use is recommended for patients who have a new event on clopidogrel, and some guidelines recommend its use combined with aspirin after stenting especially if the patient is not at risk for bleeding or felt to be at high risk of stent thrombosis.

Cangrelor

Cangrelor is similar to ticagrelor being a non-thienopyridine P2Y12 inhibitor. It has a very short half-life of 5–7 minutes and is given intravenously. In clinical trials its effectiveness was the same, slightly better than clopidogrel with similar rates of bleeding. It is also being studied to "bridge" patients who have recent coronary stents but need to come off longer-acting antiplatelet agents for surgery.

Other Platelet Antagonists

Dipyridamole

Dipyridamole blocks degradation of cAMP, resulting in modest platelet inhibition. Due to lack of consistent effect in clinical trials, single-agent dipyridamole had fallen out of favor as an antiplatelet agent. Trials using a novel-sustained release form of dipyridamole and aspirin showed greater benefit in secondary stroke prevention than aspirin alone. But this combination was no more effective than clopidogrel but had increased intracranial hemorrhage. Another issue is this pill had no benefit in cardiovascular disease. One common issue is severe headaches with starting this pill. Some patients benefit by starting with combination pills at night (along with an 81 mg aspirin in the morning) and then starting the twice daily dosing in 1 week. It should also be remembered that the effective trials utilized a special form of dipyridamole and that using the generic short-acting dipyridamole in combination with aspirin has been clearly demonstrated *not* to be effective.

Vorapaxar

This antiplatelet agent functions by inhibiting protease activated receptor 1 which is the main platelet thrombin receptor. Vorapaxar is dosed at 2.5 mg twice a day. In patients who had a myocardial infarction in the prior 2 weeks to 12 months, use of vorapaxar was shown to reduce ischemic events plus cardiovascular death but with increased bleeding. Most of the patients in this trial were also on aspirin and clopidogrel. In patients with acute coronary syndrome, the use of vorapaxar given first as a loading dose of 40 mg and then a maintenance dose leads to excess bleeding with no benefit.

Given vorapaxar half-life of 200 hours, it is unlikely that platelet transfusions will reverse the platelet inhibition caused by this drug.

Glycoprotein IIb/IIIa Inhibitors

Abciximab

Glycoprotein IIb/IIIa is a key platelet receptor that binds fibrinogen and von Willebrand protein to form the platelet aggregate. Activation of GP IIB/IIIa represents the "final common pathway" of platelet activation. No matter how the platelet is activated, the GP IIb/IIIa receptor must be activated for platelet aggregation to occur.

Abciximab is a novel antibody that blocks the GP IIb/IIIa and leads to profound suppression of platelet function. The antibody is a chimeric human-mouse antibody. Furthermore, its Fc portion is cleaved off, so it can only bind and inhibit platelet functions but will not lead to splenic uptake and thrombocytopenia. Abciximab is administered in the dose of 0.25 mg/kg bolus and then 0.125 ug/kg/min (maximum 10 mg/min) infusions for 12 hours. Abciximab needs to bind to more than 80% of the GP IIb/IIIa sites to impair platelet function. Soon after the infusion is ended, the antibody undergoes rapid redistribution, and the antiplatelet effects wear off rapidly.

Tirofiban

Tirofiban is the first of a large number of non-antibody GP IIb/IIIa inhibitors to be FDA-approved. Tirofiban is an intravenous synthetic non-peptide platelet antagonist. The dosing is weight-based with bolus of 0.4 ug/kg/min for 30 minutes and then an infusion of 0/1 ug/kg/min until resolution of the syndrome or for 12–24 hours after angiography. Patients with low

creatinine clearances (<30 mL/min) should receive half the dose.

Eptifibatide

Eptifibatide is the second non-antibody anti-GP IIb/IIIa agent available. For acute coronary syndromes, the dose is 180 ug/kg bolus followed by 2 ug/kg/min for up to 72 hours. For patients undergoing PCI, the dose is a bolus of 180 ug/kg followed by a second bolus of 180 ug/kg 10 minutes later. A continuous infusion of 2 ug/kg/min should be started after the first bolus.

Current Role of GP IIb/IIIa Inhibitors

In the pre-thienopyridine era, GP IIb/IIIa inhibitors were associated with improved outcomes in patient undergoing PCI and for those with acute coronary syndromes. Now benefit seems limited to with acute coronary syndromes who are troponin-positive or PCI patients at high risk of thrombotic complications.

GP IIb/IIIa Complications

The major side effect of these new agents is bleeding and thrombocytopenia. Bleeding is treated by giving platelet transfusions. This leads to redistribution of inhibitors and return of platelet function. In the EPIC trial, no excess bleeding was seen in patients who had to undergo an emergency bypass, but other investigators have reported severe bleeding in these patients. It may be judicious to give a platelet transfusion before bypass or early in the operation in patients who have received GP IIa/IIIa inhibitors and need an emergency bypass if excessive bleeding is noted.

Severe thrombocytopenia has been reported in 0.5–2.0% of patients receiving IIb/IIIa inhibitors. The mechanism of thrombocytopenia is unknown but is speculated to be related to conformational changes in GP IIb/IIIa induced by binding of the inhibitors.

If a patient who has received an IIb/IIIa inhibitor presents with severe thrombocytopenia, one should examine the blood smear to ensure that the low platelet count is not due to clumping of the platelets in the blood sample. If the patient has received heparin in the last 3 months, one should also consider heparin-induced thrombocytopenia in the differential.

Experience with abciximab has shown that infusion of immune globulin or the use of steroids is not helpful. The inhibitors should be promptly stopped. Platelet transfusions result in a prompt rise in platelet count if severe thrombocytopenia is present.

Aspirin

- Dose: 81–325 mg/day. Dose over 162 mg should be used for acute ischemia

Indications:

- Primary prevention of myocardial infarction
- Secondary prevention of myocardial infarction
- Secondary prevention of stroke after TIA or stroke
- Acute therapy of myocardial infarction
- Acute therapy of unstable angina
- Prevention of saphenous vein bypass thrombosis

Toxicities:
- GI upset
- Bleeding
- Drug Interactions: COX-1 inhibitors – ibuprofen, naproxen
- Reversal: Platelet transfusion (???), desmopressin

Thienopyridines

Clopidogrel

- Dose: 75 mg po once per day

Indications:

- Secondary prevention of ischemic disease in patients intolerant of aspirin or aspirin failures
- Prevention of coronary stent thrombosis in combination with aspirin

- Toxicities: Gastrointestinal upset (10%)
- Reversal: Desmopressin, platelet transfusions – two plateletpheresis units (???)

Prasugrel

- Dose 60 mg loading, 10mg daily (consider 5 mg in patients <60 kg)

Indications

- Secondary prevention of ischemic disease in patients intolerant of aspirin or aspirin failures
- Prevention of coronary stent thrombosis in combination with aspirin
- Reversal: Desmopressin, platelet transfusions – two plateletpheresis units (???)

Reversible P2Y12 Inhibitors

Ticagrelor

- Dose: 180 mg load, 90 mg BID after

Indications:

- Secondary prevention of ischemic disease in patients intolerant of aspirin or aspirin failures
- Prevention of coronary stent thrombosis in combination with aspirin
- Reversal: Desmopressin, platelet transfusions (???)

Cangrelor

- Dose: 30 ug/kg bolus then 4 ug/kg/min infusion
- Indications: PCI, bridging
- Reversal: Stopping infusions

Other Antiplatelet Agents

Sustained Release Dipyridamole/Aspirin

- Dose: 1 pill BID
- Indication: Secondary prevention of stroke
- Reversal: Desmopressin, platelet transfusion (???)

Vorapaxar (Thrombin Receptor inhibitor)

- Dose 2.5 mg bid
- Indication: Recent myocardial infarction
- Reversal:?

Glycoprotein IIb/IIIa Inhibitors

Abciximab

- Dose: 0.25 mg/kg plus 0.125 ug/kg/min (maximum 10 mg/min) for 12 hours after PCI, along with
- Heparin: 70 units/kg (maximum 7000 units) bolus with additional bolus to achieve an ACT of 200 s

Tirofiban

- Dose: 0.4 ug/kg/min for 30 minutes then an infusion of 0.1 ug/kg/min until resolution of the pain syndrome or for 12–24 hours after PCI

Eptifibatide

- Dose:Unstable angina:180 ug/kg bolus followed by 2 ug/kg/min for up to 72 hours
- PCI: 180 ug/kg bolus and then 2 ug/kg/min for 18–24 hours. Second 180 ug/kg bolus 10 minutes after the first

Toxicities common to all:

- Bleeding
- Thrombocytopenia

Suggested Reading (See Also Chap. 20)

Berger JS. Oral antiplatelet therapy for secondary prevention of acute coronary syndrome. Am J Cardiovasc Drugs. 2018;18(6):457–72.

Danielak D, Karaźniewicz-Łada M, Główka F. Ticagrelor in modern cardiology – an up-to-date review of most important aspects of ticagrelor pharmacotherapy. Expert Opin Pharmacother. 2018;19(2):103–12.

Eikelboom JW, Hirsh J, Spencer FA, Baglin TP, Weitz JI. Antiplatelet drugs: Antithrombotic Therapy and Prevention of Thrombosis, 9th ed: American College of Chest Physicians Evidence-Based Clinical Practice Guidelines. Chest. 2012;141(2 Suppl):e89S–119S. https://doi.org/10.1378/chest.11-2293.

Mega JL, Simon T. Pharmacology of antithrombotic drugs: an assessment of oral antiplatelet and anticoagulant treatments. Lancet. 2015;386(9990):281–91. https://doi.org/10.1016/S0140-6736(15)60243-4.

Ridker PM. Should aspirin be used for primary prevention in the post-statin era? N Engl J Med. 2018;379(16):1572–4.

Shah R, Rashid A, Hwang I, Fan TM, Khouzam RN, Reed GL. Meta-analysis of the relative efficacy and safety of oral P2Y12 inhibitors in patients with acute coronary syndrome. Am J Cardiol. 2017;119(11):1723–8.

Wiviott SD, Steg PG. Clinical evidence for oral antiplatelet therapy in acute coronary syndromes. Lancet. 2015;386(9990):292–302. https://doi.org/10.1016/S0140-6736(15)60213-6.

Thrombolytic Therapy

27

Thomas G. DeLoughery

The third type of antithrombotic therapy – besides inhibiting coagulation or platelets – is lysing a formed thrombosis. In normal fibrinolysis, tPA binds to fibrin and then converts plasminogen to plasmin, which lyses the clot. The ability of tPA to cleave plasminogen to plasmin is far greater when plasminogen and tPA are both bound to the fibrin clot. Moreover, when plasmin is bound to fibrin, plasmin is protected from the action of circulating alpha$_2$-antiplasmin. Any excess tPA that escapes into the plasma is rapidly inactivated by plasminogen activator inhibitor-1 (PAI-1). Any plasmin which escapes into the plasma is rapidly snuffed out by alpha$_2$-antiplasmin. Thus, active fibrinolysis is confined to the thrombus itself.

In pharmacologic fibrinolysis, the excessive quantity of endogenous plasminogen activators overwhelms the inhibitors of fibrinolysis and leads to generalized fibrinolysis. Excess plasmin can destroy any thrombi and degrades circulating fibrinogen. Although tPA is more "clot-specific" than streptokinase due to the presence of kringle regions that can bind fibrin, in practice the use of tPA has not resulted in less bleeding.

T. G. DeLoughery (✉)
Division of Hematology/Medical Oncology,
Department of Medicine, Pathology, and Pediatrics,
Oregon Health & Sciences University,
Portland, OR, USA
e-mail: delought@ohsu.edu

Agents

Streptokinase was the first thrombolytic agent to be widely used. It is derived from *Streptococcus* and has a relatively long half-life of 20 minutes. It is given as an infusion over 1 hour. Streptokinase first cleaves plasminogen by a cumbersome mechanism wherein streptokinase first binds to plasminogen. This complex then cleaves a new molecule of plasminogen to form plasmin. One unique side effect is that patients can develop antibodies to streptokinase due to prior use or due to a recent streptococcal infection.

tPA (alteplase) was one of the first drugs manufactured by recombinant DNA technology. As noted above, endogenous tPA is secreted by endothelial cells and is a direct activator of plasminogen. Currently tPA is made via recombinant DNA technology more than streptokinase but is more effective and does not have as many allergic reactions. While still used in stroke and venous thrombosis, use of thrombolytic therapy in myocardial infarctions has now shifted toward using genetically modified versions of tPA.

Urokinase (UK) is a direct activator of plasminogen. UK is not used for coronary disease but was popular for thrombolytic therapy at other sites, especially for catheter-based use. It is derived from human tissue culture media, and recombinant derivatives are in development. Currently UK is not available in the United States.

© Springer Nature Switzerland AG 2019
T. G. DeLoughery (ed.), *Hemostasis and Thrombosis*,
https://doi.org/10.1007/978-3-030-19330-0_27

Reteplase (r-PA) is a derivative of tPA that is genetically engineered by expression of only one kringle region and the protease region of tPA. These changes lengthens the half-life to 13–16 minutes. Like tPA, it is a direct plasminogen activator. The drug is administered as two boluses of 10 units each with second bolus given 30 minutes after the first bolus. Each bolus is given over 2 minutes.

Tenecteplase (TNK-tPA) has three amino acid substations which produce a plasminogen activator with longer half-life (22 minutes) and more resistance to PAI-1. It can be given as a single weight-based bolus which dramatically simplifies therapy. Currently because of the ease of use, it is the most widely used agent for thrombolytic therapy in myocardial infarctions.

Indications

Myocardial Infarction

One of the biggest advances in the treatment of myocardial infarctions was the use of thrombolytic therapy in acute myocardial infarction reducing the 1-month mortality rate by 18%. The effect is greatest if thrombolytic therapy is used early in the course of the myocardial infarction. In one trial mortality was reduced by 47% if thrombolytics were administered within 1 hour, 22.6% by 6 hours, and 10% in 6–10 hours. Patients with anterior myocardial infarctions have markedly decreased mortality when treated with thrombolytic therapy. The greatest risk of these agents is serious bleeding. The risk of death due to hemorrhage is 1.1% vs 0.4% in controls, but the increased risk of bleeding is outweighed by the reduction in myocardial infarction-related death. A patient who has had previous invasive procedures such as angiography is at risk for bleeding from arterial puncture sites. As noted in Chap. 20, the use of immediate intervention with stenting has been shown to offer improved outcomes when compared to thrombolytic therapy alone. However, if catheterization laboratories are not immediately available, the delay in care that results from waiting to transfer the patient must be weighed against the benefits of immediate thrombolytic therapy.

Stroke

Since most strokes are thrombotic in origin, it is tempting to consider thrombolytic therapy, but the serious side effect of intracranial bleeding has made researchers reluctant to consider this therapy. Studies have shown that – in carefully selected patients – if tPA therapy is given within 3 hours of stroke onset (and some patients 3–4.5 hours), there is an improvement in outcome at 6 months. Currently one should consider thrombolytic therapy for patients with stroke if they are evaluated in the very early stages of a stroke and have no major risk factors for bleeding. As noted in Chap. 21, increasingly endovascular therapy is being used for the treatment of acute stroke, but in eligible patients, thrombolytic therapy is given first.

Deep Venous Thrombosis/Pulmonary Embolism

Systemic thrombolytic therapy for deep venous thrombosis in early studies was not very successful. Early results with catheter-directed thrombolytic therapy appeared promising, but unfortunately, data from a large clinical trial shows no difference in development of post-thrombotic syndrome with this approach. However, patients with very severe DVT resulting massive edema leading to arterial compromise (phlegmasia cerulea dolens) or with disabling symptoms despite adequate anticoagulation may benefit for directed thrombolytic therapy.

For most patients with pulmonary embolism, thrombolytic therapy is not warranted as the risks outweigh the benefits. The exception remains in patients with refractory hypotension. Patients need to be screened for bleeding risks as many of the risk factors for embolism are those for bleeding (cancer, recent surgery, and older age). As with deep venous thrombosis, increasingly catheter-directed therapy for pulmonary embolism is being used, but there is little clinical trial data yet to support this.

Complications

The major complication of thrombolytic therapy is bleeding. Patients bleed at sites of previous injury due to lysis of previously formed thrombus. Patients may also have bleeding due to underlying vascular problems. A patient who suffers intracranial hemorrhage with thrombolytic therapy often has underlying cerebrovascular amyloid.

Thrombolytic therapy affects every aspect of the hemostatic system. Patients will have a low fibrinogen and elevated PT and aPTT due to destruction of factors V and VIII. Platelet dysfunction will occur due to binding of fibrinogen fragments blocking platelet receptors and also cleaving platelet receptors. Finally, there will be lysis of formed thrombi.

Patients who suffer severe bleeding after thrombolytic therapy should immediately have a PT, aPTT, fibrinogen level, and platelet count performed. Ten units of cryoprecipitate should be infused to replace fibrinogen and factor VIII. If the PT and aPTT remain elevated, two units of plasma should then be infused. If bleeding persists, platelets should be given. If the patient is having an intracranial hemorrhage, empiric therapy with cryoprecipitate, platelets, and plasma should be given.

Although reversal of the fibrinolytic state can be achieved with the use of antifibrinolytic agents, this is rarely required. The fibrinolytic state, especially with tPA, is short-lived. Infusion of fibrinogen and plasma will shorten the duration of the fibrinolytic state. Finally, reversal of fibrinolysis may result in reformation of the culprit thrombus that would then be refractory to lysis.

Thrombolytic Therapy

Streptokinase
Myocardial infarction: 1.5 million units IV over 1 hour

Urokinase
Pulmonary embolism: 4400 units/kg over 1 minute load and then 4400/kg/hour for 12 hours

Arterial thrombosis: 4000 units/minute for 4 hours and then 2000 units/minute for up to 44 hours

Tissue Plasminogen Activator (Alteplase)
Myocardial infarction: 15 mg/kg bolus, 0.75 mg/kg over 30 minutes, and then 0.5 mg/kg over the next hour

Stroke: 0.9 mg/kg (maximum 90 mg) with 10% of the dose given in 1 minute

Pulmonary embolism: 100 mg given over 2 hours

Reteplase
Myocardial infarction: two 10-unit boluses separated by 30 minutes

Tenecteplase
Myocardial infarction: weight-based bolus over 5 seconds
- <60 kg = 30 mg
- 60–69 kg = 35 mg
- 70–79 kg = 40 mg
- 80–89 kg = 45 mg
- >90 kg = 50 mg

Suggested Reading

Kluft C, Sidelmann JJ, Gram JB. Assessing safety of thrombolytic therapy. Semin Thromb Hemost. 2017;43(3):300–10.

Nakamura S, Takano H, Kubota Y, Asai K, Shimizu W. Impact of the efficacy of thrombolytic therapy on the mortality of patients with acute submassive pulmonary embolism: a meta-analysis. J Thromb Haemost. 2014;12(7):1086–95.

Sane DC, Califf RM, Topol EJ, Stump DC, Mark DB, Greenberg CS. Bleeding during thrombolytic therapy for acute myocardial infarction: mechanisms and management. Ann Intern Med. 1989;111(12):1010–22.

Vedantham S, Goldhaber SZ, Julian JA, Kahn SR, Jaff MR, Cohen DJ, Magnuson E, Razavi MK, Comerota AJ, Gornik HL, Murphy TP, Lewis L, Duncan JR, Nieters P, Derfler MC, Filion M, Gu CS, Kee S, Schneider J, Saad N, Blinder M, Moll S, Sacks D, Lin J, Rundback J, Garcia M, Razdan R, VanderWoude E, Marques V, Kearon C, Trial Investigators ATTRACT. Pharmacomechanical catheter-directed thrombolysis for deep-vein thrombosis. N Engl J Med. 2017;377(23):2240–52.

Clinical Dilemmas in Anticoagulation: Extremes of Weight, Renal Disease, Recent Bleeding, and Surgery

Thomas G. DeLoughery

Extremes of Weight

Several studies have suggested that patients who are underweight may be more at risk for bleeding since many antithrombotic agents are given as fixed doses. In underweight patients – especially under 50 kg – lower doses of the fixed-dose antithrombotic agents should be used, such as using prasugrel 5 mg or lowering the prophylactic dose of enoxaparin to 20 or 30 mg daily.

The DOACs rivaroxaban and dabigatran should be avoided in patients weighing less than 50 kg. For apixaban, there is data for use in patients less than 60 kg, and it is unclear whether this can be extrapolated to patients who weigh less than 50 kg.

Despite the epidemic of obesity, there is little guidance for use of antithrombotic drugs in these patients. For obese patients, enteric-coated aspirin should be avoided as these are not as well absorbed. All heparin products given for therapeutic intent should be dosed by actual body weight. For thrombosis prophylaxis, one can either use enoxaparin 40 mg bid for BMI of 35–50 kg/m^2, increasing to 60 mg bid for weights over 50 kg/m^2, or a regimen of 0.5 mg/kg daily, or equivalent

doses of other LMWH. For fondaparinux, one approach is to add 2.5 mg to the dose for every 50 kg in weight starting at or over 150 kg – i.e., a 150 kg patient would get 12.5 mg daily as a therapeutic dose – which is consistent with its dosing schema in lower-weight patients. There is limited data for DOACs' dosing in patients weighing over 140 kg. If these agents are used, specific levels should be drawn to ensure therapeutic levels are achieved.

Renal Disease

Anticoagulation in patients with renal disease is complicated by two issues. One issue is that many anticoagulation agents are cleared by the kidney. The second is that the presence of renal disease – even modest – can itself increase the risk of bleeding (Table 28.1).

The metabolism of antiplatelet agents is little affected by renal disease, but use of these agents is associated with increased risk of bleeding due to augmentation of the platelet defects of renal disease. Unfractionated heparin does not undergo renal metabolism, so dose adjustment is not required for abnormal renal function. However, renal disease will increase the risk of bleeding two- to threefold. Since LMWH are renally cleared, their dosing must be adjusted; most of the data is for enoxaparin. In patients on dialysis, enoxaparin dosing should be 1 mg/kg daily.

T. G. DeLoughery (✉)
Division of Hematology/Medical Oncology,
Knight Cancer Center, Oregon Health & Sciences
University, Portland, OR, USA
e-mail: delought@ohsu.edu

© Springer Nature Switzerland AG 2019
T. G. DeLoughery (ed.), *Hemostasis and Thrombosis*,
https://doi.org/10.1007/978-3-030-19330-0_28

Table 28.1 Renal dosing of antithrombotic agents

Agent	Half-life	Renal disease
Aspirin	15–30 minutes	No change in dosing
Clopidogrel	8 hours	Active metabolite renally cleared – no change in dosing
Prasugrel	7 hour	No change in dosing
Ticagrelor	7 hours	No change in dosing
Abciximab	30 minutes	No change in dosing
Tirofiban	2 hours	Decrease dose by 50% if CrCl <30 ml/min
Eptifibatide	2–3 hours	Decrease dose by 50% if CrCl <30 ml/min
Unfractionated heparin	30–150 minutes	45–225 minutes – no change in dosing
LMWH	2–8 hours	4–16 hours – decrease by 50% if CrCl <30 ml/min
Fondaparinux	17–21 hours	Should not be used if CrCl <30 ml/min
Argatroban	40 minutes	No change
Bivalirudin	25 minutes	60% dose reduction if CrCl <30 ml/min
Dabigatran	12–17 hours	If CrCl 30–50 ml/min, use 110 mg bid if available If CrCl 15–30 ml/min, use 75 mg bid Avoid if CrCl <15 ml/min
Rivaroxaban	5–9 hours	Reduce dose to 15 mg if CrCl 15–30 ml/min; avoid if <15 ml/ml.
Apixaban	9–14 hours	Decrease to 2.5 mg bid if creatinine >1.5 and weight is less than 60 kg and/or age over 80
Edoxaban	10–14 hours	If CrCl 15-30 ml/min then 30mg daily. If CrCl, 15 ml/min do not use
Warfarin	36 hours	50% reduction in CYP C2P9
Streptokinase	80 minutes	Hepatically cleared
tPA	3 minutes	Hepatically cleared
Reteplase	13–16 minutes	Hepatically cleared
Tenecteplase	15–20 minutes	Hepatically cleared

For long-term use in patients with milder renal compromise (CrCl 30–50 ml/min), the dosage should be adjusted down to 0.85 mg/kg every 12 hours. Fondaparinux is predominantly cleared via the kidneys and should be avoided in patients with creatinine clearances under 30 ml/min. For prophylactic use, a dose adjustment lowering the prophylactic dose to 1.5 mg daily may be appropriate for patients with creatinine clearance of 20–50 ml/min. There is no renal metabolism of warfarin, but data show the metabolism of warfarin is slower in dialysis patients. Lower doses should be used when initiating therapy.

All the DOACs undergo renal clearance. Dabigatran is the most dependent on renal clearance (80%), and dosage should be decreased with clearances under 50 ml/min – or an alternative agent should be chosen. For rivaroxaban (renal clearance 36%), the standard daily dose of 20 mg is reduced to 15 mg/day for clearances between 15 and 50 ml/min, and this drug should not be given if clearance is less than 15 ml/min. Edoxaban has 35% renal clearance; the standard dose of 60 mg daily is cut to 30 mg if the CrCl is 15–50 ml/

min. Edoxaban also has the unique dosing restriction of being contraindicated in atrial fibrillation stroke prophylaxis if the CrCl is more than 95 ml/min. Apixaban has the least renal metabolism (25%) and has a dosing recommendation of 5 mg bid for those on dialysis or with end-stage renal disease, with observational studies showing less bleeding than with warfarin use. Apixaban is only renally dosed (2.5 mg bid) in patients with creatinines over 1.5 mg/dl **if** the patient is over age 80 and/or if their weight is under 60 kg.

Elderly Patients and Those at Risk of Falling

Older patients have higher rates of bleeding with antithrombotic therapy; this is most often due to comorbid conditions, renal insufficiency, and polypharmacy. Counterbalancing the bleeding risk is a marked increase in thrombosis risk with aging. DOACs have been shown to have less bleeding risk in older patients and should be preferentially used over warfarin unless a contraindication is present. One common but unsubstantiated reason for denying older patients warfarin is the fear of bleeds with falls; this is the most common reason cited to deny anticoagulation to older patients. However, the data does not support this. The incidence of intracerebral hemorrhage (ICH) with falling is very low; in the May-Song-Hin paper, it was estimated a patient must fall over 295 times a year for warfarin not to be optimal therapy to prevent stroke in atrial fibrillation.

Ironically, the data is clear that the patients who are at perceived risk of falling are the most likely to benefit from anticoagulation – older, previous strokes, diabetes, etc. A crucial part of the management of these patients is also to try to correct risk factors for falling such as prescribing physical therapy and trying to reduce medications that increase the risk of falls.

Liver Disease

Aspirin is to be avoided in those with liver disease unless there is a strong indication, such as secondary prevention of myocardial infarction or presence of coronary stents, given the higher baseline risk of gastrointestinal bleeding. In patients with advanced liver disease, the use of LMWH can lead to over-anticoagulation – even if monitored by anti-Xa levels – as these levels will underestimate the heparin anticoagulation effect. Warfarin is difficult to use as many patients will have a high baseline INR. Recent studies regarding the use of DOACs have demonstrated lesser bleeding rates compared with older anticoagulants. Rivaroxaban and edoxaban have slower metabolism in patients with Child B cirrhosis and are not recommended. Dabigatran and apixaban can be used in Child B cirrhosis, but none of the DOACs should be used in more advanced liver disease (Child C cirrhosis).

Patients with Recent Bleeding

The question of when to restart anticoagulation in patients with recent bleeding is a common issue. Despite the frequency of bleeding, there are no prospective data to guide decision-making. While in some patients anticoagulation can just be stopped, others (such as those with mechanical valves, atrial fibrillation with high CHADS2 scores, or recent thrombosis) will need anticoagulation.

In patients with intracranial hemorrhage (ICH), resumption of anticoagulation was associated with lower stroke and mortality rates compared to those who never restarted anticoagulation. The use of antiplatelet agents did not improve either stroke or bleeding rates compared to no anticoagulation. Location of ICH is predictive of recurrences; lobar or "deep" (basal ganglia, thalamus, internal capsule, cerebellum, brains stem) bleeds have higher rates of rebleeding. Expert opinion and retrospective studies indicate anticoagulation need only be held for 7–14 days before restarting anticoagulation after ICH.

For those with gastrointestinal and genitourinary bleeding, the fundamental step is to look for sources of bleeding, as up to 50% of patients will be bleeding from identifiable lesions. As with ICH, studies show that patients who resume anticoagulation have fewer thromboembolic events, fewer deaths, and minimally increased risk of recurrent bleeding compared to those who did not resume anticoagulation. Studies have indicated that holding anticoagulation for 4–7 days is all that needed.

Reversal of Antithrombotic Agents (Table 28.2)

When patients taking antithrombotics are bleeding or need to go to surgery, the question of reversal is often raised. While many treatments seem logical, few have been tested in clinical trials. For antiplatelet agents, desmopressin may help improve platelet function. Platelet transfusion remains controversial as data suggest these may not improve platelet function, and the PATCH study showed transfusion is harmful for intracranial hemorrhage. For heparin and LMWH, protamine can be effective. Vitamin K and plasma/prothrombin complex concentrates (PCC) can be effective. For the DOACs, there is a specific

Table 28.2 Reversal of antithrombotic agents

Aspirin

Minor bleeding – desmopressin 0.3 mcg/kg × 1

Major bleeding – consider platelet transfusion (one apheresis unit)

Clopidogrel

Minor – desmopressin 0.3 mcg/kg × 1

Major – consider platelet transfusion; consider two units if life-threatening or brain-threatening bleeding (may not be effective)

Prasugrel

Minor – desmopressin 0.3 mcg/kg × 1

Major – consider platelet transfusion; consider two units if life-threatening or brain-threatening bleeding (may not be effective)

Ticagrelor

Minor – desmopressin 0.3 mcg/kg × 1

Major – consider platelet transfusion; consider two units if life-threatening or brain-threatening bleeding (may not be effective)

Sustained- Release aspirin/dipyridamole

Minor – desmopressin 0.3 mcg/kg × 1

Major – consider platelet transfusion

Abciximab

Major – consider platelet transfusion

Eptifibatide

Minor – desmopressin 0.3 mcg/kg × 1

Major bleeding reversal: consider platelet transfusions plus infusion of 10 units of cryoprecipitate

Tirofiban

Minor – desmopressin 0.3 mcg/kg × 1

Major bleeding reversal: consider platelet transfusions plus infusion of 10 units of cryoprecipitate

Heparin and heparin-like agents

Standard heparin

Time since last heparin dose	Dose of protamine
< 30 minutes	1 unit/100 units of heparin
30–60 minutes	0.5–0.75 units/100 units of heparin
60–120 minutes	0.375–0.5 units/100 units of heparin
> 120 minutes	0.25–0.375 units/100 units of heparin

Infusion rate should not exceed 5 mg/min. Maximum dose is 50 mg per dose

Low- Molecular- Weight Heparin

Reversal of life-threatening bleeding: Protamine – if within 4 hours of dose, give 1 mg of protamine for each 1 mg of enoxaparin or 100 units of dalteparin and tinzaparin. Repeat one-half dose of protamine in 4 hours. If 4–8 hours after dose, give 0.5 mg for each 1 mg of enoxaparin or 100 units of dalteparin and tinzaparin.

Fondaparinux

Major bleeding reversal: Protamine ineffective – rVIIa (90ug/kg) or 50 units/kg PCC may be of use.

Dabigatran

Table 28.2 (continued)

1. Idarucizumab 5 g (two 2.5 g vials)

Rivaroxaban

1. 4-factor PCC 50 units/kg *or*

2. Andexanet 800 mg bolus and 960 mg over 2 hours (if available)

Apixaban

1. 4-factor PCC 50 units/kg *or*

2. Andexanet 400 mg bolus and 480 mg over 2 hours (if available)

Edoxaban

1. 4-factor PCC 50 units/kg *or*

2. Andexanet 800 mg bolus and 960 mg over 2 hours (if available)

Warfarin

Not bleeding: goal is INR in 2–3 range

INR	Action
3–4.5	Hold dose until INR decreased
4.5–10	1.25 mg vitamin K po × 1
> 10	2.5–5 mg vitamin K po

Should see INR back in therapeutic range in 24–48 hours

Bleeding: goal is INR under 2

INR	Action
2–4.5	2.5 mg vitamin K po or IV ± FFP (15 ml/kg)
4.5–10	5 mg vitamin K ± FFP (15 ml/kg)
>10	5–10 mg vitamin K ± FFP (15 ml/kg)

FFP fresh frozen plasma

Warfarin life- or brain-threatening bleeding

4-Factor PCC

If INR 2–4: 25 units/kg (not to exceed 2500 units)

If INR 4–6: 35 units/kg (not to exceed 3500 units)

If INR > 6: 50 units/kg (not to exceed 5000 units)

Plus vitamin K 10 mg IV for all above warfarin scenarios

reversal agent for dabigatran. For Xa inhibitors, studies are ongoing to see whether PCC or the specific reversal agent andexanet is the better reversal agent. In development is ciraparantag which will be a "universal" reversal agent for all DOACs and heparin-type drugs.

Antithrombotic Therapy and Surgery

It is estimated that up to 10% of patients on antithrombotic therapy will need surgery or a procedure each year. One needs to consider both the agent the patient is taking and the bleeding risk of surgery to determine the best course of action.

Antiplatelet Agents

The most robust data on the effects of aspirin on surgical bleeding are from the POISE-2 trial and showed no difference in deaths or nonfatal myocardial infarction (HR 0.99) with or without aspirin; a mildly increased risk of major bleeding with aspirin was seen (HR = 1.23). Other studies have shown this increased risk holds true even for cardiac procedures. Recommendations are that aspirin can be stopped 3–5 days before surgery and restarted 1–2 days afterward. Patients with recent (30 days or less) cardiac events should stay on aspirin.

The P2Y12 inhibitors are thought to increase the risk of surgical bleeding more than aspirin. These agents should be stopped 7 days before surgery to allow full platelet function to return. If the ability to monitor antiplatelet effect is available (such as with VerifyNow®), one can monitor platelet function to see if surgery can be performed sooner if platelet function test results have returned to normal. As discussed below, patients with coronary artery stents will need to be on uninterrupted P2Y12 inhibitor for 3–6 months after stent placement.

In patients with drug-eluting stents, current recommendations are that surgery be delayed at least 30 days after bare metal stent placement and 3–6 months after drug-eluting stent placement.

Many nonsteroidal anti-inflammatory agents have antiplatelet properties and should be stopped before any surgery with a high risk of bleeding (Table 28.3).

Anticoagulants

Heparins

For unfractionated heparin, the IV infusion can be stopped 4 hours before the procedure while monitoring of the PTT to ensure normalization. If the patient is receiving subcutaneous heparin therapy, the last dose should be 8 hours prior.

LMWH half-life is longer, and ideally it should be held 24 hours before procedures. Given that LMWH are renally cleared, the dose should be held longer if renal dysfunction is present – 36

Table 28.3 Nonsteroidal anti-inflammatory agents and stopping time before procedures

Celecoxib
No need to hold (minimal antiplatelet effect)
Diclofenac
Stop 24 hours before
Ketoprofen
Stop 24 hours before
Ketorolac
Stop 24 hours before
Ibuprofen
Stop 24 hours before
Indomethacin
Stop 24 hours before
Meloxicam
No need to hold (minimal antiplatelet effect)
Naproxen
Stop 24 hours before
Piroxicam
Withhold for 11 days

to 48 hours, or longer, depending on the particular drug and the degree of renal impairment.

Fondaparinux's long half-life and heavy reliance on renal excretion makes it the most challenging agent to hold before surgery. For patients with normal renal function, the drug should be held 48 hours before procedures, and it should be held even longer if there is renal insufficiency.

One of the greatest risk factors for bleeding is premature resumption of heparin after surgery; resuming full therapeutic dosing at 24 hours almost doubles the risk of bleeding. For many procedures, a prophylactic dose of heparin (or LMWH) may have the best risk-benefit ratio during the first 24–72 hours after surgery.

Warfarin

For simple or low-risk bleeding procedures, the simplest option is to continue warfarin. Many cardiac procedures, such as pacemaker or ICD implantation, have shown this is the safest approach. The same is true for many non-cardiac procedures such as dental procedures and cataracts. There is also some reported experience with doing some orthopedic procedures such as total hip or knee arthroplasties while therapeutically anticoagulated with warfarin.

For many years, the standard approach to most patients on warfarin undergoing procedures was

Table 28.4 Peri-operative DOAC management for major and minor surgery

Drug	Surgery	Creatinine clearance	Days in relation to surgery					
			4	3	2	1	Surgery	
Apixaban	Major				Stop			Resume 48–72 hours postop
	Minor					Stop		Resume ~24 hours postop
Dabigatran	Major	>50 ml/min			Stop			Resume 48–72 hours postop
		≤50 ml/min	Stop					
	Minor	>50 ml/min				Stop		Resume ~24 hours postop
		≤50 ml/min			Stop			
Rivaroxaban	Major				Stop			Resume 48–72 hours postop
	Minor					Stop		Resume ~24 hours postop

Note: If CrCl <25 ml/min for apixaban or <30 ml/min for rivaroxaban, add an extra day

"bridging" with heparin. However, both observational studies and a randomized clinical trial show this is not only unnecessary but substantially increases the risk of bleeding. Currently bridging is only recommended for patients with high-risk mechanical valves, atrial fibrillation with recent stroke (some will also include CHADS2 scores >4), and recent (within 90 days) venous thromboembolic disease.

The most common bridging protocol is to stop warfarin 5 days before the procedure, wait a day, then on days 3 until 1 preoperatively administer LMWH at therapeutic dosage, with the last dose 24 hours before surgery. The night of the procedure, the patient would resume warfarin and, then 24–48 hours after surgery, would restart therapeutic subcutaneous LMWH and continue it until the INR returns to the therapeutic range.

Based on the findings of increased risks with no benefits of bridging therapy, the simplest option for most patients is to stop warfarin therapy without bridging. Warfarin can be stopped 5 days before the procedure and restarted the night of surgery. In some circumstances, prophylactic doses of LMWH should be used to reduce the risk of postoperative VTE until the INR is above 2.0.

Direct Oral Anticoagulants

Several principles hold true for DOACs. Bridging is not required for any of them. Most can be stopped 24–48 hours before procedures (Table 28.4). After a procedure, the DOAC can be restarted at 50% dose for 24 hours for complex procedures or a full dose for minor procedures.

Suggested Reading

Baharoglu MI, Cordonnier C, Al-Shahi Salman R, de Gans K, Koopman MM, Brand A, Majoie CB, Beenen LF, Marquering HA, Vermeulen M, Nederkoorn PJ, de Haan RJ, Roos YB, Investigators PATCH. Platelet transfusion versus standard care due to spontaneous cerebral haemorrhage associated with antiplatelet therapy (PATCH): a randomised, open-label, phase 3 trial. Lancet. 2016;387(10038):2605–13.

Chousou PA, Pugh PJ. Managing anticoagulation in patients receiving implantable cardiac devices. Futur Cardiol. 2018;14(2):151–64.

Devereaux PJ, Mrkobrada M, Sessler DI, Leslie K, Alonso-Coello P, Kurz A, Villar JC, Sigamani A, Biccard BM, Meyhoff CS, Parlow JL, Guyatt G, Robinson A, Garg AX, Rodseth RN, Botto F, Lurati Buse G, Xavier D, Chan MT, Tiboni M, Cook D, Kumar PA, Forget P, Malaga G, Fleischmann E, Amir M, Eikelboom J, Mizera R, Torres D, Wang CY, VanHelder T, Paniagua P, Berwanger O, Srinathan S, Graham M, Pasin L, Le Manach Y, Gao P, Pogue J, Whitlock R, Lamy A, Kearon C, Baigent C, Chow C, Pettit S, Chrolavicius S, Yusuf S, POISE-2 Investigators. Aspirin in patients undergoing noncardiac surgery. N Engl J Med. 2014;370(16):1494–503.

Douketis JD, Spyropoulos AC, Kaatz S, Becker RC, Caprini JA, Dunn AS, Garcia DA, Jacobson A, Jaffer AK, Kong DF, Schulman S, Turpie AG, Hasselblad V, Ortel TL, BRIDGE Investigators. Perioperative bridging anticoagulation in patients with atrial fibrillation. N Engl J Med. 2015;373(9):823–33.

Man-Son-Hing M, Nichol G, Lau A, Laupacis A. Choosing antithrombotic therapy for elderly patients with atrial fibrillation who are at risk for falls. Arch Intern Med. 1999;159(7):677–85.

Siontis KC, Zhang X, Eckard A, Bhave N, Schaubel DE, He K, Tilea A, Stack AG, Balkrishnan R, Yao X, Noseworthy PA, Shah ND, Saran R, Nallamothu BK. Outcomes associated with apixaban use in patients with end-stage kidney disease and atrial fibrillation in the United States. Circulation. 2018;138(15):1519–29.

Zhou Z, Yu J, Carcel C, Delcourt C, Shan J, Lindley RI, Neal B, Anderson CS, Hackett ML. Resuming anticoagulants after anticoagulation-associated intracranial haemorrhage: systematic review and meta-analysis. BMJ Open. 2018;8(5):e019672.

29

Joseph Shatzel

Cancer is a common disease; an estimated one in four people develop some form of cancer in a lifetime. Both excessive bleeding and thrombosis may be seen in cancer patients. These may be due to the direct effect of the malignant cell or to the by-products of the cancer having an effect on the hemostatic system, along with treatment-related effects that may predispose to thrombosis or bleeding.

Bleeding Syndromes

Acute Promyelocytic Leukemia (APL)

The hemostatic defects in patients with APL are multiple. Most, if not all, patients with APL have evidence of disseminated intravascular coagulation (DIC) at the time of diagnosis. Patients with APL have a higher risk of death during induction therapy when compared with patients with other forms of leukemia, mostly due to complications from coagulopathy. But, once in remission, APL patients have a significantly higher cure rate than most other forms of acute leukemia. APL is also unique among leukemias in that biological therapy

with retinoic acid and arsenic is effective in inducing remission and cure. Patients can present with pancytopenia due to leukemic marrow replacement or with diffuse bleeding due to DIC and thrombocytopenia. Life-threatening bleeding such as intracranial hemorrhage may occur at any time until the leukemia is put into remission.

Etiology

The etiology of the hemostatic defects in APL is complex and is thought to be the result of DIC, primary fibrinolysis, plus the release of other procoagulant enzymes from the leukemic cell.

The leukemic cell contains tissue factor, which can directly activate coagulation via the extrinsic pathway. In the test tube, the APL cells themselves may function as activators of coagulation and stimulate thrombin generation. Patients with APL have high levels of markers of DIC such as thrombin-antithrombin III complexes. However, patients with APL tend to have normal levels of antithrombin III, unlike patients with DIC due to other causes.

Patients with APL also show signs of increased fibrinolysis. The leukemic cells contain fibrinolytic enzymes such as urokinase. In addition, brisk fibrinolysis due to thrombin generation is also present. Inhibitors of fibrinolysis such as alpha$_2$-antiplasmin are reduced, sometimes markedly so.

J. Shatzel (✉)
Division of Hematology/Medical Oncology,
Department of Medicine and Biomedical
Engineering, Oregon Health & Sciences University,
Portland, OR, USA
e-mail: shatzel@ohsu.edu

© Springer Nature Switzerland AG 2019
T. G. DeLoughery (ed.), *Hemostasis and Thrombosis*,
https://doi.org/10.1007/978-3-030-19330-0_29

APL cells, like their non-malignant counterparts, contain a number of proteases which have been implicated in the coagulation defects of APL. These proteases can degrade von Willebrand factor and fibrinogen, which further augments the coagulation defects. In addition, the proteases may disrupt vascular integrity, leading to bleeding. Cancer procoagulant is a protease that activates factor X independent of factor VII and is found in APL and several solid tumors. Increased annexin II receptor expression on the surface of the promyelocytes binds plasminogen and its activator, tissue plasminogen activator. This increases plasmin formation, thus provoking hyperfibrinolysis.

Diagnosis

The diagnosis of APL is initially suspected based on leukemic cell morphology. The leukemic cells generally appear to be bilobed promyelocytes with prominent Auer rods. However, some patients have the microgranular form without obvious Auer rods. Demonstration of the classic translocation by directly detecting the 15:17 (q22;q12) rearrangement using fluorescent in-site hybridization or PCR is now standard for confirming the diagnosis.

When a patient is suspected of having acute leukemia, one should obtain a complete coagulation profile including PT-INR, aPTT, fibrinogen, platelet count, and D-dimers. Leukemia patients with any signs of major coagulopathy should have testing immediately sent for APL and strong consideration for empiric therapy with all-trans-retinoic acid (ATRA) to reduce the possibility of fatal bleeding. Changes in fibrinogen levels are a good marker of progress in treating the coagulation defects.

Therapy

Acute therapy for APL involves treating both the leukemia and the coagulopathy.

Currently the standard induction treatment for APL is trans-retinoic acid (ATRA) in combination with arsenic for low-risk patients and adding chemotherapy for high-risk patients. This will induce remission in over 90% of patients, and a sizable majority of these patients will be cured of their APL. ATRA therapy will also lead to early correction of the coagulation defects, often within the first week of therapy. This is in stark contrast to the chemotherapy era when the coagulation defects would become worse with therapy. Rare reports of massive thrombosis complicating therapy with ATRA exist, but the relationship to either the APL or ATRA is unknown.

Therapy for the coagulation defects consists of aggressive transfusion therapy support and possible use of other pharmacological agents to control the DIC (Table 29.1). Patients should receive frequent laboratory monitoring, up to every 6 hours, so the effectiveness of the transfusion therapy can be seen and further therapy given. One should try to maintain the fibrinogen level at over 150mg/dl; the platelet count should be maintained at 20,000 or over 50,000/uL if overt bleeding or DIC is present.

Controversy still exists over the role of heparin in the therapy of APL. Although attractive for its ability to quench thrombin, heparin use can lead to profound bleeding. One should consider the use of heparin only in certain circumstances. Patients who require large amounts of cryoprecipitate (>40 units/day) should be considered for heparin therapy. The rare patient who has thrombosis should also receive heparin. One should start with a low dose of 500 units/hr without bolus and monitor with heparin levels. Aggressive coagulation factor replacement should be used along with the heparin.

Table 29.1 Initial evaluation and management of DIC in patients with APL

1. Obtain baseline INR, aPTT, platelet count, fibrinogen, and D-dimer.
2. Based on laboratories, replace using following goals:
   INR >2 and aPTT >1.5 × normal: two units of fresh frozen plasma.
   Platelets under 50,000/ul: give one plateletpheresis unit or 6–8 platelet concentrates.
   Fibrinogen under 150 mg/dl: give 10 units of cryoprecipitate.
3. If coagulation defects are initially present, follow coagulation labs every 6 hours.
4. If patient requires over 40 units of cryoprecipitate in 24 hours or has thrombosis, consider starting heparin at 500 units/hour.

Bleeding in Other Leukemias and Myelodysplastic Syndromes

Along with the obvious thrombocytopenia due to marrow replacement, other coagulation defects may be seen in leukemias. DIC can be seen in other forms of acute leukemia apart from APL. DIC is frequently seen in acute monocytic leukemia. Patients with acute lymphocytic leukemia may also have DIC; one report showed that most patients develop signs of DIC with induction therapy.

The most common coagulation defect in acute lymphoblastic leukemia (ALL) is associated with the use of L-asparaginase. Both bleeding and thrombotic complications have been reported with the use of this effective chemotherapeutic agent. L-asparaginase decreases hepatic synthesis of many proteins, including coagulation factors, which in theory leads to risk of bleeding, but as discussed below, most often thrombosis complicates the patient's care.

Patients with chronic lymphocytic lymphoma (CLL) along with lymphoplasmacytic lymphoma (LPL or Waldenström's macroglobulinemia) or marginal zone lymphoma (MZL) may be treated with the BTK inhibitor ibrutinib. Ibrutinib inhibits platelet GPVI signaling, leading to an increase in both major and minor bleeding events.

Multiple defects are found in the platelets of patients with myelodysplastic syndrome. These include reduced platelet aggregation in response to a variety of agonists and decreased platelet stores of von Willebrand protein and fibrinogen. These patients may have severe bleeding even with platelet counts above 50,000/uL. Therapy of bleeding in myelodysplasia is often unsatisfactory, with some patients not responding even to platelet transfusions.

Myeloproliferative Syndromes

A higher incidence of bleeding is seen in many of the myeloproliferative syndromes, but the bleeding rarely results in major morbidity. One-quarter of patients with polycythemia vera experience some bleeding, but this is very rarely the cause of death. Most series report that 30% of patients with essential thrombocytosis have bleeding. Paradoxically, the risk of bleeding appears to increase with platelet counts above one million. Some patients with extreme thrombocytosis have evidence of acquired von Willebrand disease. Most bleeding in myeloproliferative syndromes consists of mucocutaneous bleeding or bruising with only a few reports of major bleeding. The use of drugs that inhibit platelet function is associated with a higher incidence of bleeding.

Despite the large number of reported in vitro abnormalities, with two exceptions, there is no one specific platelet defect that appears to explain or predict bleeding in patients with myeloproliferative syndromes. It is known that patients with platelet counts over 1,000,000/Ul can have acquired von Willebrand disease. Also, rare patients have been reported to have an acquired factor V deficiency.

Patients with markedly elevated platelet counts and acquired VWD respond to lowering the counts to below 1,000,000/ul. Platelet transfusions and/or plasma can help patients with acquired factor V deficiency. Some patients will have bleeding with no demonstrable defects; sometimes platelet transfusion or antifibrinolytic therapy with tranexamic acid can help.

Dysproteinemias

Dysproteinemia can affect many steps of the coagulation system and lead to severe bleeding. Multiple coagulation abnormalities have been described in patients with dysproteinemias (Table 29.2). The majority of bleeding complications are due to the effects of hyperviscosity.

Table 29.2 Coagulation defects associated with paraproteins

| 1. Monoclonal antibodies inhibiting coagulation factors |
| 2. Monoclonal antibodies inhibiting platelet receptors |
| 3. Monoclonal antibodies inhibiting fibrin formation |
| 4. Amyloid deposits adsorbing factor X |
| 5. Amyloid deposits adsorbing alpha$_2$ antiplasmin |

First, the physical structure of the fibrin clot may be abnormal due to increased serum globulins. Polymerization of fibrin is impaired in some patients with circulating light chains, which is suggested by prolonged thrombin or reptilase times. Myeloma proteins have also been shown to inhibit the thrombin time in normal plasma. The site for factor XIII activity on fibrin strands can be blocked by an abnormal protein.

Platelet abnormalities are less well defined in patients with myeloma although prolonged bleeding times have been described. Presumably both defects are due to inhibition of platelet function by abnormal proteins.

The abnormal protein can bind to coagulation factors leading to inhibition of factor function, especially of factor VIII. Monoclonal proteins with specificity toward platelet GP IIb/IIIa have been reported. These patients may have mild to no thrombocytopenia but have a very severe bleeding diathesis.

Therapy for the hemostatic defects in the dysproteinemic syndromes includes removal of the offending protein, either by reducing the synthesis through treating the plasma cell dyscrasia or by intensive plasmapheresis. In several patients, return of normal hemostasis was correlated with a substantial reduction in the monoclonal protein concentration.

Patients with systemic amyloidosis, either primary or that associated with myeloma, often demonstrate a marked increase in easy bruisability and other bleeding symptoms. In one study of 337 patients, abnormal bleeding and coagulation tests were seen in 28 and 51%, respectively. Among other studies, the most common defects in coagulation testing of patients with amyloid was an elevation in the thrombin time which is seen in 30–80% of cases. An increased prothrombin time was seen in 20–24% of cases and an increased aPTT in up to 70%.

Factor X deficiency was first reported to be associated with amyloidosis in 1962; subsequent studies have shown that the clotting factor is adsorbed onto amyloid proteins. Splenectomy, plasmapheresis, and treatment with melphalan and prednisone have been reported to reduce the amyloid burden and to increase the factor X levels.

In patients with factor X deficiency receiving bone marrow transplant, improvement in factor X levels was seen in those patients who responded to the transplant.

Another cause of bleeding in patients with systemic amyloidosis is systemic fibrino(geno) lysis. The euglobulin clot lysis time is shortened with striking decreases in α_2-PI, plasminogen, and circulating plasmin-antiplasmin complexes. Some patients have also been reported to have elevated plasma levels of tissue-type plasminogen activator. The mechanisms responsible for the fibrinolytic state are not known. Hypotheses include increased release of plasminogen activators, decreased plasminogen activator inhibitors, blood vessels infiltrated with amyloid, decreased α_2-PI because of its adsorption onto amyloid fibrils, or perhaps amyloid liver disease. The use of fibrinolytic inhibitors such as tranexamic acid has both corrected laboratory tests of fibrinolysis and reduced bleeding symptoms.

Acquired Factor Deficiencies

Acquired von Willebrand disease (VWD) occurs most often in hematological malignancies – lymphomas, myeloproliferative syndromes, myeloma, and monoclonal gammopathies – but can be seen with Wilms' tumors and with the use of certain drugs such as ciprofloxacin. Patients with acquired VWD can present as type 1 (decreased total von Willebrand protein) or type 2 (loss of high-molecular-weight multimers) disease. The most common cancers associated with acquired VWD are lymphoproliferative disorders and – as noted above – myeloproliferative neoplasms. Patients with acquired VWD can have variable responses. Desmopressin is effective in many patients with acquired VWD type 1 and 2, but the effectiveness and duration of effect are often reduced. For bleeding patients, high doses of the von Willebrand concentrate Humate P are indicated with careful monitoring of levels. For patients with very strong inhibitors that factor concentrates cannot overcome or severe life-threatening bleeding, rVIIa may prove useful.

Factor VIII deficiency due to autoantibodies is the most frequent acquired coagulation factor deficiency complication in older cancer patients. Patients will have a prolonged aPTT, a positive screening test for a factor inhibitor, and a low factor VIII level. For severe or life-threatening bleeding, recombinant VIIa, factor VIII inhibitor bypass agent (FEIBA), or the newly approved recombinant porcine factor VIII are all acceptable treatments to provide hemostasis. Immunosuppression is used to eliminate the autoantibody. Steroids are first-line therapy, but often oral cyclophosphamide and rituximab are added. Ridding the patient of the inhibitor does not require successful tumor treatment and should be attempted before major procedures such as surgical cancer resection.

Cancer and Thrombosis

Thrombosis can be the presenting sign of cancer. As many as 10–20% of older patients who present with a deep venous thrombosis will be found to have cancer on initial evaluation. Furthermore, over the next 2 years as many of 25% of patients will develop cancer. Certain signs are more worrisome for cancer as an underlying cause of the thrombosis. Patients with warfarin-refractory thrombosis, idiopathic bilateral deep vein thrombosis, or both arterial and venous thrombosis seem to be at particular risk for having an underlying malignancy.

One question that commonly arises is whether a patient with idiopathic thrombosis should be aggressively worked up for cancer. This question was addressed in a prospective clinical trial (the SOME trial) which found that routine CT scanning in patients with idiopathic thrombosis did not provide a clinically significant benefit. Current recommendations are age-appropriate cancer screening and aggressive work-up of any worrisome signs – such as guaiac positive stools. Another common issue is the finding of an "incidental" pulmonary embolism on a CT obtained for tumor staging or evaluation of response to chemotherapy. Despite the "incidental" nature of finding the thrombosis, the prognosis is presumed to be similar to clinically detected thrombosis, and these need to be aggressively treated.

Rare patients can present with thrombosis and associated disseminated intravascular coagulation. Patients with tumor-related DIC have thrombosis with low platelets and an abnormal coagulation profile. These patients may also develop a non-bacterial thrombotic endocarditis (NBTE) and have multiple arterial embolic events.

The cancers most frequently associated with thrombosis are adenocarcinoma of the lung and gastrointestinal cancers, especially pancreatic adenocarcinoma. Primary brain tumors are also associated with a higher risk of thrombosis. Thrombosis rates for breast and prostate cancer are not as extreme. Clinical scoring systems, such as the Khorana Score, can be used to predict the likelihood of thrombosis based on certain clinical factors.

The etiology of the thrombosis may be direct activation of factor VII by tumor-expressed tissue factor. A direct activator of factor X has also been implicated. Patients with cancer have elevations of inflammatory cytokines that can further augment the hypercoagulable state.

Treatment of the cancer can also lead to thrombosis. Chemotherapy – especially cisplatinum, fluorouracil, and asparaginase – increases the risk of thrombosis perhaps due to endothelial damage. Biological agents such as thalidomide and lenalidomide also increase thrombosis risk. Surgery for cancer patients increases the risk of thrombosis, so much so that 4 weeks of thromboprophylaxis after certain cancer surgeries has proven to be beneficial. Hormonal therapy such as tamoxifen or some of the newly approved CDK inhibitors is also associated with an increased thrombotic risk.

Cancer-related thrombosis requires aggressive anticoagulation. For over a decade, the initial therapy for cancer-associated thrombosis was low-molecular-weight heparin (LMWH). Four randomized trials have shown that 3–6 months of therapy with LMWH is superior to warfarin in cancer patients. Recently three major clinical trials have suggested the DOACs edoxaban, rivaroxaban, and apixaban can also be safely used to treat cancer-related thrombosis. Each trial showed that the respective DOAC was noninferior to LMWH at prevention of recurrent thrombosis. Some trials did suggest there may be an increased rate of GI bleeding in patients with upper GI malignancies as compared to LMWH.

Patients who failed warfarin or a DOAC need to be treated indefinitely with LMWH. Rare patients who fail LMWH may benefit from raising the dose by 25% or by changing to fondaparinux.

Brain tumors or brain metastases are not a contraindication to anticoagulation. The only exceptions are brain metastases from thyroid, melanoma, renal, or choriocarcinoma as these tumor metastases have a high rate of bleeding. It should be remembered that placement of an inferior vena cava filter without concurrent anticoagulation is associated with an unacceptable rate of complications, including death from massive thrombosis.

Myeloproliferative Syndromes

Thrombosis is the most common cause of death in the myeloproliferative syndromes. Although many patients will have markedly elevated blood counts, patients with essential thrombocytosis may have thrombotic complications when the platelet count is in the 4–600,000/uL range. Patients with polycythemia rubra vera are also at increased risk of thrombosis when their hematocrits are over 45%. The thrombosis may be due to small vessel events, perhaps in part from increased viscosity, or to large vessel thrombosis. Patients with myeloproliferative syndromes have a higher risk of thrombosis even with relatively normal blood counts, suggesting an intrinsic defect in the blood cells leading to thrombosis.

Patients with myeloproliferative syndromes may have thrombosis in any location, but thromboses at two certain sites should raise concern about an underlying myeloproliferative syndrome. Patients with Budd-Chiari and other visceral vein thromboses have a high incidence of underlying myeloproliferative syndromes. Patients with essential thrombocytosis can also have platelet occlusion of the small digital vessels leading to erythromelalgia. These patients will have swollen, red, and very painful digits. The patients may only have slightly elevated platelet counts and are often misdiagnosed with arthritis. One helpful diagnostic clue is that these patients will respond dramatically to a single aspirin per day.

Certain patients, especially those with Budd-Chiari syndrome, may have an "occult" myeloproliferative syndrome with perhaps no evidence of any hematological disorder on the peripheral smear or bone marrow aspirate. These patients may have genetic evidence of myeloproliferative disease with positive testing for the JAK2 or CALR mutation.

The diagnosis of a myeloproliferative syndrome is easy in patients with very abnormal blood counts. However, many patients with hepatic vein or other unusual thrombosis will have only mildly elevated blood counts or normal counts. In these patients, genetic testing for JAK2, CALR, or rarely cMPL mutations can be diagnostic.

Therapy of Thrombosis in Myeloproliferative Syndromes

Intravenous heparin followed by a DOAC or warfarin is indicated for most patients with acute venous thromboembolism complicating the myeloproliferative disorders. Catheter-based thrombolytic therapy should be considered in patients who have acute occlusion of the hepatic or portal veins, especially in the event of progressive liver dysfunction. Long-term oral anticoagulants are usually recommended for prevention of recurrent thromboses. In a few instances, liver transplantation has been successful in treating liver failure due to Budd-Chiari syndrome.

Antiplatelet therapy, usually with aspirin, is recommended for the prevention and treatment of cerebral, coronary artery, or peripheral vascular thrombosis. Low doses of aspirin (81 mg/d) are preferable in patients with myeloproliferative disease because the risk of bleeding with aspirin is dose-related. There is some evidence that dosing at 81 mg twice a day may offer improved antiplatelet effect. There are currently no data concerning the use of newer agents such as clopidogrel, but this may be reasonable for patients allergic to aspirin.

In addition to antithrombotic therapy, treating elevated blood counts is also important. For patients with thrombocytosis, hydroxyurea (1 g daily to start) is the preferred therapy as trials have shown antithrombotic benefit. For younger patients who have concerns about hydroxyurea, pegylated interferon starting at 45–90 ug is another consideration. In patients with myelofibrosis, or PV patients who have failed hydroxyurea, the JAK inhibitor ruxolitinib is a new therapeutic option which has shown improvements in symptom burden and improved survival in patient with myelofibrosis. Meta-analysis also suggests ruxolitinib may decrease the risk of venous and arterial thrombosis. For patients with polycythemia, reduction of the hematocrit to under 45% with phlebotomy, hydroxyurea, ruxolitinib, or interferon is crucial.

Another issue is whether to reduce platelet counts or to give aspirin to patients with myeloproliferative disorders who do not have a history of thrombosis. Platelet reduction with hydroxyurea should be considered in asymptomatic older subjects (>65 years) if they have atherosclerosis, risk factors for arterial disease, or symptoms of vascular ischemia, particularly if they have a JAK2v617f mutation. Also important is controlling reversible risk factors such as smoking and elevated cholesterol. All patients with polycythemia should have their hematocrits reduced to less than 45%. Low-dose aspirin therapy is appropriate for most patients as a primary preventative antithrombotic agent. The exception would be patients with high platelet counts and acquired von Willebrand disease.

Paroxysmal Nocturnal Hemoglobinuria (PNH)

PNH remains a poorly understood clonal hematopoietic disorder that leads to complement driven intravascular hemolysis. One of the leading causes of morbidity and mortality in patients with PNH is thrombosis. Patients can present with venous or arterial thrombosis. Also, like myeloproliferative syndromes, PNH is associated with a high incidence of visceral vein thrombosis at presentation. The cause of the hypercoagulable state is unknown, but complement-activated platelets have been implicated. In two large series, the rate of thrombosis in PNH was 28–39%, with thrombosis leading to death in 58%. The introduction of the complement inhibitor eculizumab has led to control of the hemolysis in most patients with PNH, and there is strong evidence it also reduces thrombosis rates. Eculizumab should be used in any patient with PNH who has had thrombosis, severe hemolysis, or a significant PNH clone (>50%). Recently, the longer-acting ravulizumab was also FDA approved after every 8-week ravulizumab was shown to be noninferior to every 2-week eculizumab.

Catheter Thrombosis

Central venous catheters are essential to many aspects of cancer therapy. The incidence of clinically apparent thrombosis from central venous catheters is estimated to be 5–30%. The signs of catheter thrombosis are nonspecific and the incidence of thrombosis is thought to be underestimated. Catheter thrombosis can also be a sign of heparin-induced thrombocytopenia (HIT) since heparin is often used to ensure patency.

Patients with thrombosis often notice arm pain and swelling. Diagnosis is made by Doppler. Some patients may only have central vein thrombosis and may require venography or CT angiography to make the diagnosis. Rates of incidental catheter thrombosis reported in studies that performed routine screening ultrasounds are as high as 50%. Accordingly, many patients have the diagnosis found while undergo scanning for other reasons.

The best therapy is not well defined. If the catheter is functional and required for cancer therapy, it may stay in place as long as anticoagulation is initiated. While some guidelines recommend 3 months of anticoagulation following catheter removal, increasing data regarding peripherally inserted central catheters suggest that simply removing the catheter may be the safest approach as the risk of bleeding with anticoagulation is high. Anticoagulation is reserved for the severely symptomatic. For thrombosis with tunneled lines, anticoagulation should be given unless the risk of bleeding is substantial. Prevention of catheter thrombosis is difficult as prophylaxis has not been shown to be beneficial.

Chemotherapeutic Agents

Adjuvant chemotherapy for breast cancer has been associated with an increased risk of both arterial and venous thromboembolism (in 5–7% of patients). The thrombogenic stimulus is not clear, but this could reflect vascular damage by the chemotherapeutic agents or perhaps a reduction in protein C or protein S concentrations. Several commonly used hormonal therapies for breast cancer also carry thrombotic risk. The selective estrogen receptor modulators tamoxifen and raloxifene both increase thrombotic risk as compared to placebo in the adjuvant setting. In metastatic breast cancer patients, the newly improved CDK inhibitors appear to increase thrombotic risk to varying degrees. Abemaciclib in particular carries a black box warning for thrombosis.

L-asparaginase – an effective therapy for acute lymphocytic leukemia – is associated with high rates of thrombosis. The overall rate of thrombosis in children is 5% but may be as high as 36% if asymptomatic thromboses are included and can range from 5% to 18% in adult. The rate of potentially devastating CNS thrombosis is approximately 1–2% of patients with childhood ALL and up to 4% of adults. Thrombosis usually occurs 2–3 weeks after the start of a course of therapy. Most patients recover, although several deaths have been reported and others are left with debilitating neurologic defects.

The pathogenesis of the thrombotic complications of L-asparaginase may be related to decreased levels of antithrombin III, protein C, protein S, and plasminogen via general inhibition of hepatic protein synthesis by L-asparaginase.

Prior to using heparin to treat thrombosis, measurement of fibrinogen should be performed and kept at levels greater than 150 mg/dl during anticoagulation. Platelets need to be kept greater than 50,000/uL.

There remains no consensus on prevention of thrombosis given varying results of clinical trials. Most would recommend checking aPTT, PT-INR, antithrombin, and fibrinogen at the start of asparaginase therapy and then perhaps every other day for a total of 7 days after each dose. If PEG-asparaginase is used, monitoring may need to be longer given the 5–6-day half-life. Debate remains about the effectiveness of either antithrombin or anticoagulation for thrombosis prophylaxis. Increasing data suggest varying doses of LMWH may be effective at thrombosis prevention. Data on the use of DOACs for prophylaxis are minimal to date.

The anti-myeloma agents thalidomide and lenalidomide are both associated with substantial rates of thrombosis that can be as high as 36–75%. The incidence is higher with the use of dexamethasone and with chemotherapy, especially doxorubicin. These agents may have a direct toxic effect on the vascular endothelium promoting a prothrombotic state. Aspirin appears useful for thrombosis prevention in low-risk patients, while those who have had previous thrombosis, those who are receiving dexamethasone or chemotherapy, or those with central lines may benefit from warfarin or LMWH prophylaxis. Clinical trials are underway to assess DOACs in this area.

Thrombotic microangiopathies (TM) can be associated with medications such as calcineurin inhibitors, mitomycin, and thienopyridines. With calcineurin inhibitors, the TM occurs within days after the agent is started with the appearance of a falling platelet count, falling hematocrit, and rising serum LDH level. Some cases have been fatal, but often the TM resolves with decreasing the calcineurin inhibitor's dose or changing to another agent.

Now, the most common anti-neoplastic drug causing TM is gemcitabine with an incidence of 0.1–1%. The appearance of the TM syndrome associated with gemcitabine can be delayed, and the condition often is fatal. Severe hypertension often precedes the clinical appearance of the

TM. The use of plasma exchange is controversial, and there are increasing reports of the use of short courses of the complement inhibitor eculizumab.

Bone Marrow Transplantation

Hepatic veno-occlusive disease (VOD or sinusoidal obstruction syndromes) is a relatively common complication of stem cell transplantation and is seen in 1–50% of patients, but the frequency seems to vary widely based on the regimen used and from center to center. The clinical syndrome includes weight gain, hepatic tenderness, and jaundice soon after transplantation which can progress to liver failure and the hepatorenal syndrome. Early thrombosis of the hepatic venules leading to obstruction and eventual fibrosis is the most commonly accepted mechanism for VOD. Pre-existing liver dysfunction, especially hepatitis C, prior therapy with gemtuzumab ozogamicin, the use of vancomycin in the pre-transplant period, and advanced age are some of the important risk factors for development of the disorder. Conditioning regimens that include busulfan also increase the incidence, and the risk also appears to be higher in patients undergoing allogeneic rather than autologous transplantation.

Multiple coagulation defects have been demonstrated in patients at risk of VOD. Elevated levels of plasminogen activator inhibitor-1 have been suggested as a noninvasive test for VOD. Factor V Leiden mutation and the prothrombin 20210 mutation have also been reported as potential risk factors. Elevated levels of prothrombotic cytokines such as TNF and IL-6 have been shown to be elevated in patients with VOD.

Despite the role of thrombosis in pathogenesis of VOD, studies using traditional antithrombotic therapy have been disappointing; the use of defibrotide – an oligonucleotide with multiple anti-inflammatory actions – has been promising, leading to its recent FDA approval. The approval is based off of a multi-institutional phase III study of 102 patients with transplant-related VOD which demonstrated improved 100-day survival as compared to historical controls.

TMs can complicate both autologous and allogeneic bone marrow transplants. The incidence ranges from 15% for allogeneic to 5% for autologous bone marrow transplants. Several types of TMs are recognized in bone marrow transplantations. One is "multi-organ fulminant" which occurs early (20–60 days), has multi-organ system involvement, and is often fatal. Another type of TM is similar to calcineurin inhibitors' TMs. A "conditioning" TM, which occurs 6 months or more after total body irradiation, is associated with primary renal involvement. Finally, patients with systemic CMV infections can present with a TM syndrome related to vascular infection with CMV. The etiology of bone marrow transplant-related TM appears to be different from that of "classic" TTP since alterations of ADAMTS13 have not been found in BMT-related TTP implicating therapy-related vascular damage. The therapy of bone marrow transplant TM is uncertain. Patients should have their calcineurin inhibitors' doses decreased. Although plasma exchange is often tried, response is poor in those with fulminant or conditioning-related TM. Emerging data suggests that, similar to chemotherapy-induced TMs, eculizumab may be a useful therapeutic agent.

Suggested Reading

Barbui T, Finazzi G, Falanga A. Myeloproliferative neoplasms and thrombosis. Blood. 2013;122(13):2176–84.

Choudhry A, DeLoughery TG. Bleeding and thrombosis in acute promyelocytic leukemia. Am J Hematol. 2012;87(6):596–603.

Kraaijpoel N, Carrier M. How I treat cancer-associated venous thromboembolism. Blood. 2019;133(4):291–8.

Leebeek FW. Update of thrombosis in multiple myeloma. Thromb Res. 2016;140(Suppl 1):S76–80.

Patel HK, Khorana AA. Anticoagulation in cancer patients: a summary of pitfalls to avoid. Curr Oncol Rep. 2019;21(2):18.

Patriquin CJ, Kiss T, Caplan S, Chin-Yee I, Grewal K, Grossman J, Larratt L, Marceau D, Nevill T, Sutherland DR, Wells RA, Leber B. How we treat paroxysmal nocturnal hemoglobinuria: a consensus statement of the Canadian PNH Network and review of the national registry. Eur J Haematol. 2019;102(1):36–52.

Shatzel J, Scherber R, DeLoughery TG. Bleeding and thrombosis in hematologic neoplasia. In: Neoplastic diseases of the blood. Switzerland: Springer; 2018. p. 1263–89.

Hemostasis and Thrombosis in Pregnancy

30

Molly M. Daughety
and Bethany T. Samuelson Bannow

Thrombocytopenia in Pregnancy

Thrombocytopenia is common in pregnancy. It is often benign and does not require intervention, but rarely, it can represent a dangerous syndrome that requires management as outlined below.

Gestational Thrombocytopenia

Gestational thrombocytopenia is the most common cause of thrombocytopenia in pregnancy and accounts for approximately 70–80% of cases (Burrows and Kelton 1993; Gernsheimer et al. 2013; Boehlen et al. 2000; Sainio et al. 2000). While the exact pathophysiology is unclear, expanded plasma volume and expedited clearance are possible explanations. Gestational thrombocytopenia is characterized by mild to moderate thrombocytopenia that typically presents in the second or third trimester in a woman with no prior history of thrombocytopenia.

M. M. Daughety (✉)
Division of Hematology and Oncology, Duke University Medicine Center, Durham, NC, USA

B. T. Samuelson Bannow
Division of Hematology and Oncology, Duke University Medicine Center, Durham, NC, USA

The Hemophilia Center, Oregon Health & Science University, Portland, OR, USA

Platelet counts typically range between 130 and 150 × 10^9/L. If platelet counts drop below 100 × 10^9/L, gestational thrombocytopenia is considered less likely and further workup to evaluate for an alternative etiology is advised (Gernsheimer et al. 2013; Reese et al. 2018). Two other important features are (1) spontaneous resolution within 1–2 months of delivery and (2) the neonate who is born with normal platelet counts (James 2011). The diagnosis of gestational thrombocytopenia is clinical, and the recommended treatment is observation with platelet count monitoring at every routine prenatal visit and then a follow-up platelet count 1–3 months after delivery to ensure resolution (Gernsheimer et al. 2013).

Immune Thrombocytopenic Purpura

Immune thrombocytopenic purpura (ITP) is the second most common cause of isolated thrombocytopenia in pregnancy, occurring at a rate of approximately 3% (Gernsheimer et al. 2013). It is somewhat difficult to differentiate from gestational thrombocytopenia since both are a diagnosis of exclusion. However, ITP in pregnancy typically presents with platelet counts <100 × 10^9/L and can develop at any time during pregnancy (Gernsheimer et al. 2013). Additionally, antibodies may cross the placenta and cause neonatal alloimmune thrombocytopenia (NAIT). A history of ITP in the patient is helpful, but not always present. Lastly, ITP in pregnancy does not always spontaneously resolve with delivery.

Treatment of ITP in Pregnancy

Treatment of ITP in pregnancy is not always necessary. In the first and second trimester, women who are asymptomatic with platelets >30 × 10⁹/L do not require treatment until delivery is imminent. However, if these patients develop symptomatic bleeding, platelets <30 × 10⁹/L or have a planned procedure, low-dose steroids, or IVIG are recommended. When delivery is imminent, treatment may be required to achieve a platelet goal of ≥50 × 10⁹/L to allow for emergent cesarean section or ≥80–100 × 10⁹/L for epidural, if needed. Of note, ITP during pregnancy is not a contraindication to vaginal delivery.

For severe cases of ITP that are refractory to steroids and IVIG, splenectomy may be considered in the second trimester. There is minimal safety data on anti-D immunoglobulin and azathioprine in pregnancy, and these agents should only be considered as last resort (Michel et al. 2003; Alstead et al. 1990; Price et al. 1976). Other commonly used agents in nonpregnant patients with ITP (mycophenolate mofetil, cyclophosphamide, cyclosporine A, rituximab, thrombopoietin receptor agonists, and dapsone) are *not* recommended.

Thrombotic Microangiopathy

When thrombocytopenia in pregnancy is accompanied by microangiopathic hemolytic anemia, three syndromes must be considered: (1) preeclampsia/HELLP, (2) thrombotic thrombocytopenic purpura (TTP), and (3) atypical hemolytic uremic syndrome (aHUS). These conditions can be life-threatening, and each requires unique treatment to reduce associated morbidity and mortality.

Preeclampsia/HELLP

Preeclampsia is defined by new onset HTN and proteinuria after the 20th week of gestation.

HELLP (hemolysis, elevated liver function tests, low platelets) is often considered a severe variant and is defined as preeclampsia with any of the following abnormalities: blood pressure >160/110 mmHg, platelet count <100 × 10⁹/L, impaired liver function, creatinine >1.1 mg/dL, pulmonary edema, or cerebral disturbances (George et al. 2015). Thrombocytopenia is usually the first sign of HELLP, and signs of microangiopathic hemolysis are often seen on smear, although not required for diagnosis. HELLP syndrome can result in severe maternal and fetal complications including disseminated intravascular coagulopathy, organ failure, and death (Haram et al. 2009). The cornerstone of treatment for HELLP is blood pressure management and delivery of the fetus.

Thrombotic Thrombocytopenic Purpura

TTP is a rare thrombotic microangiopathy (TMA) caused by a deficiency of ADAMTS13 – a metalloprotease responsible for cleaving von Willebrand factor multimers. Most often, this is due to an acquired inhibitor to ADAMTS13 activity, but the condition can also be inherited. Classical TTP is defined as ADAMTS13 activity of <10%, but because the results of this assay may not be available for several days, the diagnosis of TTP and the initiation of plasma exchange is often based on clinical suspicion in the presence of microangiopathic hemolytic anemia, elevated LDH, and thrombocytopenia without another clinically apparent etiology (George et al. 2015). Initial management of TTP in pregnancy is the same as the general population with plasma exchange daily until platelets and LDH return to near normal levels; then it is gradually tapered off (Gernsheimer et al. 2013). If TTP occurs in the first trimester, regular plasma exchange guided by blood counts can be performed.

Atypical Hemolytic Uremic Syndrome

Atypical HUS is a complement-mediated TMA caused by congenital defects of the alternative pathway of the complement system. It is almost clinically indistinguishable from TTP, but it is not caused by ADAMTS13 deficiency (ADAMTS13 level is >10%) or shiga toxin. The mainstay of treatment for aHUS is eculizumab, and there is data to suggest it is safe to use during pregnancy (Canigral et al. 2014; Kelly et al. 2015).

Acute Fatty Liver of Pregnancy

Lastly, a rare and life-threatening cause of thrombocytopenia in pregnancy that must be considered in the appropriate clinical scenario is acute fatty liver of pregnancy (AFLP). The incidence is not well defined, and estimates in the literature vary widely. ALFP is triggered by microvesicular fatty infiltration of maternal hepatocytes that leads to acute liver failure and can result in the death of both the mother and fetus. The initial presenting symptoms are often non-specific and include nausea, vomiting, and abdominal pain, on average around the 36th week of gestation (Knight et al. 2008). Disease progression is characterized by significant liver enzyme elevations and signs of hepatic dysfunction such as encephalopathy, coagulopathy, and hypoglycemia. The diagnosis of AFLP is one based on clinical symptoms and laboratory signs; liver biopsy is a last resort in a patient with an uncertain diagnosis and in which management would be affected by confirmation. Early recognition, prompt delivery, and supportive care are critical to improve maternal and fetal outcomes. If rapid improvement of liver function does not occur after delivery, evaluation for liver transplant is recommended as it confers the best chance for survival (Ockner et al. 1990; Riely et al. 1987).

Hemorrhage in Pregnancy

Postpartum Hemorrhage

Postpartum hemorrhage (PPH) is the leading cause of mortality during childbirth, accounting for 35% of maternal deaths worldwide (Victora et al. 2016). Ninety-nine percent of deaths from PPH occur in low- and middle-income countries, while only 1% of deaths from PPH occur in

developed countries (Haeri and Dildy 2012). Primary PPH is defined as blood loss of >1000 mL in the first 24 hours after delivery (Committee on Practice B-O 2017). The most common cause of primary PPH is uterine atony followed by retained placenta and genital tract trauma. Oxytocin and other uterotonic agents are commonly used to prevent PPH in the general obstetric population. More recently, tranexamic acid was shown in a randomized placebo-controlled trial (WOMAN trial) to significantly reduce the risk of bleeding-associated death in women with PPH (1·5% vs 1·9%, [RR] 0·81, [95% CI 0·65–1·00]; $p = 0.045$) (Shakur et al. 2010). For patients who are refractory to medical therapy, uterine artery embolization, local tamponade, and surgical hysterectomy are procedural alternatives.

Delayed Postpartum Hemorrhage

Secondary or delayed postpartum hemorrhage is defined as PPH that occurs between 24 hours and 6 weeks after delivery (Committee on Practice B-O 2017). While uncommon in women with intact hemostatic systems, women with known bleeding disorders are at increased risk. A hematologist should be involved in the management of pregnancies complicated by von Willebrand disease (vWD), hemophilia carriers, as well as other rare bleeding disorders in order to ensure that appropriate monitoring and prophylaxis against bleeding is implemented. In this section, we will outline the pathophysiology and appropriate treatment of each disorder during pregnancy.

Von Willebrand Disease

vWD is the most common inherited bleeding disorder, occurring in up to 1% of the population; however, only a small fraction of those affected are symptomatic (Sadler et al. 2000). Von Willebrand factor (vWF) is critical in primary hemostasis as it serves as a bridge between platelets and injured endothelial tissue; it also aids in fibrin clot formation by functioning as a carrier protein to factor VIII (Wagner 1990). vWD results when there is a quantitative (type I and type III) or a qualitative (type II) deficiency in vWF. During pregnancy, estrogen upregulates the production of most clotting factors, including vWF and factor VIII, so diagnosis during pregnancy may be difficult and a preconception workup is most reliable. Women with type 2B vWD may also develop thrombocytopenia in the setting of increased levels of dysfunctional vWF. It is recommended to check vWF labs around 34–36 weeks of gestation to develop a delivery plan. In most cases, a minimum vWF level of 50 IU/dL is recommended for epidurals and vaginal delivery (Tuohy et al. 2011). If levels are below this or if the patient has had bleeding complications, some may recommend targeting vWF levels ≥50 IU/dL close to delivery and for 3–5 days following delivery (Tuohy et al. 2011). vWF concentrate is the preferred therapy in pregnancy and for postpartum hemorrhage. The use of desmopressin (DDAVP) is controversial due to concerns over maternal hyponatremia and placental insufficiency; however, this has not been shown in any prospective clinical trial and surveys of hematologists show that it is routinely used (Kujovich 2005). Of note, vWF levels tend to return to prepregnancy levels within 7–21 days of delivery (James et al. 2015). As such, we recommend monitoring for postpartum hemorrhage up to 3 weeks after delivery.

Hemophilia

Hemophilia is an X-linked inherited bleeding disorder that results from deficiency of clotting factor VIII (hemophilia A) or clotting factor IX (hemophilia B). This mostly affects males, but women with one affected X chromosome can have lower levels of factor VIII or IX and may require attention during significant hemostatic challenges like childbirth. Hemophilia carriers can have a range of factor activity levels, so this should be checked at least once during pregnancy and repeated close to delivery if low (<40%) to determine if factor replacement is needed (Kadir et al. 2013). Like VWF, FVIII levels increase throughout pregnancy and thus may rise to or above the normal range even in women with lower baseline levels. FIX levels do not increase

in pregnancy. Since 50% of male children born to hemophilia carriers will be affected by the syndrome, it is recommended to do noninvasive gender determination testing, either by ultrasound or by testing maternal blood for a Y chromosome-specific sequence from free circulating fetal DNA (Chalmers et al. 2011). If the gender is determined to be male, definitive diagnostic testing for hemophilia is advised to help guide intrapartum management. Chorionic villus sampling and amniocentesis during the first trimester are options for early diagnosis; however, the risks of miscarriage are around 1–2% and 0.5–1%, respectively (Ludlam et al. 2005). For women wishing to avoid the risks associated with early diagnosis, third trimester amniocentesis is an option and is typically performed between 35 and 36 weeks of gestation due to a 1% risk of inducing labor (Chalmers et al. 2011).

The optimal mode of delivery for a fetus at risk of or with known hemophilia is a matter of debate, and recommendations and opinions vary. In general, invasive monitoring procedures, such as intrapartum scalp electrodes and fetal scalp blood sampling, and delivery with forceps and ventouse extraction should be avoided due to the increased risk of intracranial and extracranial hemorrhage (Chalmers et al. 2011). We recommend that the decision regarding vaginal delivery versus cesarean section should primarily be based on maternal indications. Hemophilia carrier status is not a contraindication to vaginal delivery. For women who require factor replacement, factor concentrates should be continued for 3–4 days postpartum to achieve a trough >50 IU/dL (Kadir et al. 2013).

Rare Bleeding Disorders

There are many rare bleeding disorders that may require attention during pregnancy. These include inherited deficiencies of coagulation factors I, II, V, VII, X, XI, and XII, which represent 5% of all inherited bleeding disorders. An extensive discussion about the treatments of each of these is outside the scope of this chapter. But, in general, clinically relevant factor deficiencies are treated with fresh frozen plasma or factor concentrates. Importantly, fibrinogen plays a key role in placental implantation and maintenance during pregnancy, so recognition and treatment of hypofibrinogenemia should be initiated as early as possible in pregnancy.

Thrombosis in Pregnancy

Acute Venous Thromboembolism

Pulmonary embolism (PE) remains the leading cause of maternal death in developed countries, resulting in an estimated 1–3 maternal deaths per 100,000 live births (Lu et al. 2017; Heit et al. 2005; Bates et al. 2012). The incidence of venous thromboembolism (VTE) is estimated to be between 0.5 and 2.2 per 1000 patients (Heit et al. 2005; Gherman et al. 1999; Lindqvist et al. 1999; Simpson et al. 2001; James et al. 2006; Andersen et al. 1998; Jacobsen et al. 2008; McColl et al. 1997) five times higher than the nonpregnant population. Thrombotic risk is highest in the 6–12 weeks following delivery, with the risk of deep venous thrombosis (DVT) and PE being 5 and 15 times higher, respectively, compared to the antepartum period (Heit et al. 2005; Kamel et al. 2014).

Diagnosis of Acute VTE
Pregnancy causes a hypercoagulable state due to elevated levels of estrogen and progesterone which results in an upregulation in the levels of clotting factors (including fibrinogen, II, VII, VIII, IX, and XII) and a decrease in the levels of anticoagulants (protein C, protein S, and antithrombin III) (Bremme 2003; James et al. 2014). This makes blood clots not only more common in pregnancy but also more difficult to diagnose, since D-dimer is physiologically elevated in pregnancy and is not validated as a clinical prediction tool in this population. For suspected DVTs, compression ultrasound (CUS) is the first diagnostic test of choice, with reported 95% sensitivity and >95% specificity for symptomatic proximal DVTs (Polak and Wilkinson 1991). If CUS is positive for DVT, prompt therapeutic

anticoagulation is warranted. If the initial CUS is negative, however, further investigation with serial CUS, Doppler ultrasound, or MRI is recommended, especially if clinical suspicion of a proximal DVT (i.e., iliac vein) remains high.

The preferred diagnostic test for PE in pregnancy is controversial and guidelines from multiple societies vary (Konstantinides et al. 2014; Chan et al. 2014; Leung et al. 2011; McLintock et al. 2012). In women suspected of having a PE *without* lower extremity DVT symptoms, computed tomographic pulmonary angiography (CTPA) is our preferred first test over ventilation perfusion scintigraphy due to its superior diagnostic sensitivity and specificity and because of the substantially reduced fetal radiation dose of CTPA when compared to ventilation perfusion scintigraphy (Winer-Muram et al. 2002; Russell et al. 1997; British Thoracic Society Standards of Care Committee Pulmonary Embolism Guideline Development G 2003; Hayashino et al. 2005; Quiroz et al. 2005). However, ventilation perfusion scans are preferred by some societies because it avoids the high radiation dose delivered to female breast tissue by CTPA, which can increase the patient's lifetime risk of breast cancer (Einstein et al. 2007). Ultimately, the decision will depend on what is available at the institution at the time the patient presents and a shared decision-making conversation between the patient and her provider.

Treatment of Acute VTE
Therapeutic dose low molecular weight heparin (LMWH) is the preferred anticoagulant treatment of VTE during pregnancy with consensus among major international guidelines (Bates et al. 2016). When compared to unfractionated heparin (UFH), LMWH has a lower bleeding risk, a lower risk of heparin-induced thrombocytopenia (HIT), less osteoporosis, and more predictable pharmacokinetics (Lu et al. 2017). Unlike warfarin, studies suggest that LMWH does not cross the placenta (Andrew et al. 1985; Dimitrakakis et al. 2000) and observational data suggests that there is no increase in incidence of embryopathies or fetal demise with LMWH (Bar et al. 2000). Direct oral anticoagulants should not be used

during pregnancy due to inadequate safety data in humans (Beyer-Westendorf et al. 2016).

At the time of delivery, therapeutic LMWH should be held at least 24 hours prior to vaginal delivery or cesarean section to allow for regional anesthesia. Therapeutic anticoagulation can be safely resumed 4–6 hours after vaginal delivery and 6–12 hours after cesarean delivery (Bates et al. 2012). Therapeutic anticoagulation should be resumed no sooner than 12 hours after epidural removal (Horlocker et al. 2010). If significant bleeding precludes the reinitiation of anticoagulation, attempts should be made to achieve prompt hemostasis to allow resumption of anticoagulation as soon as possible.

After delivery, it is recommended to anticoagulate mothers using LMWH or warfarin with a LMWH bridge. For these women, breastfeeding can be safely initiated immediately postpartum, while on the LMWH and/or warfarin. Although anti-factor Xa levels have been detected in breast milk, it is in low concentrations and unlikely to cause any untoward effects in the child (Richter et al. 2001). Warfarin appears to lack any breast milk excretion (Orme et al. 1977). DOACs are not currently recommended in breast-feeding women due to inadequate safety data.

For pregnant women with acute VTE, full-dose subcutaneous LMWH is recommended throughout pregnancy and for at least 6 weeks postpartum. Patients may transition to warfarin (target INR 2.0–3.0) postpartum with a minimum total duration of 3 months (Bates et al. 2012).

Management of Prior VTE

Postpartum Prophylaxis

Anticoagulation during the antepartum and postpartum period is not reserved for VTE events that occur during pregnancy. For pregnant women with a prior episode of VTE, *6 weeks of anticoagulation postpartum* with low- or intermediate-dose LMWH or warfarin (target INR 2.0–3.0) is recommended to prevent recurrent VTE postpartum (Bates et al. 2012).

Antepartum Prophylaxis

In these women with prior VTE, antepartum management is delineated based on risk of recurrence. For women with a *low risk* of recurrent VTE (i.e., single episode of VTE due to a transient risk factor unrelated to pregnancy or estrogen), the guidelines recommend clinical monitoring during the antepartum period and the standard 6 weeks of postpartum prophylaxis detailed above. For women with an *intermediate to high risk* of recurrent VTE (i.e., multiple unprovoked VTEs, pregnancy- or estrogen-related VTE), the guidelines recommend low- or intermediate-dose LMWH during the antepartum period and the standard 6 weeks of postpartum prophylaxis detailed above (Bates et al. 2012). The optimal dosing of LMWH for thromboprophylaxis in pregnant women with a moderate to high risk of recurrent VTE is unclear, but a randomized controlled trial is currently underway to answer this question (Bleker et al. 2016).

Congenital Thrombophilias

With scientific advancements, there has been a greater appreciation of and a broader diagnosis of congenital causes of thrombophilia. These include but are not limited to mutations in factor V Leiden (FVL) mutation and the prothrombin G20210A gene and deficiencies in protein S, protein C, and antithrombin III (ATIII). Some estimate that inherited thrombophilias are present in up to 50% of the venous thrombotic events that occur during pregnancy and in the postpartum period (Greer 1999), but the presence of thrombophilias does not always lead to a thrombotic event.

Antepartum and Postpartum Prophylaxis

Attempts have been made to quantify the relative risk of VTE in pregnancy in the presence of these congenital thrombophilias. In general, the relative risk of VTE is considered highest among patients with homozygous FVL and prothrombin 20210GA gene mutations, combined FVL and prothrombin gene mutation heterozygotes, and

ATIII deficiency. Thus, CHEST guidelines recommend, for pregnant women with no prior VTE but with a family history of VTE who are known to be homozygous for FVL or prothrombin 20210GA mutation, *antepartum prophylaxis with low- or intermediate-dose LMWH and 6 weeks of postpartum prophylaxis* (Bates et al. 2012). ACOG guidelines include combined FVL and prothrombin gene mutation heterozygotes and ATIII deficiency in this group of high-risk thrombophilias and recommend antepartum LMWH and postpartum prophylaxis for 6 weeks for these patients, as well (James 2011). For pregnant women with all other thrombophilias with no prior VTE but with a family history of VTE, *antepartum clinical vigilance and postpartum prophylaxis for 6 weeks is recommended* (James 2011; Bates et al. 2012).

Screening for Congenital Thrombophilias

There has long been a concern about thrombophilias complicating pregnancy and leading to increased rates of fetal loss. However, this is based on mostly case-control studies or observational studies with methodological limitations. A recent randomized trial of antepartum thromboprophylaxis in women with thrombophilia showed no benefit in terms of reducing the risk of VTE, pregnancy loss, or placenta-mediated pregnancy complications (Rodger et al. 2014), and guidelines recommend against screening women with a history of pregnancy complications for inherited thrombophilias (Bates et al. 2012).

Acquired Thrombophilia: Antiphospholipid Syndrome

Diagnosis of APS

Unlike congenital thrombophilias, there is strong evidence of an association between antiphospholipid syndrome (APS) and poor pregnancy outcomes. APS is an acquired thrombophilia caused by an autoimmune disorder characterized clinically by venous or arterial thrombosis, or recurrent first trimester miscarriages, or fetal death in the second or third trimester, or preterm birth due to severe preeclampsia or placental insufficiency that occurs in the presence of antiphospholipid antibodies (Miyakis et al. 2006). The antiphospholipid antibodies used for laboratory diagnosis are lupus anticoagulant, anticardiolipin ELISA (IgG or IgM, medium or high titers >99th percentile), and anti-ß2-microglobulin ELISA (IgG or IgM, medium or high titers >99th percentile), which must be present on two or more separate occasions, at least 12 weeks apart (Miyakis et al. 2006).

Antepartum and Postpartum Management of APS

In contrast to inherited thrombophilias, studies have shown benefit with antepartum thromboprophylaxis with heparin (either UFH or LWMH) plus aspirin in terms of preventing pregnancy loss in women with APS (Mak et al. 2010; Empson et al. 2005). Guidelines recommend the use of antepartum prophylactic or intermediate-dose UFH or prophylactic dose LMWH combined with low-dose aspirin in pregnant women with APS (Bates et al. 2012). Postpartum thromboprophylaxis in patients with persistent APS antibodies but without prior thrombosis is of unclear benefit and randomized controlled trials are needed to establish a standard of care. A reasonable practice based on current evidence would be to consider postpartum prophylaxis with LMWH for at least 6 weeks postpartum or until the patient returns to her long-term oral anticoagulant therapy.

Suggested Reading

Alstead EM, Ritchie JK, Lennard-Jones JE, Farthing MJ, Clark ML. Safety of azathioprine in pregnancy in inflammatory bowel disease. Gastroenterology. 1990;99(2):443–6.

Andersen BS, Steffensen FH, Sorensen HT, Nielsen GL, Olsen J. The cumulative incidence of venous thromboembolism during pregnancy and puerperium--an 11 year Danish population-based study of 63,300 pregnancies. Acta Obstet Gynecol Scand. 1998;77(2):170–3.

Andrew M, Boneu B, Cade J, Cerskus AL, Hirsh J, Jefferies A, et al. Placental transport of low molecular weight heparin in the pregnant sheep. Br J Haematol. 1985;59(1):103–8.

Bar J, Cohen-Sacher B, Hod M, Blickstein D, Lahav J, Merlob P. Low-molecular-weight heparin for thrombophilia in pregnant women. Int J Gynaecol Obstet. 2000;69(3):209–13.

Bates SM, Greer IA, Middeldorp S, Veenstra DL, Prabulos AM, Vandvik PO. VTE, thrombophilia, antithrombotic therapy, and pregnancy: antithrombotic therapy and prevention of thrombosis, 9th ed: American College of Chest Physicians Evidence-Based Clinical Practice Guidelines. Chest. 2012;141(2 Suppl):e691S–736S.

Bates SM, Middeldorp S, Rodger M, James AH, Greer I. Guidance for the treatment and prevention of obstetric-associated venous thromboembolism. J Thromb Thrombolysis. 2016;41(1):92–128.

Beyer-Westendorf J, Michalski F, Tittl L, Middeldorp S, Cohen H, Abdul Kadir R, et al. Pregnancy outcome in patients exposed to direct oral anticoagulants - and the challenge of event reporting. Thromb Haemost. 2016;116(4):651–8.

Bleker SM, Buchmuller A, Chauleur C, Ni Ainle F, Donnelly J, Verhamme P, et al. Low-molecular-weight heparin to prevent recurrent venous thromboembolism in pregnancy: rationale and design of the Highlow study, a randomised trial of two doses. Thromb Res. 2016;144:62–8.

Boehlen F, Hohlfeld P, Extermann P, Perneger TV, de Moerloose P. Platelet count at term pregnancy: a reappraisal of the threshold. Obstet Gynecol. 2000;95(1):29–33.

Bremme KA. Haemostatic changes in pregnancy. Best Pract Res Clin Haematol. 2003;16(2):153–68.

British Thoracic Society Standards of Care Committee Pulmonary Embolism Guideline Development G. British Thoracic Society guidelines for the management of suspected acute pulmonary embolism. Thorax. 2003;58(6):470–83.

Burrows RF, Kelton JG. Fetal thrombocytopenia and its relation to maternal thrombocytopenia. N Engl J Med. 1993;329(20):1463–6.

Canigral C, Moscardo F, Castro C, Pajares A, Lancharro A, Solves P, et al. Eculizumab for the treatment of pregnancy-related atypical hemolytic uremic syndrome. Ann Hematol. 2014;93(8):1421–2.

Chalmers E, Williams M, Brennand J, Liesner R, Collins P, Richards M, et al. Guideline on the management of haemophilia in the fetus and neonate. Br J Haematol. 2011;154(2):208–15.

Chan WS, Rey E, Kent NE, Group VTEiPGW, Chan WS, Kent NE, et al. Venous thromboembolism and antithrombotic therapy in pregnancy. J Obstet Gynaecol Can. 2014;36(6):527–53.

Committee on Practice B-O. Practice bulletin no. 183: postpartum hemorrhage. Obstet Gynecol. 2017;130(4):e168–e86.

Dimitrakakis C, Papageorgiou P, Papageorgiou I, Antzaklis A, Sakarelou N, Michalas S. Absence of transplacental passage of the low molecular weight heparin enoxaparin. Haemostasis. 2000;30(5):243–8.

Einstein AJ, Henzlova MJ, Rajagopalan S. Estimating risk of cancer associated with radiation exposure from 64-slice computed tomography coronary angiography. JAMA. 2007;298(3):317–23.

Empson M, Lassere M, Craig J, Scott J. Prevention of recurrent miscarriage for women with antiphospholipid antibody or lupus anticoagulant. Cochrane Database Syst Rev. 2005;(2):CD002859.

George JN, Nester CM, McIntosh JJ. Syndromes of thrombotic microangiopathy associated with pregnancy. Hematology Am Soc Hematol Educ Program. 2015;2015:644–8.

Gernsheimer T, James AH, Stasi R. How I treat thrombocytopenia in pregnancy. Blood. 2013;121(1):38–47.

Gherman RB, Goodwin TM, Leung B, Byrne JD, Hethumumi R, Montoro M. Incidence, clinical characteristics, and timing of objectively diagnosed venous thromboembolism during pregnancy. Obstet Gynecol. 1999;94(5 Pt 1):730–4.

Greer IA. Thrombosis in pregnancy: maternal and fetal issues. Lancet. 1999;353(9160):1258–65.

Haeri S, Dildy GA. Maternal mortality from hemorrhage. Semin Perinatol. 2012;36(1):48–55.

Haram K, Svendsen E, Abildgaard U. The HELLP syndrome: clinical issues and management. A review. BMC Pregnancy Childbirth. 2009;9:8.

Hayashino Y, Goto M, Noguchi Y, Fukui T. Ventilation-perfusion scanning and helical CT in suspected pulmonary embolism: meta-analysis of diagnostic performance. Radiology. 2005;234(3):740–8.

Heit JA, Kobbervig CE, James AH, Petterson TM, Bailey KR, Melton LJ. Trends in the incidence of venous thromboembolism during pregnancy or postpartum: a 30-year population-based study. Ann Intern Med. 2005;143(10):697–706.

Horlocker TT, Wedel DJ, Rowlingson JC, Enneking FK, Kopp SL, Benzon HT, et al. Regional anesthesia in the patient receiving antithrombotic or thrombolytic therapy: American Society of Regional Anesthesia and Pain Medicine evidence-based guidelines (third edition). Reg Anesth Pain Med. 2010;35(1):64–101.

Jacobsen AF, Skjeldestad FE, Sandset PM. Incidence and risk patterns of venous thromboembolism in pregnancy and puerperium--a register-based case-control study. Am J Obstet Gynecol. 2008;198(2):233 e1–7.

James A. Committee on Practice B-O. Practice bulletin no. 123: thromboembolism in pregnancy. Obstet Gynecol. 2011;118(3):718–29.

James AH, Jamison MG, Brancazio LR, Myers ER. Venous thromboembolism during pregnancy and the postpartum period: incidence, risk factors, and mortality. Am J Obstet Gynecol. 2006;194(5):1311–5.

James AH, Rhee E, Thames B, Philipp CS. Characterization of antithrombin levels in pregnancy. Thromb Res. 2014;134(3):648–51.

James AH, Konkle BA, Kouides P, Ragni MV, Thames B, Gupta S, et al. Postpartum von Willebrand factor levels in women with and without von Willebrand disease and implications for prophylaxis. Haemophilia. 2015;21(1):81–7.

Kadir RA, Davies J, Winikoff R, Pollard D, Peyvandi F, Garagiola I, et al. Pregnancy complications and obstetric care in women with inherited bleeding disorders. Haemophilia. 2013;19(Suppl 4):1–10.

Kamel H, Navi BB, Sriram N, Hovsepian DA, Devereux RB, Elkind MS. Risk of a thrombotic event after the 6-week postpartum period. N Engl J Med. 2014;370(14):1307–15.

Kelly RJ, Hochsmann B, Szer J, Kulasekararaj A, de Guibert S, Roth A, et al. Eculizumab in pregnant patients with paroxysmal nocturnal hemoglobinuria. N Engl J Med. 2015;373(11):1032–9.

Knight M, Nelson-Piercy C, Kurinczuk JJ, Spark P, Brocklehurst P, System UKOS. A prospective national study of acute fatty liver of pregnancy in the UK. Gut. 2008;57(7):951–6.

Konstantinides SV, Torbicki A, Agnelli G, Danchin N, Fitzmaurice D, Galie N, et al. 2014 ESC guidelines on the diagnosis and management of acute pulmonary embolism. Eur Heart J. 2014;35(43):3033–69, 69a-69k.

Kujovich JL. von Willebrand disease and pregnancy. J Thromb Haemost. 2005;3(2):246–53.

Leung AN, Bull TM, Jaeschke R, Lockwood CJ, Boiselle PM, Hurwitz LM, et al. An official American Thoracic Society/Society of Thoracic Radiology clinical practice guideline: evaluation of suspected pulmonary embolism in pregnancy. Am J Respir Crit Care Med. 2011;184(10):1200–8.

Lindqvist P, Dahlback B, Marsal K. Thrombotic risk during pregnancy: a population study. Obstet Gynecol. 1999;94(4):595–9.

Lu E, Shatzel JJ, Salati J, DeLoughery TG. The safety of low-molecular-weight heparin during and after pregnancy. Obstet Gynecol Surv. 2017;72(12):721–9.

Ludlam CA, Pasi KJ, Bolton-Maggs P, Collins PW, Cumming AM, Dolan G, et al. A framework for genetic service provision for haemophilia and other inherited bleeding disorders. Haemophilia. 2005;11(2):145–63.

Mak A, Cheung MW, Cheak AA, Ho RC. Combination of heparin and aspirin is superior to aspirin alone in enhancing live births in patients with recurrent pregnancy loss and positive anti-phospholipid antibodies: a meta-analysis of randomized controlled trials and meta-regression. Rheumatology (Oxford). 2010;49(2):281–8.

McColl MD, Ramsay JE, Tait RC, Walker ID, McCall F, Conkie JA, et al. Risk factors for pregnancy associated venous thromboembolism. Thromb Haemost. 1997;78(4):1183–8.

McLintock C, Brighton T, Chunilal S, Dekker G, McDonnell N, McRae S, et al. Recommendations for the diagnosis and treatment of deep venous thrombosis and pulmonary embolism in pregnancy and the postpartum period. Aust N Z J Obstet Gynaecol. 2012;52(1):14–22.

Michel M, Novoa MV, Bussel JB. Intravenous anti-D as a treatment for immune thrombocytopenic purpura (ITP) during pregnancy. Br J Haematol. 2003;123(1):142–6.

Miyakis S, Lockshin MD, Atsumi T, Branch DW, Brey RL, Cervera R, et al. International consensus statement on an update of the classification criteria for definite antiphospholipid syndrome (APS). J Thromb Haemost. 2006;4(2):295–306.

Ockner SA, Brunt EM, Cohn SM, Krul ES, Hanto DW, Peters MG. Fulminant hepatic failure caused by acute fatty liver of pregnancy treated by orthotopic liver transplantation. Hepatology. 1990;11(1):59–64.

Orme ML, Lewis PJ, de Swiet M, Serlin MJ, Sibeon R, Baty JD, et al. May mothers given warfarin breast-feed their infants? Br Med J. 1977;1(6076):1564–5.

Polak JF, Wilkinson DL. Ultrasonographic diagnosis of symptomatic deep venous thrombosis in pregnancy. Am J Obstet Gynecol. 1991;165(3):625–9.

Price HV, Salaman JR, Laurence KM, Langmaid H. Immunosuppressive drugs and the foetus. Transplantation. 1976;21(4):294–8.

Quiroz R, Kucher N, Zou KH, Kipfmueller F, Costello P, Goldhaber SZ, et al. Clinical validity of a negative computed tomography scan in patients with suspected pulmonary embolism: a systematic review. JAMA. 2005;293(16):2012–7.

Reese JA, Peck JD, Deschamps DR, McIntosh JJ, Knudtson EJ, Terrell DR, et al. Platelet counts during pregnancy. N Engl J Med. 2018;379(1):32–43.

Richter C, Sitzmann J, Lang P, Weitzel H, Huch A, Huch R. Excretion of low molecular weight heparin in human milk. Br J Clin Pharmacol. 2001;52(6): 708–10.

Riely CA, Latham PS, Romero R, Duffy TP. Acute fatty liver of pregnancy. A reassessment based on observations in nine patients. Ann Intern Med. 1987;106(5):703–6.

Rodger MA, Hague WM, Kingdom J, Kahn SR, Karovitch A, Sermer M, et al. Antepartum dalteparin versus no antepartum dalteparin for the prevention of pregnancy complications in pregnant women with thrombophilia (TIPPS): a multinational open-label randomised trial. Lancet. 2014;384(9955):1673–83.

Russell JR, Stabin MG, Sparks RB, Watson E. Radiation absorbed dose to the embryo/fetus from radiopharmaceuticals. Health Phys. 1997;73(5):756–69.

Sadler JE, Mannucci PM, Berntorp E, Bochkov N, Boulyjenkov V, Ginsburg D, et al. Impact, diagnosis and treatment of von Willebrand disease. Thromb Haemost. 2000;84(2):160–74.

Sainio S, Kekomaki R, Riikonen S, Teramo K. Maternal thrombocytopenia at term: a population-based study. Acta Obstet Gynecol Scand. 2000;79(9):744–9.

Shakur H, Elbourne D, Gulmezoglu M, Alfirevic Z, Ronsmans C, Allen E, et al. The WOMAN trial (World Maternal Antifibrinolytic Trial): tranexamic acid for the treatment of postpartum haemorrhage: an international randomised, double blind placebo controlled trial. Trials. 2010;11:40.

Simpson EL, Lawrenson RA, Nightingale AL, Farmer RD. Venous thromboembolism in pregnancy and the puerperium: incidence and additional risk factors from a London perinatal database. BJOG. 2001;108(1):56–60.

Tuohy E, Litt E, Alikhan R. Treatment of patients with von Willebrand disease. J Blood Med. 2011;2:49–57.

Victora CG, Requejo JH, Barros AJ, Berman P, Bhutta
    Z, Boerma T, et al. Countdown to 2015: a decade of
    tracking progress for maternal, newborn, and child
    survival. Lancet. 2016;387(10032):2049–59.
Wagner DD. Cell biology of von Willebrand factor. Annu
    Rev Cell Biol. 1990;6:217–46.

Winer-Muram HT, Boone JM, Brown HL, Jennings SG,
    Mabie WC, Lombardo GT. Pulmonary embolism in
    pregnant patients: fetal radiation dose with helical
    CT. Radiology. 2002;224(2):487–92.

Hemorrhage and Thrombosis in Women

31

Bethany T. Samuelson Bannow

Hemorrhagic Complications

Heavy Menstrual Bleeding

Due to the routine challenges of menstruation and pregnancy, women with bleeding disorders present earlier and more often with symptoms compared to their male counterparts. A commonly reported initial symptom is that of heavy menstrual bleeding (HMB), previously referred to as menorrhagia, or other abnormal uterine bleeding (AUB). HMB is defined as menstrual blood loss of >80 mL per cycle. As this definition is impractical in the clinical setting, the clinician may rely on a more pragmatic combination of predictors of HMB, including iron deficiency (low ferritin), passing of clots >1 inch in diameter, and frequent changing of protection (more than once per hour). Other common features include prolonged menses (flow lasting longer than 7 days), the need to wear more than one form of protection at a time (e.g., pad and tampon), and the need to awaken to change pads or tampons overnight (Warner et al. 2004).

B. T. Samuelson Bannow (✉)
The Hemophilia Center, Oregon Health & Science University, Portland, OR, USA

Division of Hematology and Oncology, Duke University Medicine Center, Durham, NC, USA
e-mail: samuelsb@ohsu.edu

Approximately one third of women will seek treatment for HMB at some point.

HMB can be seen in a variety of settings. Rates of HMB from 20–30%, and occasionally as high as 60–70%, have been reported in women on anticoagulant therapy. Other etiologies include anatomic causes (fibroids or polyps), irregular ovulation (particularly in the first 1–3 years postmenarche and in the perimenopausal period), pregnancy-related (miscarriage, ectopic pregnancy), pelvic inflammatory disease, endometriosis, and cancers (particularly in postmenopausal patients). Up to a quarter of women with HMB are believed to have an underlying bleeding diathesis. The workup of HMB should include a careful history with attention to potential medication effects (antiplatelet agents or anticoagulants), trauma, signs and symptoms of anemia, risk factors or features of ovulatory dysfunction (e.g., polycystic ovarian syndrome), or malignancy (postmenopausal bleeding, abnormal Papanicolaou tests, and/or known human papillomavirus infection). A careful family history should also be taken for diagnoses or symptoms of bleeding disorders. Laboratory evaluation for underlying disorders of hemostasis and a gynecologic evaluation should also be considered in certain situations.

Laboratory Workup

Initial laboratory workup of a patient with HMB and suspected bleeding disorder should include a complete blood count (CBC) with attention to total hemoglobin and mean corpuscular volume (MCV) for evidence of iron deficiency anemia as well as total platelet count and ferritin level. If there is suspicion for an underlying bleeding disorder, a basic coagulation panel including prothrombin time (PT), activated partial thromboplastin time (APTT) and fibrinogen, von Willebrand factor (VWF) antigen and activity, and factor VIII (FVIII) should also be ordered. It should be noted that VWF and FVIII are acute phase reactants and therefore false negatives may be seen in the setting of illness or stress. Estrogen therapies, in rare cases, may also lead to normalization of values in patients with mild von Willebrand disease (VWD). If clinical suspicion is substantial in a patient with normal levels at a single point in time, repeat testing is advisable. If testing of all these parameters falls within the normal range and the clinician strongly suspects an underlying bleeding disorder, particularly in patients with evidence of other mucocutaneous bleeding, platelet studies including aggregometry should be considered as up to 47% of women with HMB may have decreased aggregation with one or more agonists (Philipp et al. 2003).

Gynecologic Workup

In addition to the careful medical history outlined above, a referral to gynecology should be considered. Additional features of the menstrual history may be elicited, including regularity of cycles and age of menarche, sexual history including risk of pregnancy and/or sexually transmitted infections (STIs), symptoms of thyroid dysfunction, or hyperandrogenism. Additional evaluation may include pelvic examination, a pregnancy test, Papanicolaou (pap) testing, endometrial biopsy, and/or testing for STIs as indicated. Either transabdominal or transvaginal ultrasound may be useful to identify uterine abnormalities depending on the age and comfort level of the patient.

Management

In addition to potential medical complications, such as iron deficiency and/or anemia, HMB is associated with a significant decrease in quality

Table 31.1 Treatment strategies for heavy menstrual bleeding

First-line therapies
Hormonal management
Levonorgestrel IUS/etonogestrel subcutaneous implant
Combined hormonal contraceptives[a]
Second-line therapies
Tranexamic acid (start with menses, continue 5 days)
Aminocaproic acid
Third-line therapies (for women with diagnosed bleeding disorders and refractory bleeding)
Stimate® (intranasal desmopressin)
Factor infusions
Therapies for women who have completed childbearing
Endometrial ablation
Hysterectomy
Adjunctive therapies
Iron supplementation for iron deficiency with or without anemia
NSAIDs[b]

[a]Omission of placebo weeks may be beneficial
[b]Only in patients without underlying bleeding disorders

of life, as well as missed work and school days, for many patients. Fortunately there are a wide variety of options for management, including hormonal therapies, prohemostatic agents, and surgical/procedural interventions. The primary goal of treatment in most cases is to reduce blood loss and subsequent effects. A general approach to management is outlined in Table 31.1 and therapeutic options are discussed in detail below.

The levonorgestrel intrauterine system (LNG-IUS) has proven to be exceptionally effective in the treatment of HMB, with a 71–95% reduction in menstrual blood loss. The etonogestrel subdermal implant is similarly effective. Both of these methods may result in intermittent or frequent spotting, in which case alternative therapies may be considered. However, given high rates of amenorrhea (40–60% with the IUD, 20–70% with the implant) and excellent contraceptive efficacy (>99%), these are often excellent options for women with HMB (Adeyemi-Fowode et al. 2017; Di Carlo et al. 2015).

Many women also experience good results with the introduction of combined oral contraceptives (OCPs), which have been shown to reduce blood loss by 35–69% and can be administered continuously without breaks to prevent menses altogether and thus interference of HMB with school, work, or personal functions. Occasionally this may lead to breakthrough bleeding, in which case planned, infrequent breaks may be timed for patient convenience. This option may be preferable for nulliparous women and adolescents who are uncomfortable with the idea of LNG-IUS or dermal implant placement. The effects of contraceptive patches and vaginal rings on HMB have not been well studied.

In certain circumstances, most often in women with known hemostatic defects and HMB refractory to hormone therapy, prohemostatic agents may be used as an alternative or additional therapy. Antifibrinolytics are good choices in many patients, with tranexamic acid (1300 mg three times daily) administered at the onset of menses, being the most commonly prescribed agent. Courses are typically restricted to 5 days and may be repeated with each cycle. Aminocaproic acid is another alternative but has a less convenient dosing schedule and higher pill burden and is not as well studied in HMB. Of potential concern with antifibrinolytic use is thrombotic risk, particularly in combination with estrogen-containing contraceptives. Package labeling indicates the use of combination hormonal contraception as a contraindication to the use of tranexamic acid. However, increased risk of thrombosis has never been established in clinical trials and large studies of tranexamic acid in high-risk populations, such as postpartum hemorrhage patients and trauma patients, have failed to demonstrate any significant increase in rates of thrombosis. In patients with otherwise uncontrolled HMB resulting in symptomatic anemia and no history of thrombosis, the benefits of this combination are likely to outweigh risks.

Factor replacement, including FVIII and VWF, and/or desmopressin may rarely be useful and necessary in patients with von Willebrand disease and other disorders of hemostasis. The efficacy of desmopressin is often limited by tachyphylaxis and patients require testing of response in advance as well as education on the risks, signs, and symptoms of hyponatremia. Of note, if intranasal desmopressin is used (which is likely to be preferable method of administration), care should be taken to ensure that the appropriate dose for hemostatic control is used (150mcg, marketed as Stimate®), rather than the lower enuresis dosing (typically 10–40mcg). Combination VWF/FVIII concentrates may be infused in the clinic or at home but are expensive and inconvenient. Other factor concentrates or blood components may be necessary for major uterine bleeding in patients with specific defects of hemostasis, including acquired or congenital thrombocytopenias, rare factor deficiencies, hypofibrinogenemia, or afibrinogenemia. These agents should be limited to girls and women who are unable to achieve adequate control of HMB with any of the previously discussed options.

Surgical therapies for HMB include endometrial ablation and hysterectomy. Endometrial ablation is often initially successful but many women ultimately require additional surgery, whether repeat ablation or hysterectomy, a finding that is far less common in women undergoing hysterectomy (relative risk of 14.9 at 1 year). Hysterectomy does carry additional risk of postoperative complications, requires a longer recovery period, and may pose additional risks to women with underlying disorders of hemostasis, but is a definitive and permanent solution to HMB. Uterine artery embolization may be helpful for women with fibroids but has not been studied for other forms of HMB. Surgical options should be limited to patients who have completed childbearing as all are associated with future infertility.

Adjunctive Therapies

Iron deficiency, with or without anemia, is a common complication of AUB and HMB. Deficiencies can be further worsened during pregnancy and the postpartum period. Supplementation with oral iron or, if required, IV iron is strongly recommended and has been associated with improved outcomes, particularly in school-age children.

Nonsteroidal anti-inflammatory drugs (NSAIDs) are often useful for management of menstrual cramping and have been demonstrated to decrease menstrual bleeding in some patients

(10–52%). They are typically contraindicated, however, in patients with underlying bleeding disorder due to increased risk of bleeding from other sites. Caution should be exercised in patients with non-menstrual bleeding (epistaxis or other mucocutaneous bleeding) or a family history of bleeding pending a workup for an underlying bleeding disorder.

Special Populations

Girls and women who are carriers of hemophilia A or B may also present with HMB. In such cases factor levels may be found to be significantly less than 50% of expected due to skewed lyonization (increased inactivation of the normal factor gene). HMB may also be seen, however, in carriers with apparently "normal" or "adequate" levels of factor either for one of the many other reasons outlined above or due to an imperfect correlation between bleeding symptoms and factor levels, leading to higher rates of bleeding among hemophilia carriers than previously appreciated (Plug et al. 2006). In these cases, in addition to the above recommended workup, specific factor levels (FVIII or FIX as appropriate) should be checked. If identified, these deficiencies have further implications, including potentially increased risk of bleeding with invasive procedures and pregnancy, a 50% chance of hemophilia in each male offspring, and a 50% chance of hemophilia carriership in each female offspring.

Girls and women who require anticoagulant therapy often experience HMB which can be particularly difficult to control. Switching agents may result in decreased bleeding in certain patients, particularly those on rivaroxaban which may have a higher rate of HMB as compared to apixaban or warfarin (Martinelli et al. 2016). In many cases the LNG-IUS or the subdermal implant may provide the dual benefit of reduced HMB and highly effective contraception (important for preventing pregnancy while on potentially teratogenic anticoagulants and due to the increased risk of recurrent thrombosis in pregnancy and the postpartum period). In patients averse to these therapies or who do not achieve adequate control despite them, estrogen-

containing therapies may be considered while the patient is on therapeutic anticoagulation without an apparent increase in recurrence of thrombosis. All estrogen-containing therapies should be discontinued at least 1 month prior to planned discontinuation of anticoagulation, and increased risk of thrombosis may persist for up to 3 months after discontinuation of the estrogen-containing agent.

Thrombotic Complications

Estrogen-Associated Thrombosis

Estrogen-containing contraceptives, such as OCPs, have long been associated with an increased risk of venous thromboembolism (VTE). The relative risk of thrombosis for those on OCPs is increased two- to fourfold. However, given that the baseline risk of thrombosis in young women is only about 2–3:10,000, the use of OCPs leads to only one extra thrombosis per 1666 women. The risk of thrombosis is highest with estrogen doses of ≥50 mcg (seen in "first-generation" formulations) and is also slightly increased in "third-generation" pills that contain desogestrel, gestodene, and norgestimate or pills that use drospirenone. Risk is lowest in levonorgestrel-containing combinations containing 30mcg or less of estradiol, although the absolute risk remains small.

This higher risk of thrombosis is further exaggerated with contraceptive rings and patches which are associated with a risk of VTE roughly twice that of therapy with OCPs. Progesterone-only pills (minipills) do not appear to have an increase of thrombosis at the cost of considerably decreased contraceptive efficacy. Injectable depot progesterone has, however, been associated with a 2.2–3.6-fold increased risk of thrombosis. Neither the levonorgestrel IUD nor etonogestrel subdermal implants have been associated with increased risk of thrombosis and are useful contraceptive options for women with thrombophilia with the potential benefit of managing HMB associated with anticoagulation.

Pathophysiology

There are many changes in the hemostatic system with the increased estrogen levels that "shift" women toward a hypercoagulable state. Levels of procoagulant proteins such as factors VII and VIII and fibrinogen increase. Decrements in the natural anticoagulants to levels commonly associated with thrombosis are also seen. Lower levels of antithrombin III and free protein S are common. These natural changes are synergistic with any underlying hypercoagulable states. Up to 60% of women who develop thrombosis while pregnant will be found to have factor V Leiden (FVL). Women with FVL (particularly in the homozygous state) are more likely to have thrombosis with any estrogen exposure. Since estrogens raise the level of factor VIII, women may be more dependent on protein C to degrade factor V and control hemostasis. If the ability to degrade factor V is impaired, this may promote a hypercoagulable state.

Management

Upon making the diagnosis of VTE in a woman on estrogen-containing therapy, anticoagulation should be administered immediately. Any of the direct oral anticoagulants (DOACs) will be a reasonable first choice although it should be noted that, as opposed to rivaroxaban and apixaban, dabigatran and edoxaban require a 5–10-day lead in period of parenteral anticoagulant, which may be highly inconvenient particularly in a patient who is eligible for outpatient therapy. Either rivaroxaban or apixaban may be started immediately, with attention to increased dosing in the initial period (15 mg BID for 21 days for rivaroxaban, 10 mg BID for 7 days for apixaban). Following this initial period, rivaroxaban can be dosed once daily, with a meal, which may be preferable for otherwise healthy young women who find it difficult to remember a twice daily dose. Rivaroxaban may, however, result in higher rates of HMB (hazard ratio of 2.1 compared to vitamin K antagonists) compared to apixaban (hazard ratio of 1.18 compared to vitamin K antagonists) and therefore may not be the agent of choice for a woman with heavy periods in the nonanticoagulated state.

Due to the extremely low risk of recurrence of estrogen-associated thrombosis (<1% at 1 year and 6% at 5 years compared to 5% and 17% of women with non-estrogen-associated thrombosis) (Eischer et al. 2014), duration of anticoagulation is generally limited to 3 months in the absence of ongoing estrogen exposure (including pregnancy). Discontinuation of estrogen-containing therapies is strongly recommended. Also due to the low risk of recurrence, results of thrombophilia workup generally do not impact the management of these events and therefore are not routinely recommended. In certain patients with atypical thrombosis (i.e., arterial or splanchnic vein) or other concerning signs/symptoms (e.g., abnormal complete blood count parameters, unexplained weight loss, physical exam abnormalities), additional evaluation such as limited thrombophilia workup for antiphospholipid antibodies, paroxysmal nocturnal hemoglobinuria, myeloproliferative neoplasm, and/or appropriate cancer screening may be advisable.

Use of Estrogen Therapies in Patients with a History of Thrombosis

Contraception

Women who have had a previous thrombosis and are not currently anticoagulated should not use estrogen-containing OCPs, patches, or vaginal rings. Prevention of unplanned pregnancy is, however, paramount given increased risks to both the mother and fetus (see Chap. 30 for a discussion of pregnancy management in patients with a history of thrombosis). Relative risk of thrombosis and expected failure rate of various forms of contraceptives are described in Table 31.2.

Progesterone-only therapy is preferred in patients with a history of VTE, with the LNG-IUS and etonogestrel subdermal implant offering effective pregnancy prevention without additional risk of thrombosis. While the progesterone-only pill does not appear to increase risk of thrombosis, it has a relatively high rate of failure (>9%), substantially increased by missed (or even delayed) doses. Barrier contraception is similarly safe from a thrombotic risk standpoint and has an

Table 31.2 Relative risk of thrombosis and efficacy of various contraceptive methods

Contraceptive method	Relative risk of thrombosis	Unintended pregnancy at 1 year
None/barrier	*ref*	12–85%
Combined OCPs	1.9–4.2	0.1–8%
Combined patch	7.9	9%
Vaginal ring	6.5	9%
Levonorgestrel IUD	0.3–0.9[a]	0.2%
Etonogestrel implant	1.4[a]	0.05%
Progestin-only pills	0.9–1.0[a]	9%
Depot medroxyprogesterone	2.2–3.6	6%

[a]Not statistically significant compared to no contraceptives

added benefit of reducing sexually transmitted infections but is variably effective for contraception (2% annual failure rate with perfect use, 18% with typical use). Depot medroxyprogesterone is effective for contraception but not recommended in patients with a history of thrombosis due to increased risk of recurrence. Surgical options including tubal ligation or vasectomy (for women with only one male partner) are also highly effective without long-term increased thrombotic risk, although appropriate care must be taken in the perioperative period to reduce risk of recurrent thrombosis or bleeding in the anticoagulated woman. As always, a minimum period of 3 months is recommended between the diagnosis of VTE and elective surgery.

After the LNG-IUS and subdermal implant, estrogen-containing OCPs are one of the most effective nonsurgical forms of contraception (0.1% annual failure rate with perfect use, 8% with typical use). In rare cases, these therapies may be required either as the preferred or only effective form of contraception or for management of a separate gynecologic issue such as HMB. If started in the setting of ongoing anticoagulation use and discontinued 1 or more months prior to discontinuation of anticoagulation, the risk of recurrent thrombosis does not appear to be substantially increased by OCPs.

The use of estrogen-containing therapies in a patient known to have factor V or other thrombophilia but without a history of thrombosis is controversial. Although the risk is probably low, most would recommend against it in favor of progesterone-only options discussed above. These options are also preferable for women with first-degree relatives with unprovoked or estrogen-associated VTE.

Hormone Replacement Therapy

Hormone replacement therapy (HRT) may be required in specific situations either to manage severe symptoms after natural menopause or to combat adverse effects of early menopause in patients with primary ovarian failure or who experience surgical menopause at a young age. Avoidance of oral estrogens is highly recommended, given strong evidence of increased risk of recurrence (10.7% in patients on HRT compared to 2.3% in patients on placebo) (Hoibraaten et al. 2000). This is also true of patients with specific known thrombophilias (FVL or prothrombin gene mutation). Transdermal estrogen, however, does not appear to be associated with a significantly increased risk for VTE development among women without a history of thrombosis, including those with known thrombophilia, but safety in patients with a history of thrombosis is unknown. This must, however, be combined with progestin therapy in women with a uterus due to the dramatically increased risk of uterine cancer associated with unopposed estrogen use. Long-term effects on cardiovascular risks (arterial thrombosis) are unknown. Vaginal preparations (including the cream, ring, and tablet) do not appear to increase serum estrogen levels above the menopausal range and are not associated with increased risk of VTE and should be used preferentially for genitourinary symptoms of menopause although will not address systemic symptoms such as hot flashes. The safety of systemic HRT for women with a history of thrombosis already on anticoagulation is unknown but presumed to be reduced compared to patients not on anticoagulation.

Summary

Heavy menstrual bleeding is a common diagnosis in reproductive-aged women that can be associated with a number of adverse effects including iron deficiency anemia and decreased quality of life. An appropriate level of suspicion for underlying bleeding disorders in women with this diagnosis is necessary but in most cases symptoms can be well managed by hormonal methods with occasional need for antifibrinolytic therapy. Iron therapy should be offered to deficient women.

Venous thromboembolism is an uncommon diagnosis in young women but risk is increased in the setting of increased estrogen states including combined hormonal contraceptives, pregnancy, and the use of hormone replacement therapy. Women who experience these events are at a low risk of recurrence outside of these states but such states must either be avoided in the future or managed with appropriate anticoagulant prophylaxis. The LNG-IUS and etonogestrel subdermal implants are excellent options for contraceptives in these patients due to high efficacy for prevention of pregnancy without increasing the risk of recurrent VTE.

Suggested Reading

Adeyemi-Fowode OA, Santos XM, Dietrich JE, Srivaths L. Levonorgestrel-releasing intrauterine device use in female adolescents with heavy menstrual bleeding and bleeding disorders: single institution review. J Pediatr Adolesc Gynecol. 2017;30:479–83. https://doi.org/10.1016/j.jpag.2016.04.001.

Di Carlo C, Guida M, De Rosa N, Sansone A, Gargano V, Cagnacci A, Nappi C. Bleeding profile in users of an etonogestrel sub-dermal implant: effects of anthropometric variables. An observational uncontrolled preliminary study in Italian population. Gynecol Endocrinol. 2015;31:491–4. https://doi.org/10.3109/09513590.2015.1018163.

Eischer L, Eichinger S, Kyrle PA. The risk of recurrence in women with venous thromboembolism while using estrogens: a prospective cohort study. J Thromb Haemost. 2014;12:635–40. https://doi.org/10.1111/jth.12528.

Hoibraaten E, Qvigstad E, Arnesen H, Larsen S, Wickstrom E, Sandset PM. Increased risk of recurrent venous thromboembolism during hormone replacement therapy--results of the randomized, double-blind, placebo-controlled estrogen in venous thromboembolism trial (EVTET). Thromb Haemost. 2000;84:961–7.

Martinelli IL, Anthonie WA, Middeldorp S, Levi M, Beyer-Westendorf J, van Bellen B, Bounameaux H, Brighton TA, Cohen AT, Trajanovic M, Gebel M, Lam P, Wells PS, Prins MH. Recurrent venous thromboembolism and abnormal uterine bleeding with anticoagulant and hormone therapy use. Blood. 2016;127:1417–25. https://doi.org/10.1182/blood-2015-08-665927.

Philipp CS, Dilley A, Miller CH, Evatt B, Baranwal A, Schwartz R, Bachmann G, Saidi P. Platelet functional defects in women with unexplained menorrhagia. J Thromb Haemost. 2003;1:477–84.

Plug I, Mauser-Bunschoten EP, Brocker-Vriends AH, van Amstel HK, van der Bom JG, van Diemen-Homan JE, Willemse J, Rosendaal FR. Bleeding in carriers of hemophilia. Blood. 2006;108:52–6. https://doi.org/10.1182/blood-2005-09-3879.

Warner PE, Critchley HO, Lumsden MA, Campbell-Brown M, Douglas A, Murray GD. Menorrhagia I: measured blood loss, clinical features, and outcome in women with heavy periods: a survey with follow-up data. Am J Obstet Gynecol. 2004;190:1216–23. https://doi.org/10.1016/j.ajog.2003.11.015.

Pediatric Thrombosis

32

Kristina Haley

Introduction

Thrombosis is a rare event in the pediatric population, but the incidence has increased over the last decade and current estimates indicate an incidence of approximately 0.07–0.49 per 10,000 children in developed countries or 4.9–21.9 per 10,000 hospital admissions (Mahajerin and Croteau 2017; Takemoto et al. 2014; Setty et al. 2012). Pediatric thrombosis occurs in a bimodal distribution, with a first peak in the neonatal period and a second peak in the adolescent years. However, when normalized for hospital admissions and discharges, the incidence of thrombosis increases with age (Mahajerin and Croteau 2017; Setty et al. 2012). In general, pediatric thrombosis is a tertiary care problem with more events occurring in children with chronic care conditions such as congenital heart defects, renal disease, or malignancies as well as in children admitted to the ICU, who have experienced trauma, or who have central venous catheters. The vast majority of pediatric thrombosis are provoked or associated with an underlying condition (Setty et al. 2012; Jaffray and Young 2018). Treatment of thrombosis in the pediatric population requires special consideration due to the unique characteristics of the developing hemostatic system, the likelihood that affected children will go on to live for decades after their thrombotic event, and the risk of anticoagulation in a young and active patient. Treatment guidelines for pediatric thrombosis are available in the CHEST guidelines, edition 9, as well as the American Society of Hematology 2018 guidelines for management of venous thromboembolism: treatment of pediatric venous thromboembolism (Monagle et al. 2012, 2018).

Ranges of Normal

The hemostatic system is developmentally regulated, resulting in qualitative and quantitative differences in coagulation factors, fibrinolytic proteins, and platelet function in an age-dependent manner (Jaffray and Young 2013). The term "developmental hemostasis" has been applied to the period of time when the hemostatic system exists in an evolving balance of pro- and anticoagulant functions. Most coagulation protein levels are low at birth and slowly rise to adult range over the first year of life. Levels of antithrombin and proteins C and S are significantly lower at birth with protein C levels remaining lower than adult range until the teenage years (Jaffray and Young 2013). It is important when interpreting laboratory values in younger patients to use age-specific normal ranges.

K. Haley (✉)
Department of Pediatrics, Division of Pediatric Hematology/Oncology, Oregon Health & Sciences University, Portland, OR, USA
e-mail: haley@ohsu.edu

© Springer Nature Switzerland AG 2019
T. G. DeLoughery (ed.), *Hemostasis and Thrombosis*,
https://doi.org/10.1007/978-3-030-19330-0_32

Deep Venous Thrombosis and Pulmonary Embolism

Venous thromboembolism (VTE) remains a rare event in childhood, but the incidence is increasing. The vast majority of pediatric VTEs are provoked, and at least one risk factor is identified in the majority of VTEs (Mahajerin and Croteau 2017; Setty et al. 2012; Jaffray and Young 2018). Risk factors associated with VTE in pediatric patients include chronic disease processes such as congenital heart disease, inflammatory bowel disease, or malignancy (Mahajerin and Croteau 2017; Setty et al. 2012; Jaffray and Young 2018; Branchford et al. 2012). Additional risk factors associated with pediatric thrombosis include immobility, systemic or localized infection, admission to the ICU, prolonged hospitalization (>5 days), mechanical ventilation, obesity, exogenous hormone use, surgery, and presence of a central venous line (Branchford et al. 2012). Inherited thrombophilias such as factor V Leiden, protein C deficiency, protein S deficiency, antithrombin deficiency, or prothrombin gene mutation may increase risk in synergy with acquired risk factors in patients with provoked thrombosis (van Ommen and Nowak-Gottl 2017; Tormene et al. 2002; Mahajerin et al. 2014).

The most important aspect of diagnosing DVT and PE in children is having a high index of suspicion since this is a rare event in the pediatric population. Similar to adults, patients will present with pain, swelling, and warmth of the overlying skin in the affected extremity or with persistent chest pain or shortness of breath when a pulmonary embolism is present (Jaffray and Young 2018). For children with a central line, they may present with recurrent central line malfunction. In addition, they may present with complications of occlusion like SVC syndrome (Jaffray et al. 2017).

Although pediatric studies are lacking, the use of Doppler ultrasound remains the first choice for diagnostic testing (Jaffray and Young 2018). Proximal upper central vein thromboses can be challenging to visualize with Doppler ultrasound, and echocardiography, CT angiograms, and MRA are sometimes employed when the clinical

suspicion for a proximal upper central vein thrombosis is high but the Doppler is negative. A CT pulmonary angiography scan is the diagnostic imaging of choice for young children for whom there is a high suspicion of PE as V/Q scans can be challenging to obtain in an uncooperative young child (Zaidi et al. 2017). In an older child, however, a V/Q scan may be employed as the first-line step in investigating a PE. If the V/Q scan is negative, though, and clinical suspicion remains high, further evaluation with a CT may be needed.

There is limited data regarding the utility of D-dimers in the pediatric population, and the negative predictive value of a D-dimer has not been validated in children (Zaidi et al. 2017). Until this data is made more robust, D-dimers should be used with caution, even in the adolescent population. The role of testing for inherited thrombophilia is controversial in the pediatric age group and results rarely affect acute or chronic therapy decisions, particularly in provoked thrombosis. Current guidelines recommend against thrombophilia testing in provoked thrombosis (Chalmers et al. 2011). There may be some utility in evaluating for inherited thrombophilia in pediatric patients with unprovoked VTE, but results are unlikely to change management (Jaffray and Young 2018). However, results of testing may help understand pathophysiology in unprovoked thrombosis. Testing for antiphospholipid antibodies (lupus anticoagulant, anti-cardiolipin IgG and IgM, and anti-beta2-glycoprotein IgG and IgM) at diagnosis of VTE and again at 12 weeks from diagnosis if initial testing is positive in unprovoked VTE is also helpful in determining length of therapy. The role of this testing in provoked VTE is less clear. A baseline CBC, PT/INR, PTT, and renal/liver function should be obtained prior to initiating anticoagulation in pediatric patients.

The risks of embolization or thrombosis-related mortality are important considerations in the pediatric age group; however; these events are relatively rare in this population. VTE mortality rates of 11.4 per 1000 child-years are reported, and all-cause mortality in pediatric patients with VTE is estimated to be 9–17% (Mahajerin and Croteau 2017). The mortality attributed to the

VTE itself, though, is low at 1.5–2.2% (Mahajerin and Croteau 2017). The more common deleterious outcome of pediatric VTE is post-thrombotic syndrome and resultant abnormal venous anatomy and chronic venous insufficiency. Post-thrombotic syndrome (PTS) is less commonly reported in pediatric patients with VTE as compared to adults with VTE with 12.4% of children with VTE reported to have PTS (Mahajerin and Croteau 2017). However, the incidence of PTS is likely underreported owing to low index of suspicion and short-term follow-up. The pediatric patient will likely live for decades following their thrombotic event; thus, preventing this long-term complication that can have significant impact on quality of life and healthcare costs is vital. Restoring normal vascular flow through clot resolution is an important goal of anticoagulation.

Treatment recommendations for pediatric VTE are available in the form of a variety of guidelines, and the American Society of Hematology 2018 guidelines provide the most up-to-date recommendations (Monagle et al. 2012, 2018). However, these guidelines are generally derived from weak evidence, are often extrapolated from adult data, and are frequently based on expert opinions. The guidelines do provide a framework for treatment, though, and they are typically employed in the treatment of pediatric VTE. Due to the unique features of the developing hemostatic system as well as the pediatric specific balance of risk and benefit involved in pediatric VTE management, treatment of pediatric VTE should be carried out in coordination with a pediatric hematologist if one is available.

Treatment in the neonatal population is guided by the extent of thrombosis as well as symptoms, and there are circumstances when reimaging is recommended rather than initiating anticoagulation immediately, particularly if the risk of bleeding with anticoagulation is too high in very premature infants. However, the majority of neonatal VTEs are managed with anticoagulant therapy (Monagle et al. 2012). For children with provoked thrombosis, 3 months of anticoagulation is generally the standard of care (Monagle et al. 2012, 2018). If the provoking factor remains present, ongoing anticoagulation until the provoking factor(s) have been removed may be considered. However, in children with unprovoked thrombosis, therapy is extended to 6–12 months and at times indefinitely (Monagle et al. 2012, 2018). Studies are currently ongoing to determine the optimal duration of anticoagulation for provoked pediatric thrombosis. The role of prophylaxis for neonates and children has not been clearly established, but risk-based prophylaxis should be at least considered in the older adolescent population as well as children with recurrent thrombosis (Branchford et al. 2012).

Catheter-Related Thrombosis

As in adults, the use of catheters in children is associated with a high rate of venous thrombosis, and central venous catheters (CVCs) are the most common risk factor for VTE development in children (van Ommen et al. 2001). The highest rate of CVC-related thrombosis occurs in children less than 1 year of age and likely reflects the smaller diameter vessels of the infant. In addition, CVC-related thromboses are more likely to occur in patients with malignancy, critical illness, congenital heart disease, systemic infection, total parenteral nutrition, trauma, and in patients admitted to the Neonatal Intensive Care Unit (Jaffray et al. 2017). Central line occlusion or frequent central line infections are sometimes the first sign of thrombosis and should increase suspicion for a VTE. In neonates with catheter-related thrombosis, thrombocytopenia may be the presenting sign.

The umbilical arteries and vein are unique sites used for catheterization in newborns. In autopsy findings, 20–65% of neonates who have an umbilical line at the time of demise have evidence of thrombosis (Veldman et al. 2008). Estimates of symptomatic VTE in infants with umbilical lines are wide-ranging. Long-term complications include renal disease, portal hypertension, and varices. Thrombosis of the umbilical artery is more rare (Veldman et al. 2008) but may be associated with severe complications such as renal or mesenteric artery thrombosis, renal failure, or death (Ergaz et al. 2012).

Treatment of CVC-related thrombosis is different in pediatric patients than in adult patients (Monagle et al. 2012, 2018). Current guidelines (2018) recommend against removal of functioning CVC when a thrombosis is present if the patient requires ongoing venous access. However, if the CVC is not needed or is not functioning, the guidelines recommend removal. If the line is removed, the guidelines recommend delaying removal of the CVC until after initiation of anticoagulation. The recommended duration of anticoagulation for CVC-associated VTE is 3 months or shorter. If the CVC remains present if other provoking factors remain present after the 3 months of anticoagulation, extended anticoagulation may be considered (Monagle et al. 2012, 2018). Arterial line thrombosis mandates the removal of the line. If significant ischemia occurs, catheter-directed thrombolytic therapy should be considered (Monagle et al. 2012, 2018).

Abdominal Venous Thrombosis

Abdominal VTE is less common than extremity vein thrombosis in the pediatric patient. However, 12–17% of pediatric VTE is intra-abdominal and the IVC is the most common vessel affected (Kumar and Kerlin 2017). IVC thromboses are most often the result of extension of a proximal lower extremity thrombosis. A rare finding in a pediatric patient is congenital IVC agenesis or atresia (prevalence of 0.6%), but it should be considered in a pediatric patient presenting with a seemingly unprovoked proximal lower extremity DVT (Kumar and Kerlin 2017).

Renal vein thrombosis is most common during the first month of life and the majority occur in the first week of life. Conditions that predispose to renal vein thrombosis are cyanotic heart disease, dehydration, sepsis, and umbilical vein catheterization (Kumar and Kerlin 2017). Thrombocytopenia, hematuria, renal dysfunction, and flank mass are common presenting signs. Diagnosis can be made by ultrasound or by vascular imaging (Kumar and Kerlin 2017). Therapy remains controversial in neonates. In renal vein thrombosis without IVC invasion,

conservative therapy is recommended with frequent reimaging and initiation of anticoagulation if extension occurs. For RVT associated with IVC invasion, anticoagulation is recommended (Monagle et al. 2018).

Portal vein thrombosis is uncommon in the pediatric population. In neonates, where it is more common than older children, it is frequently associated with umbilical vein catheterization (Kumar and Kerlin 2017). In older children, it has been associated with liver transplantation, intra-abdominal infections, splenectomy, sickle cell disease, and antiphospholipid antibodies, but in >50%, the underlying etiology is not identified. In adolescents with an unprovoked portal vein thrombosis, evaluation for paroxysmal nocturnal hemoglobinuria and Janus tyrosine kinase 2 (JAK2) mutations may be useful (Kumar and Kerlin 2017). Optimal treatment is not well studied, but anticoagulation is recommended by current guidelines for pediatric portal vein thrombosis if it is occlusive, in a patient who is post liver transplant, and if it is idiopathic. However, the guidelines suggest against anticoagulation in those with nonocclusive portal vein thrombosis. If cavernous transformation is present, anticoagulation may increase the risk for variceal bleeding and is generally not indicated (Monagle et al. 2012, 2018).

Pediatric Stroke

The incidence of childhood acute ischemic stroke (AIS) is about 2.4/100,000/year, but exact numbers are difficult to determine (Felling et al. 2017). The incidence of perinatal AIS is much higher, with estimates of one per 2500–4000 live births (deVeber et al. 2017). The perinatal period is one of the highest risk times for AIS in an individual's life. For pediatric AIS, the risk of AIS decreases with age until mid-adolescence. Outside of the perinatal period and the first year of life, the risk for AIS is very low (Felling et al. 2017).

Risk factors for perinatal AIS can be attributed to the mother, placenta, or the neonate, and the etiology of perinatal AIS is typically thought to be multifactorial. Specific risk factors include maternal fever, prolonged rupture of membranes, low APGAR scores, placental thrombosis, neonatal acidosis, neonatal fever, neonatal sepsis, and neonatal congenital heart disease (Felling et al. 2017; deVeber et al. 2017). There is a very low recurrence rate of perinatal AIS, which supports the idea that the pathophysiology is linked to the pregnancy, placenta, or features of the newborn period (Felling et al. 2017). It is not uncommon to identify a thrombophilic condition in a neonate with AIS; however, the presence or absence of a thrombophilia is unlikely to change management. Treatment of neonatal or perinatal AIS is generally supportive, and anticoagulation or antiplatelet therapy is rarely employed (deVeber et al. 2017). However, some circumstances may indicate a need for anticoagulation or antiplatelet therapy, such as presence of other VTE, congenital heart disease, or a cardioembolic source, and involvement of a pediatric hematologist in treatment decisions can be helpful (Monagle et al. 2012, 2018).

There are many risk factors for childhood AIS, and the risk factors vary substantially from the adult population. Risk factors include arteriopathies, congenital heart disease, sickle cell disease, malignancy, collagen vascular disease, rheumatologic disorders, and thrombophilias (acquired and congenital) (Felling et al. 2017). Arteriopathies are recognized as a common risk factors in pediatric patients, and arterial abnormalities are found in 40–80% of children with AIS who undergo vascular imaging (Felling et al. 2017). Cerebral arteriopathy may be linked to infectious causes. Varicella infection is associated with a transient cerebral arteriopathy, especially within 1 year of varicella diagnosis (Felling et al. 2017). However, with vaccination, varicella-associated vasculopathy is a less common cause of childhood stroke than it used to be. Newer studies have identified other herpes viruses as an associated factor in the development of pediatric AIS. Arterial dissection may be more common in pediatric patients than in adult patients (Felling et al. 2017). Congenital, as well as acquired, heart disease is another important risk factor for childhood AIS, and this population is reported to

have a 16-fold increased risk of AIS compared to the general population. While childhood AIS has a low risk of recurrence (Felling et al. 2017; deVeber et al. 2017), patients with associated congenital heart disease are at a higher risk of AIS recurrence than those who have AIS due to other causes. Sickle cell disease is another important risk factor for childhood AIS. Chronic transfusion therapy in children identified at high risk for stroke based on transcranial Doppler velocity is an effective primary prevention management strategy but is not available in all parts of the world (Felling et al. 2017). Patients with sickle cell disease should be considered at high risk for AIS, especially if they are experiencing an acute illness, an acute sickle cell event, infection, or severe anemia.

The CHEST guidelines provide recommendations for treatment of childhood AIS (Monagle et al. 2012). The general approach, in addition to supportive care as managed by neurologists and the intensive care unit, is anticoagulation for arterial dissection and cardioembolic causes and aspirin for other causes as long as no intracranial hemorrhage is identified (Monagle et al. 2012). Aspirin therapy is recommended to be continued for 2 years following an AIS (Monagle et al. 2012). For cardioembolic causes of AIS, anticoagulation for at least 3 months is recommended (Monagle et al. 2012). For AIS associated with arterial dissection, anticoagulation is recommended for at least 6 weeks with ongoing evaluation of vasculature. Additional treatment based on the etiology may be indicated as in sickle cell disease.

Childhood AIS has significant long-term complications, with significant neurologic deficits being reported in 31–51% of patients with childhood AIS (Felling et al. 2017). Emotional and behavioral challenges are common. Older children are more likely to have long-term effects of AIS than younger children. Recurrence is generally uncommon. In the Canadian registry of AIS, 1% of neonates and 12.6% of older children experienced recurrent AIS or transient ischemic attacks. The majority of patients with recurrent AIS had their recurrence within the first 3 months. There was a smaller portion of children in the

Canadian registry that had recurrence beyond 1 year (deVeber et al. 2017).

The incidence of cerebral sinus venous thrombosis (CSVT) is approximately 0.6/100,00 children per year, with 30–50% of CSVT cases occurring in the newborn period (Ichord 2017). CSVT is predominantly associated with underlying conditions such as dehydration, head and neck infection, trauma, recent CNS surgery, or iron deficiency anemia (Ichord 2017). CSVT results in outflow obstruction, venous congestion, edema, and ultimately infarction with or without associated hemorrhage (Ichord 2017). Symptoms of CSVT are variable and depend on the age of the patient and the contributing factors to thrombosis development. Neonates may present with decreased level of consciousness and/or seizures (Ichord 2017). Older children typically present with decreased level of consciousness, headache, and vomiting (Ichord 2017). The exam may be notable for impaired mental status, papilledema, sixth nerve palsy, or a bulging fontanelle in a neonate (Ichord 2017). Diagnosis is optimally done using MRI and MR venography, which will identify the thrombosis as well as any associated brain injury (Ichord 2017). Anticoagulation is indicated in the treatment of CSVT, and hemorrhage is not an absolute contraindication to treatment as the hemorrhage is likely a result of the venous obstruction (Monagle et al. 2012, 2018). The duration of treatment with anticoagulation is at least 3 months, but 6–12 months of anticoagulation may be more appropriate in unprovoked CSVT or in CSVT that has not resolved after 3 months of treatment. The majority of children survive the acute CSVT and approximately 50% go on to live normal lives; however, up to 40% will go on to have neurologic deficits.

Homozygous Protein C or S Deficiency

Homozygous protein C or S deficiency should be suspected when purpura fulminans occurs hours to days after delivery (Price et al. 2011). Other presenting symptoms include blindness due to retinal thrombosis and hemorrhage, central nervous system hemorrhage, severe disseminated intravascular coagulation (DIC), and large vessel thrombosis (Takemoto et al. 2014). Diagnosis is made by proving absence of protein C or S in the neonate (utilizing age-specific reference ranges) and by demonstrating that the parents are heterozygous for protein C or S deficiency (Price et al. 2011). Treatment is aimed at replacing the missing protein, and typically fresh frozen plasma is given (10–20 ml/kg) every 6–12 hours (Price et al. 2011). Protein C concentrate is available and offers more specific therapy (Manco-Johnson et al. 2016). There is no concentrate available for protein S. Once the patient has stabilized and all skin lesions have healed, long-term replacement with FFP or protein C concentrate plus or minus anticoagulation is prescribed.

Pediatric Use of Antithrombotic Agents

Antiplatelet Therapy

Despite the need for and use of antiplatelet therapy in children, little data exists regarding dosing of these agents (Monagle et al. 2001). In the neonatal population, particularly, differences in platelet function may affect antiplatelet therapy. For mechanical valves, aspirin doses in the range of 6–20 mg/kg/day have been used (Monagle et al. 2001). Lower doses (1–5 mg/kg/day) have been employed in individuals with Blalock-Taussig (BT) shunts, other endovascular shunts, and some ischemic strokes (Monagle et al. 2001). Little data exists on dosing ticlopidine, clopidogrel, or GP IIb/IIIa inhibitors in children (Monagle et al. 2001).

Heparin and Heparin-Induced Thrombocytopenia

Use of standard heparin is challenging in infants because of their low levels of antithrombin and other differences in the coagulation system (Monagle et al. 2001). Frequently, treatment with heparin is initiated with a bolus dose of 75 units/kg. Maintenance dosing should be based on measurement of the anti-Xa level with a goal of 0.3–0.7 IU/mL but typically is around 28 units/kg/h for children under 1 year of age and 20 units/kg/h for older children (Monagle et al. 2001; Samuel et al. 2016; Malec and Young 2017).

Heparin-induced thrombocytopenia (HIT) can occur in neonates and children, but it is very rare. Due to the need for frequent catheterization with attendant heparin exposure, HIT should be considered in children with congenital heart disease with recurrent thrombosis or with new thrombocytopenia.

Low Molecular Weight Heparin

Low molecular weight heparin (LMWH) offers several advantages in children, especially in ease of dosing and monitoring (Table 32.1). Neonates require higher doses than older children. The best-studied agent in pediatric patients is enoxaparin, with the dosing of 1 mg/kg/q12 hours for age over 2 months and 1.5–1.75 mg/kg/q12 for under 2 months (Malec and Young 2017). Anti-Xa levels should be checked 4 hours after the second or third dose with a goal level of 0.5–1.0 IU/ml (Monagle et al. 2001; Malec and Young 2017). In the neonatal population where a patient's weight may be changing in short periods of time, care should be taken to evaluate weight-based dosing with significant increases or decreases of weight in order to ensure that the drug is in the therapeutic window. Fondaparinux is also utilized in the pediatric population and has the advantages of once-daily dosing, no risk of HIT, and no risk of osteoporosis (Malec and Young 2017).

Table 32.1 Pediatric dosing of heparin and LMWH heparin

Standard heparin
Bolus: 75 units/kg
Maintenance
<1 year: 28 units/kg/h
>1 year: 20 units/kg/h
Adjust to aPTT range that reflects heparin level of 0.35–0.70 anti-Xa units
Enoxaparin
Treatment dose
<2 months: 1.5 mg/kg every 12 hours
>2 months–adult: 1.0 mg/kg every 12 hours

Table 32.2 Pediatric dosing of warfarin

Day 1: Warfarin 0.2 mg/kg	
Day 2–4 protocol	
INR	Action
1.1–1.3	Repeat day 1 dose
1.4–1.9	50% of day 1 dose
2.0–3.0	50% of day 1 dose
3.1–3.5	25% of day 1 dose
>3.5	Hold until INR <3.5, then 50% of previous dose
Maintenance guidelines	
INR	Action
1.1–1.3	Increase dose by 20%
1.4–1.9	Increase dose by 10%
2.0–3.0	No change
3.1–3.5	Decrease by 10%
>3.5	Hold until INR <3.5, then 20% of previous dose

Warfarin

Despite often having lower levels of vitamin K-dependent proteins, children typically require more warfarin per unit of body weight than adults (Streif et al. 1999). Age-based starting points for doses are available (Table 32.2): 2 months to 1 year, 0.2 mg/kg; 1–5 years, 0.09 mg/kg; 6–10 years, 0.07 mg/kg; and 11–18 years, 0.06 mg/kg. Warfarin can be difficult in a young infant or child due to variability in their dietary intake, and for acute anticoagulation, LMWH is generally preferred (Malec and Young 2017). If a patient is placed on warfarin, the INR should be monitored closely to keep it in range for the disease being managed.

Thrombolytic Therapy

The role of thrombolytic therapy in pediatric thrombosis is controversial and has not been well studied. The most studied thrombolytic agent in children is tissue plasminogen activator (tPA). Current guidelines suggest against the use of thrombolysis in pediatric deep vein thrombosis and submassive pulmonary embolism (Monagle et al. 2012). However, the guidelines suggest the use of thrombolysis in PE with hemodynamic compromise (Monagle et al. 2012). While limited data exists regarding the use of thrombolysis in pediatric patients, there are circumstances where thrombolysis may be employed, particularly at centers with experienced interventional radiologists or cardiologists as well as an intensive care unit and pediatric hematologists (Tarango and Manco-Johnson 2017).

New Oral Anticoagulants

The new oral anticoagulants have not yet been studied in the pediatric population, but they may provide an excellent opportunity for improved anticoagulation in this population (Malec and Young 2017).

Suggested Reading

Branchford BR, Mourani P, Bajaj L, Manco-Johnson M, Wang M, Goldenberg NA. Risk factors for in-hospital venous thromboembolism in children: a case-control study employing diagnostic validation. Haematologica. 2012;97(4):509–15.

Chalmers E, Ganesen V, Liesner R, et al. Guideline on the investigation, management and prevention of venous thrombosis in children. Br J Haematol. 2011;154(2):196–207.

deVeber GA, Kirton A, Booth FA, et al. Epidemiology and outcomes of arterial ischemic stroke in children: the Canadian Pediatric Ischemic Stroke Registry. Pediatr Neurol. 2017;69:58–70.

Ergaz Z, Simanovsky N, Rozovsky K, et al. Clinical outcome of umbilical artery catheter-related thrombosis - a cohort study. J Perinatol. 2012;32(12):933–40.

Felling RJ, Sun LR, Maxwell EC, Goldenberg N, Bernard T. Pediatric arterial ischemic stroke: epidemiology, risk factors, and management. Blood Cells Mol Dis. 2017;67:23–33.

Ichord R. Cerebral sinovenous thrombosis. Front Pediatr. 2017;5:163.

Jaffray J, Young G. Developmental hemostasis: clinical implications from the fetus to the adolescent. Pediatr Clin N Am. 2013;60(6):1407–17.

Jaffray J, Young G. Deep vein thrombosis in pediatric patients. Pediatr Blood Cancer. 2018;65(3).

Jaffray J, Bauman M, Massicotte P. The impact of central venous catheters on pediatric venous thromboembolism. Front Pediatr. 2017;5:5.

Kumar R, Kerlin BA. Thrombosis of the abdominal veins in childhood. Front Pediatr. 2017;5:188.

Mahajerin A, Croteau SE. Epidemiology and risk assessment of pediatric venous thromboembolism. Front Pediatr. 2017;5:68.

Mahajerin A, Obasaju P, Eckert G, Vik TA, Mehta R, Heiny M. Thrombophilia testing in children: a 7 year experience. Pediatr Blood Cancer. 2014;61(3):523–7.

Malec L, Young G. Treatment of venous thromboembolism in pediatric patients. Front Pediatr. 2017;5:26.

Manco-Johnson MJ, Bomgaars L, Palascak J, et al. Efficacy and safety of protein C concentrate to treat purpura fulminans and thromboembolic events in severe congenital protein C deficiency. Thromb Haemost. 2016;116(1):58–68.

Monagle P, Michelson AD, Bovill E, Andrew M. Antithrombotic therapy in children. Chest. 2001;119(1 Suppl):344S–70S.

Monagle P, Chan AKC, Goldenberg NA, et al. Antithrombotic therapy in neonates and children: antithrombotic therapy and prevention of thrombosis, 9th ed: American College of Chest Physicians evidence-based clinical practice guidelines. Chest. 2012;141(2 Suppl):e737S–801S.

Monagle P, Cuello CA, Augustine C, et al. American Society of Hematology 2018 guidelines for management of venous thromboembolism: treatment of pediatric venous thromboembolism. Blood Adv. 2018;2(22):3292–316.

Price VE, Ledingham DL, Krumpel A, Chan AK. Diagnosis and management of neonatal purpura fulminans. Semin Fetal Neonatal Med. 2011;16(6):318–22.

Samuel S, Allison TA, Sharaf S, et al. Antifactor Xa levels vs. activated partial thromboplastin time for monitoring unfractionated heparin. A pilot study. J Clin Pharm Ther. 2016;41(5):499–502.

Setty BA, O'Brien SH, Kerlin BA. Pediatric venous thromboembolism in the United States: a tertiary care complication of chronic diseases. Pediatr Blood Cancer. 2012;59(2):258–64.

Streif W, Andrew M, Marzinotto V, et al. Analysis of warfarin therapy in pediatric patients: a prospective cohort study of 319 patients. Blood. 1999;94(9):3007–14.

Takemoto CM, Sohi S, Desai K, et al. Hospital-associated venous thromboembolism in children: incidence and clinical characteristics. J Pediatr. 2014;164(2):332–8.

Tarango C, Manco-Johnson MJ. Pediatric thrombolysis: a practical approach. Front Pediatr. 2017;5:260.

Tormene D, Simioni P, Prandoni P, et al. The incidence of venous thromboembolism in thrombophilic children: a prospective cohort study. Blood. 2002;100(7):2403–5.

van Ommen CH, Nowak-Gottl U. Inherited thrombophilia in pediatric venous thromboembolic disease: why and who to test. Front Pediatr. 2017;5:50.

van Ommen CH, Heijboer H, Buller HR, Hirasing RA, Heijmans HS, Peters M. Venous thromboembolism in childhood: a prospective two-year registry in The Netherlands. J Pediatr. 2001;139(5):676–81.

Veldman A, Nold MF, Michel-Behnke I. Thrombosis in the critically ill neonate: incidence, diagnosis, and management. Vasc Health Risk Manag. 2008;4(6):1337–48.

Zaidi AU, Hutchins KK, Rajpurkar M. Pulmonary embolism in children. Front Pediatr. 2017;5:170.

Index

Printed in the United States
By Bookmasters